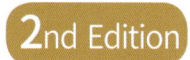

Safe Filler Injection
Technique Demonstration
using live imaging tools

Seung Min Oh | Bong Cheol Kim

DAEHAN

Foreword

People's desire to look young and beautiful is universal regardless of their age and gender. Filler procedures allow people to easily achieve these desires within a short period of time, and therefore are becoming increasingly popular. In the past, filler procedures were known for filling and smoothing wrinkles; however, recently, they are being additionally used for volumizing and augmenting sunken areas.

The basic criteria for fillers require that they do not cause severe foreign body reactions and remain for a certain period of time without being absorbed by the body too quickly. Due to these characteristics, it has become possible to construct beautiful faces, but at the same time, concerns about various side effects have been raised. While using fillers, we have constantly deliberated on the safe and efficient use of such a fine tool for patients.

These concerns have been resolved to a certain extent through the exchange of clinical experiences among many experienced doctors at conferences, seminars, and small discussion meetings. However, there are still questions remaining. In this book, knowledge gained through experiences and facts ascertained through studies about least-investigated areas are presented. You will find summaries of valuable experiences and new ideas from articles, books and discussions among senior doctors and colleagues.

Among the many questions considered, the most concerning were about the organization of vasculature and its physiology within a live body, rather than in a cadaver or an anatomical illustration. This is important as we want to avoid vascular accidents associated with filler procedures. Although the anatomical illustrations or cadaver studies have provided us with a great insight we failed to completely resolve these questions. After much thought, we have proposed utilizing MRI scans and CT angiography obtained from live bodies. With the help of many doctors, we have had the opportunity to test this approach and have summarized the results in this book. One surprising discovery is that organization of blood vessels within our body is not only very complicated, but also in many cases different from what is portrayed in illustrations.

Our desire to share such valuable information with doctors has led to the publication of this book. Some of the information in this book may be incomplete, focusing primarily on our own personal clinical experiences without sufficient scientific evidence. This book also addresses some questions that still need to be resolved. However, as information should not be simply disregarded until all questions have been perfectly addressed, we have decided to take a step forward and start documenting all that we have found so far. Moreover, this book also demonstrates several new attempts that have not been tested previously.

> **1. We demonstrate the vasculature and depth of actual blood vessels based on imaging acquired from live bodies.**

Firstly, we demonstrate a novel approach, which is the use of MRI and CT scans of live bodies. This method provides an upgraded treatment scheme leading to improved treatment results as doctors can visualize the precise depth and location of blood vessels in relation to bones, muscles and skin. This is especially useful in areas at risk for vascular accidents.

> **2. We explain filler procedures in detail.**

Secondly, we provide detailed explanations on how to use cannulas and needles. Readers can obtain more information on how to achieve satisfactory and safe results in the danger zones.

> **3. We recommend appropriate fillers for each area according to filler characteristics.**

Thirdly, in order to provide instruction on the appropriate filler selection for each area, we considered various questions and investigated the characteristics of fillers. As a result, clinicians may wisely select appropriate fillers for each area using this research. We look forward to additional research and theses on the characteristics of fillers and the way they change after being injected into the body.

> **4. We added the results of the filler dissolution tests**

Fourthly, we added experimental results for filler dissolution as well as newly proven research.

We have summarized a lot of information in this book. In areas where questions remain, these sections simply end by stating what needs to be found. However, we expect that many doctors will be able to engage in active discussions about fillers based on this book. We wish for our efforts to contribute to doctors' safe and beautiful filler procedures.

March 2017
One breezy day,
Co-authors **Seung Min Oh** and **Bong Cheol Kim**

Words of Appreciation

It has already been three years since we published the first edition of "Safe Filler Injection Technique Demonstrations Using Live Imaging Tools". In those years we have further deepened our knowledge on filler techniques and nurtured them by conducting numerous scientific studies.

We genuinely hope that we provide a safe and rational guide to many other clinicians and researchers by means of our book. These days, we feel gratified to see various clinicians cite our book in their books and presentations. This was a part of the reason why we rushed to publish the second edition to fulfill the deficiency of the previous edition and deliver novel materials.

I would like to express my deepest appreciation to all of you who have showed interests in our work. We will keep going and try our best to contribute on making the ideal filler treatment that is safe and effective.

Co-authors Seung Min Oh and Bong Cheol Kim

Author's Profile

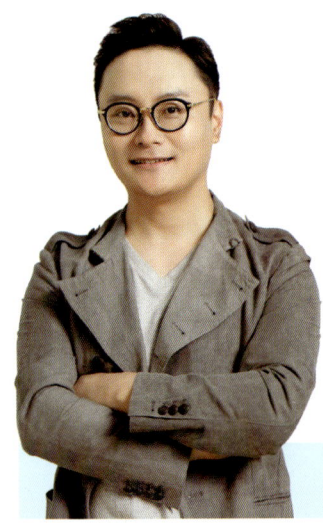

Seung Min Oh

Director of ON Clinic

College of Medicine, Seoul National University,

Internship - Seoul National University Hospital

Residency - Seoul National University Hospital, Seoul

Medical MBA, Kyung Hee University

President of OK Medi. Co. Ltd.

Executive board member of the Korean Association for Laser, Dermatology and Trichology

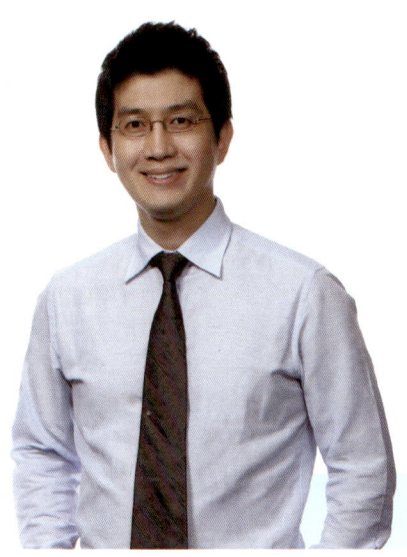

Bong Cheol Kim

Director of Lamar Isu Clinic

College of Medicine, Cheonnam National University

Internship - Samsung Medical Center (Seoul)

Residency - Samsung Medical Center (Seoul)

Executive board member of the Korean Association for Laser,

Dermatology and Trichology

CONTENTS

Part 1
Filler Types and Choosing Fillers

1. Types of Fillers ... 4

2. Characteristics of Each Filler ... 6

   1. Characteristics of HA Fillers ... 7
      1) Physical Characteristics of HA Fillers ... 7
         (1) Cross-linking ... 11
         (2) Cross-linking Ratio ... 11
         (3) Gel Hardness ... 14
         (4) HA Degradation ... 14
         (5) Viscoelasticity ... 15
         (6) Filler Concentration and the Relative Degree of Hydration ... 16
         (7) Filler Injection and Anti-Oxidant Substances ... 17
         (8) Fillers that Harden after Injection ... 19
         (9) Spread of Fillers ... 21
         (10) Cohesiveness ... 22
      2) HA Filler from Physician's Perspective ... 25
      3) Summary of Characteristics of Fillers ... 27
   2. Characteristics of Calcium Fillers ... 35
   3. Characteristics of Fillers Composed of Polycaprolactone (PCL) ... 39

3. Categorization of the Filler Market ... 43

4. Filler Selection ... 44

   1. Standards for Filler Selection ... 44
   2. Filler Selection and Safety ... 46

Part 2
Basic Introduction

1. Design Method 52
  1. Designing the Whole and Parts 52
  2. Design Considering Facial Expressions 53
  3. Tricks for Safe Procedures 54

2. Filler Administration with Cannulas 57
  1. Puncturing Method for Cannula Insertion 59
  2. Method of Using Cannula Depending on the Depth 60
  3. Cannula Advancement and Separation of Tissue 63

3. Basic Method of Using a Needle 65
  1. Method of Using a Needle 65
  2. Considerations of Bevel Location in Procedures 67
  3. Post Dermal Subcision Injection Method 68
  4. Perpendicular Pulling Injection Method 69
  5. Perpendicular Injection of a Large Bolus 70

4. No Bleeding Technique 71

5. Molding 76
  1. What is Molding? 76
  2. Molding Method for Each Facial Area 84
     1) Molding Under Eyes (the Smile Line) 84
     2) Under Eye Guider 85
     3) Nasolabial Folds and Cheeks 86
     4) Massage after Injection 86

6. Dissolution Test 88
  1. How to Use Hyaluronidase 88
  2. An Experiment for Melting HA Fillers 90

Part 3
Basic Anatomy

1. The Vasculature 107
1. The Facial Artery & Vein 107
2. Variations in the Facial Artery 109
3. The Supratrochlear Artery (STA) & Supraorbital Artery (SOA) 109
4. Superficial Temporal Artery (SfTA) 110
5. The External Carotid Artery & Internal Carotid Artery 111
6. Palpation of the Artery 112
7. Visual Inspection of Veins 113

2. Nerves 114
1. CN V (Trigeminal Nerve) – Sensory 114
2. CN VII (Facial Nerve) – Motor 116

3. Fat Compartments 118
1. Superficial Fat 118
2. Deep Fat 119

4. Muscles 120
1. Muscles around the Eyes 120
2. Muscles around the Mouth 120
3. Muscles of the Nose 121

5. The SMAS & Retaining Ligaments 122
1. The SMAS (Superficial Musculo-Aponeurotic System) 122
2. The Retaining Ligaments 125
   1) True Retaining Ligaments 125
   2) False Retaining Ligaments 126

Part 4
Filler Treatment for Each Facial Area

Upper Face

1. Forehead 130
2. Glabella 148
3. Temples 160

Mid Face

4. Nose 178
5. Nasolabial Folds 190
6. Cheek (Upper Cheek and Lower Cheek) 210
7. Dark Circles 230
8. Lower Eyelid Pretarsal Augmentation 248
9. Sunken Eyes 254

Lower Face

10. Chin 260
11. Marionette Line 268
12. Lips 274

Part 5
Filler Complications

1. Filler Complications and Interventions — 284
1. Bruising and Hematoma — 285
2. Erythema — 286
3. Edema — 287
4. Neovascularization — 288
5. PIH — 288
6. Nodule — 288
7. Infection — 290
8. Skin Necrosis (Blood Vessel Complications) — 291

2. Mechanism and Treatment of Skin Necrosis — 294
1. Predisposing Factors of Skin Necrosis — 294
2. Factors Affecting the Extent of Skin Necrosis — 295
3. Symptoms of Skin Necrosis — 295
4. Treatment of Skin Necrosis — 297
5. Notes for Preventing Necrosis during Procedures — 301
6. Tips for Early Discovery and Treatment of Necrosis — 303
7. Factors Affecting the Prognosis of Skin Necrosis — 303

3. Other Blood Vessel Complications — 304
1. Blindness and Cerebral Infarct — 304
2. Pulmonary Embolism — 306

Safe Filler Injection Technique Demonstration
– using live imaging tools

Part
1

Filler Types and Choosing Fillers

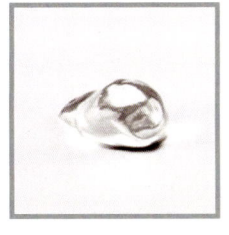 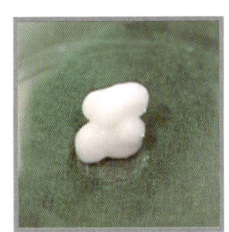 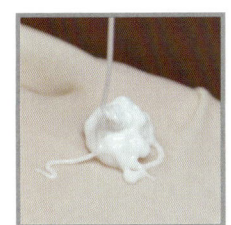

Safe Filler Injection Technique Demonstration
- using live imaging tools

Part 1: Filler Types and Choosing Fillers

1. Types of Fillers

2. Characteristics of Each Filler

   1. Characteristics of HA Fillers

      1) Physical Characteristics of HA Fillers
- (1) Cross-linking
- (2) Cross-linking Ratio
- (3) Gel Hardness
- (4) HA Degradation
- (5) Viscoelasticity
- (6) Filler Concentration and the Relative Degree of Hydration
- (7) Filler Injection and Anti-Oxidant Substances
- (8) Fillers that Harden after Injection
- (9) Spread of Fillers
- (10) Cohesiveness

      2) HA Filler from Physician's Perspective

      3) Summary of Characteristics of Fillers

   2. Characteristics of Calcium Fillers

   3. Characteristics of Fillers Composed of Polycaprolactone (PCL)

3. Categorization of the Filler Market

4. Filler Selection

   1. Standards for Filler Selection

   2. Filler Selection and Safety

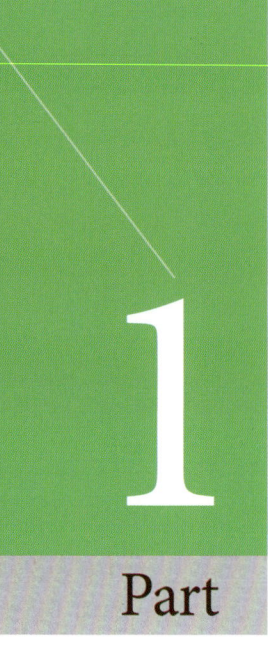

Filler Types and Choosing Fillers

1. Types of Fillers

● ● ●   Due to frequent use and excessive market supply, there are approximately 100 types of fillers in the country. Compared to the time when there were not many choices, it has become difficult for physicians to choose the type of filler to use.

Due to the rules of the filler market, if they are bought in large amounts, they can be bought at a lower cost. However, there are so many competing products and questions raised in relation to these new products that rather than using just one type of product, there is a tendency to attempt using various fillers, even in the middle of a process.

It is almost impossible to know all the characteristics of the approximately 100 fillers there are to choose from. Accordingly, we think it is necessary to categorize these filler characteristics into a few groups based on important standards. Thereafter, physicians may choose their preferred fillers from the filler groups with common characteristics.

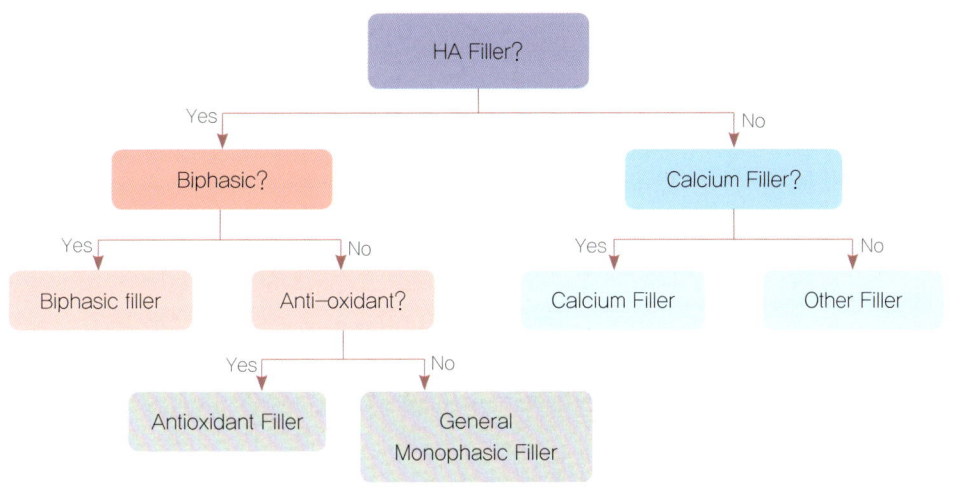

Fig. 1-1 **Choosing Fillers**

When choosing fillers, one can go through the following steps. At the turning point in the middle, a decision should be made based on personal preferences for important items.

It seems reasonable to choose a filler based on systematic categories according to characteristics. In order to fulfill the most important purpose, which is patient satisfaction after each procedure, it is important to know the basic characteristics of fillers.

In order to learn about the characteristics of various fillers, the algorithm shown in Fig. 1-1 above is useful; however, since there are so many types, in reality, other methods are often used. In most cases, a professional learns about the characteristics of the fillers on his or her list first, and use them first-hand to comprehend their characteristics to decide whether to use them.

Summary of Conditions for an Ideal Filler	1. Safe 2. Effective 3. Long retention time 4. Cost-effective

2. Characteristics of Each Filler

● ● ●　　In order to learn about the characteristics of fillers, some clarifications must be made about what constitutes an ideal filler. In general, ideal fillers are safe, long-lasting, efficacious, and are cost-effective.

It is certain that safety is the most important condition for any product used in the body regardless of it being a medical device or not. Safety is assured in the process of product approval before doctors can determine at a clinical site. Of course, there are exceptional cases; however, we do not especially need to be concerned about the safety of fillers that could be encountered clinically.

From the perspective of patients getting a filler procedure, pain, swelling and economic cost could be considered. Therefore, it can be expected that the greater longevity of fillers would benefit both the patient and the practitioner. patient However, due to concerns regarding side effects that may arise as time passes for permanent or long-term fillers, a long duration period may not necessarily be ideal.

Table 1-1 Characteristics of Fillers (For Each HA Product)

Type	Characteristics	Antioxidant	Type	Characteristics	Antioxidant
Restylane	Biphasic		Bellast	Monophasic	
Juvederm	Monophasic		Yvoire	Biphasic	
Stylage	Monophasic	Yes	Teosyal	Monophasic	Yes
Glytone	Monophasic	Yes	the CHAEUM	Monophasic	
Neuramis	Monophasic				

Table 1-2 Standards for Understanding the Characteristics of Fillers

Sequence	Characteristics	Contents
1	Cross-linking	Convert HA from liquid to gel
2	Cross-linking Ratio	Important characteristic of filler properties
3	Gel Hardness	Main factor for maintaining shape
4	Decomposition of HA	Deciding factor for duration period
5	Viscoelasticity	The most important characteristic for deciding filler properties
6	Concentration and Degree of Hydration of Filler	Related to properties of filler
7	Filler Injection and Anti-oxidant Materials	Related to duration period of filler
8	Hardness After Injecting Filler	Related to shape maintenance and touch-up timing
9	Spreading of Filler	Shape maintenance and duration period
10	Cohesiveness	

1 Characteristics of HA Fillers

1) Physical Characteristics of HA Fillers

■ Standards for Understanding Characteristics of Fillers

Through cross-linking, hyaluronic acid (HA) is converted from a liquid to gel state. HA in a liquid state is not only absorbed easily but also not shape-retainable. Through cross-linking, a solid structure is developed that retains resistance against hyaluronidase. In general, hardness, consistency, viscosity, etc., which are used to describe the physical characteristics of HA filler materials, are all substantially related to the degree and method of cross-linking.

In general, there are 15 g of free HA in the skin, and per day, about 5 g of it is melted away by hyaluronidase. Thus, the half-life of this compound is about one to two days, and it all disappears within one week. If it becomes solidified through cross-linking, it would not be absorbed as easily and gain various filler characteristics. BDDE, which is used in cross-linking, is generally known as a harmful substance. It is not toxic when bound within a filler; however, if it remains free after the combining reaction, it is toxic to the body. Therefore, completely removing any remains of BDDE after the manufacturing process is very important for reducing unexpected side effects after the procedure.

HA fillers produced by cross-linking generally have a duration period of six months to one year and six months, depending on the degree of cross-linking and the particle size. Decomposition of fillers happens due to hyaluronidase that exists naturally. Free radicals that initially damage the structure of HA fillers renders fillers to dissolve easily in reaction to hyaluronidase. In order to maintain the duration period of the filler stably, it may be important to consider how to protect fillers from free radicals. By using mannitol or vitamins that have anti-oxidant functions, anti- oxidant HA fillers in which the HA is prevented from decomposing due to free radicals may have improved durability and stability.

Finally, if criteria for an ideal filler include being safe, easy to shape and durable for a long period of time, cross-linking, which significantly affects the degree of hardness and durability, plays an important role in the quality of fillers. Each company has a characteristic approach for cross-linking and consequently, various types of compounds such as biphasic, monophasic monopolified or monophasic polydensified are created. However, from the perspective of actually choosing fillers, rather than the physical and biochemical characteristics on a particle level, convenience or feeling for the user on a macro-level is more important. Therefore, when choosing fillers, explanations by companies are important, but it is also important to comprehend how users actually feel. This book focuses on sharing the experiences of the authors on such information.

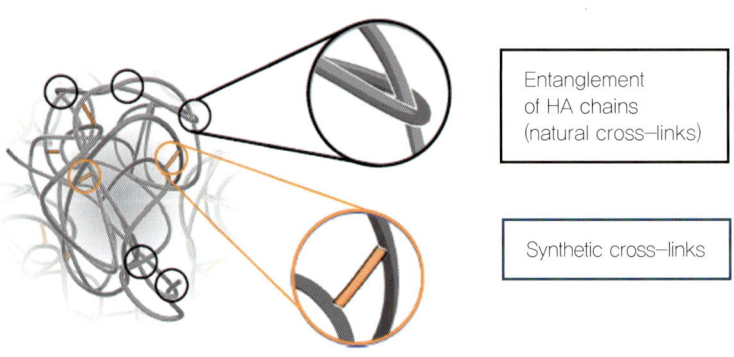

Fig. 1-2 NASHA technique of Restylane. Restylane is the first developed filler and has long history

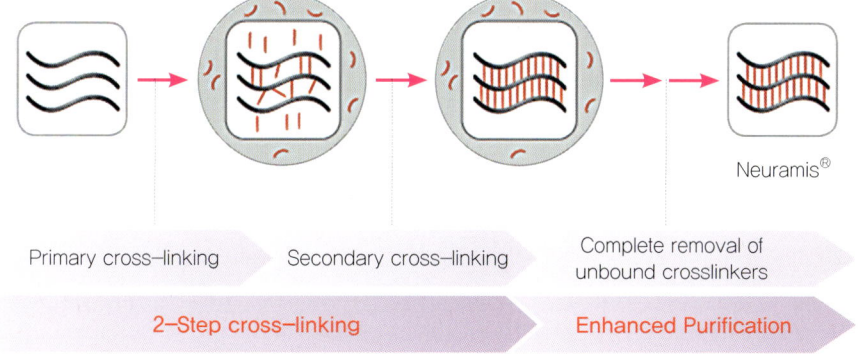

Fig. 1-3   **Neuramis, Medytox.** A newly developed Korean monophasic filler

It would not be difficult to choose a product which has proved its safety, been commercialized completely and been on the market for a certain period of time. However, depending on the treatment area or procedural method, there is definitely a need for more appropriate fillers. We hope that this book will provide some assistance in expanding the scope of choices and clarifying the standards for choice. The quality of fillers recommended in this book may not necessarily be adequate from a physician's perspective because, as mentioned later, each physician may have different standards for selecting fillers.

Although high-priced fillers may have comparative advantages in many areas, it may not necessarily always be right to use them.

Safe Filler Injection Technique Demonstration – using live imaging tools

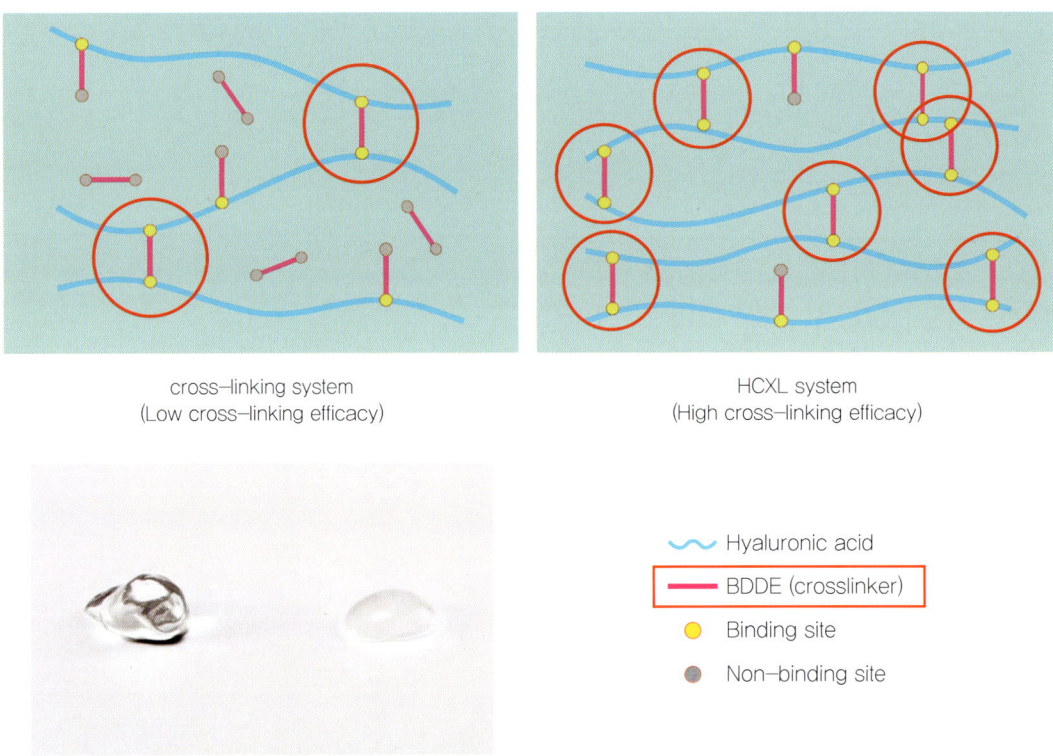

Fig. 1-4   Bellast of Dong Kook Pharm

(1) Cross-linking

■ Summary: Cross-linking Method for Each HA Filler Product

HA fillers are generally categorized as either biphasic or monophasic. The fundamental difference between these is present in the particle structure, but the difference felt by a physician in reality is in viscoelasticity. Each company provides stability by combining free HA in various forms. It is difficult to say which method is the best. Fillers can be appropriate or inappropriate depending on each physicianphysician's preferences, each patientpatient's physical characteristics and the characteristics of the area of the procedure.

By looking into the structure of the particles in the fillers shown above, it can be seen that companies use various additional techniques beyond merely making three-dimensional structures using BDDE and stabilization. 1st picture shows the structure of Restylane, Galderma(Fig. 1-2), 2nd picture shows of Neuramis, Medytox(Fig. 1-3), 3rd picture shows Bellast, Dong Kook Pharm monophasic filler(Fig. 1-4), Apart from the difference at the molecular level, we want to see this from a clinical perspective.

(2) Cross-linking Ratio

There is no clear standard for the most ideal degree of cross-linking. The higher the cross-linking ratio, the firmer a filler becomes, while viscosity and durability also increase. Considering that an ideal filler is supposed to be effective and long-lasting, one could easily conclude that increasing the cross-linking ratio would be good. However, BDDE and DVS, which are used for this cross-linking process, are fundamentally toxic. Therefore, although there are advantages to raising the cross-linking ratio, the likelihood of complications increases. The hydrophilic property would be reduced and a foreign substance or immunity reaction may occur.

BDDE and DVS slow down the decomposition of fillers due to enzymes or free radicals by binding to the hydroxyl groups of hyaluronic acid. In this case, the degree of cross-linking refers to the percentage calculated by the number of cross-linkers per 100 disaccharide units.

Safe Filler Injection Technique Demonstration – using live imaging tools

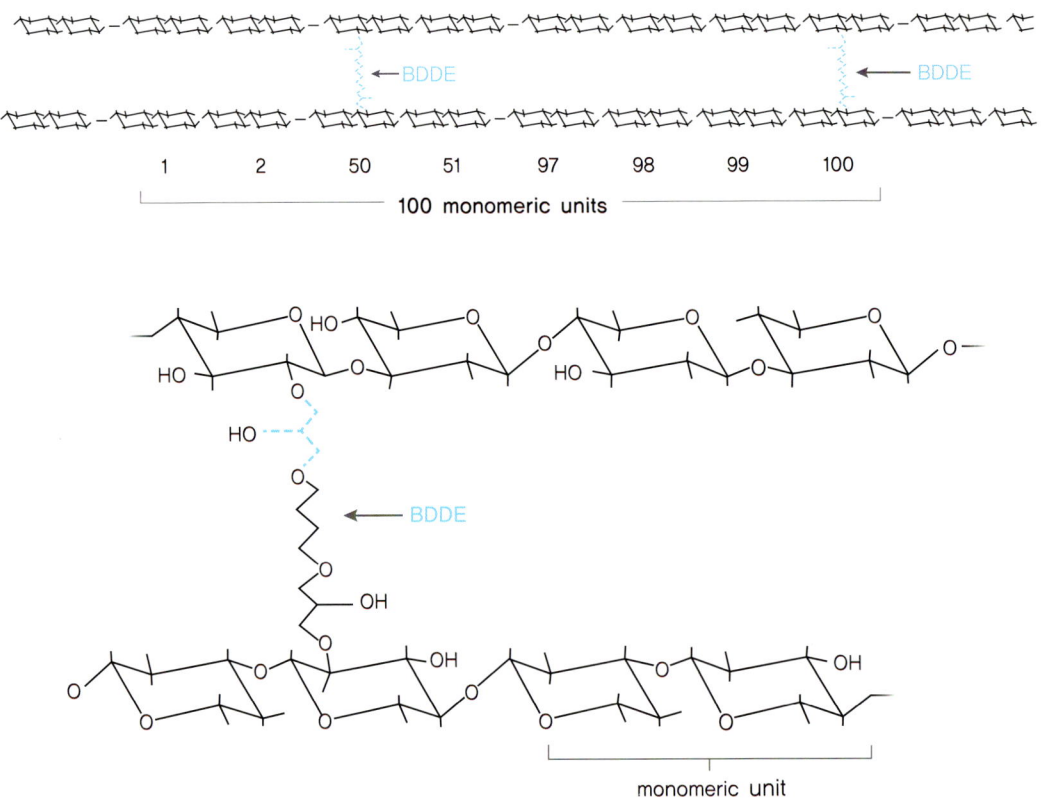

Fig. 1-5　Cross-linking Ratio Example of 2%

Table 1-3	Summary of Cross-linking Characteristics
Cross-linker Residue	Extremely harmful to the body BDDE (1,4-butanediol diglycidyl ether) DVS (di-vinyl sulfone)
Cross-linking Ratio	If 2%, two cross-linkers for 100 monomers Correlation with gel hardness The most ideal cross-linking ratio is unknown If the cross-linking ratio is high, durability increases but hydrophilia decreases Immunity reaction may develop or rejection may occur

A filler with the lowest possible cross-linking ratio while maintaining an acceptable level of viscoelasticity, hardness, and lifting capacity would be considered an ideal filler. Restylane, for example, is known to contain the same concentration of hyaluronic acid as other hyaluronic acid intradermal fillers but has a very low cross-linking rate. This can be explained by the natural cross-linking concept (Refer to Fig. 1-2). Cross-linking is a necessary process in the production of hyaluronic acid fillers.

The term modification efficiency encompasses the aforementioned concept. The modification efficiency values of the different HA products have been provided in the graph below (Fig. 1-6). The family of products manufactured employing the NASHA technique have relatively high modification efficiency rates.

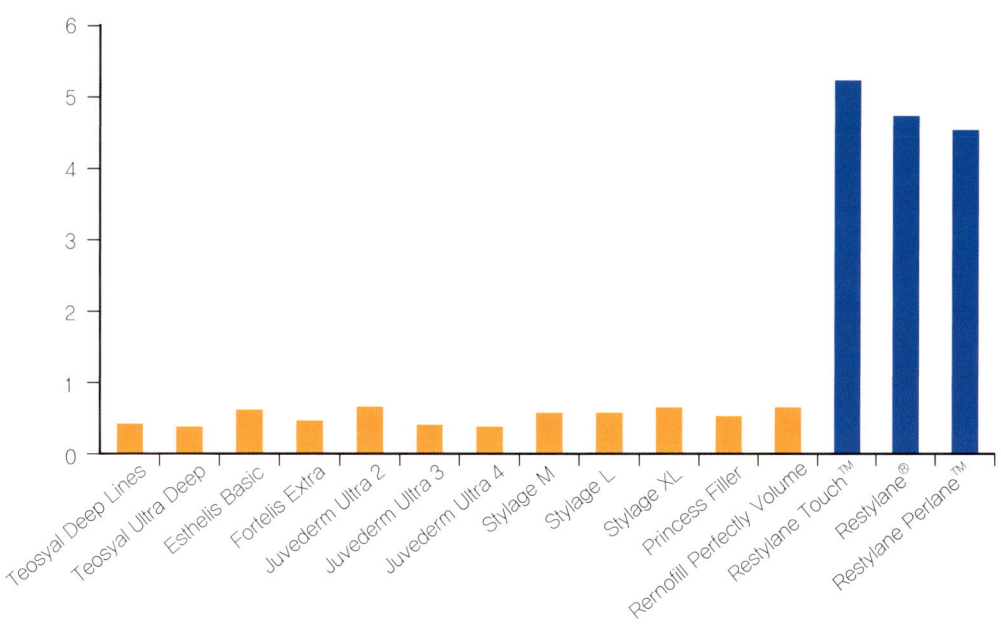

Fig. 1-6 The modification efficiency for different HA-fillers

(3) Gel Hardness

Gel hardness refers to the degree of hardness of hyaluronic acid. The harder this substance is, the better it will hold shape, making it more effective. However, since fillers are injected through a small-gauge needle into human body, it could be difficult to inject hard fillers. The hardness of gel is indicated by strength marked with G′.

Gel hardness is affected by the HA concentration, degree of cross-linking, amount of uncross-linked HA and manufacturing process. Various filler characteristics are interrelated and affect each other. If one aspect is made overly strong, this will cause side effects.

(4) HA Degradation

In the event the surface area of HA particles or lumps expands, the surface area exposed to enzymes that break down HA expands as well. Therefore, in order to satisfy one criterion of an ideal filler, a long duration period, it would be helpful to have the particles in a gel be as big and consistent as possible. In reality, with biphasic HA fillers, products with long duration periods are made by enlarging particle size.

On one hand, if the decomposition process is closely observed, a breakdown process due to free radicals in addition to enzymes can be found. As free radicals are small in size, they may be able to freely go inside the filler through pores naturally formed by HA folds. On the other hand, as enzymes are larger in size, they may be able to dissolve fillers only from the outside in which they come into contact.

Based on various research, consistency in filler particle size does not result in big differences in the speed of filler decomposition. There is not much difference in the speed of decomposition and absorption among fillers with varying size particles.

In conclusion, large particle size may help extend the longevity of fillers; however, consistency in particle size seems to have a lesser effect on longevity.

Nowadays, not only the natural degradation of fillers, but also the solvation process by hyaluronidase has become a hot topic of interest. This is due to the increased use of hyaluronidase in case of filler complication. This topic will be further discussed in detail in a later chapter.

(5) Viscoelasticity

■ Characteristics

- Degree of Stickiness (cohesiveness)
- Related Characteristics
    - Degree of cross-linking
    - Crossed vs non-crossed ratio
    - Sizing method
    - Average gel particle size
    - Size distribution
    - Manufacturing process
- Consistent sizes via sieving
    - Viscoelasticity increase

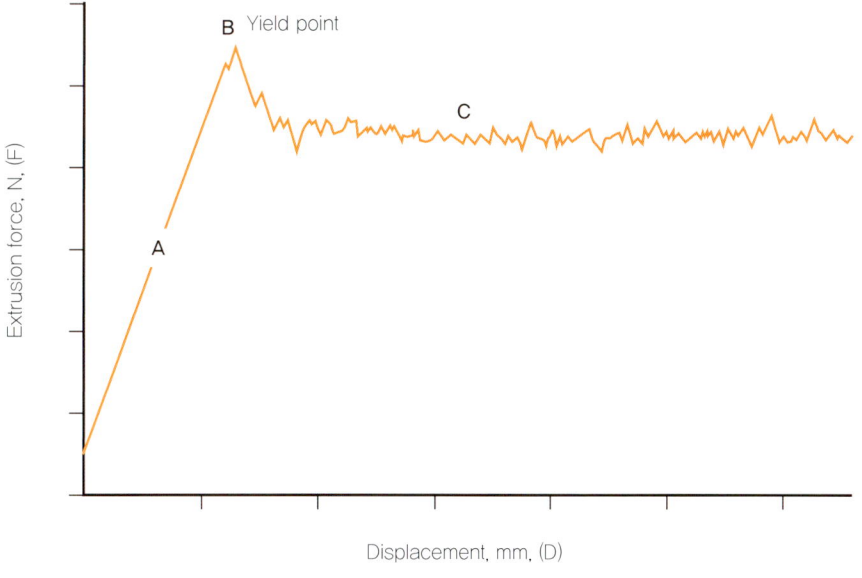

Fig. 1-7 **Strength Required for Injecting Fillers.** When exerting strength on the pistol for injecting fillers, strength increases proportionally up to a certain point and hits a peak at the yield point. After that, strength required slightly decreases and holds at a certain level.

The viscoelasticity of fillers is important for molding and maintaining shapes. Basically, fillers with high viscoelasticity have an excellent ability to maintain shapes, so they are used mainly for lifting purposes to create volume. These fillers demonstrate their strength when injected in a large amount into the deep subcutaneous layer. On the other hand, fillers with low viscoelasticity that are easily spread out are advised to be injected into the dermal layer or upper subcutaneous layer in order to mold finely.

The viscoelasticity of fillers is correlated with other physical characteristics: cross-linking method and ratio, manufacturing process, particle size, consistency, and etc. Therefore, it is difficult to make viscoelasticity as desired by adjusting only one of these characteristics..

As shown in Fig. 1-7, the strength required for injecting a filler through a pistol increases proportionally up to a certain level and reaches a peak at the yield point. The required strength then decreases slightly and only a certain amount of strength is required thereafter.

In presence of high viscoelasticity or large and consistent particle size, more strength is required for injection, causing inconvenience to users. By mixing free HA as a lubricant, which is presumed to slightly reduce viscoelasticity, the shooting process can be relieved.

However, since free HA is easily absorbed, a dramatic decrease in the volume injected can occur, which also implies a short durability. Therefore, manufacturing technology has been evolvingin such a way that free HA is used as little as possible for lubricating purposes, while at the same time the shooting process is being improved. Recently developed monophasic HA fillers are based on technology where no free HA is present.

(6) Filler Concentration and the Relative Degree of Hydration

In theory, HA and water are determined to combine very strongly when cross-linked weakly. This is due to the polyanionic characteristic of a HA molecule as well as the characteristics of hydrogen bonding.

When fillers are injected, the most ideal condition is for them to be set in shape right after injection, but some swelling is experienced in reality. This swelling may be due to tissue damage caused by the procedure, but mainly because of the concentration of commercialized HA being slightly higher than its parallel status. The concentration generally used for filler procedures, 20-24 mg/mL, usually causes absorption of water and increases volume from the time of initial adjustment.

The recent trend for fillers is to improve deficient areas by adding volume in the subcutaneous layer and below rather than improving wrinkles by injecting products into the dermal layer, so the tendency for fillers to cause the additional water absorption after a procedure may serve as an advantage.

However, since there is a risk of over- or under-adjustment, maintenance of initial volume is desired.

Moreover, it is not easy to distinguish whether swelling after injection is caused by tissue damage or bleeding rather than water absorption. Thus, the ideal type of filler would maintain volume from the time of injection. One recently developed filler has been released as a stably hydrated product. As it maintains its original state, without further absorption of water, there is little change to the mass, as has been proved through biopsy.

Authors have conducted various experiments for melting or diluting HA fillers and discovered some astonishing results.

They found that different HA products attract water at different levels. While some products absorb saline completely and formulate HA gel with new concentration, others partially maintain their original HA filler property to a certain level without affably bonding with water.

These studies have provided significant facts for understanding and selecting fillers, which will be explained more in depth later in the "An Experiment for Melting HA Fillers part.

(7) Filler Injection and Anti-Oxidant Substances

As monophasic and biphasic fillers are manufactured to be structurally different at the particle level, their properties differ as well. In reality however, physicians are not be able to distinguish these differences at the particle level at the clinical site. Physicians understand the clinical differences by touching and using the products.

Biphasic fillers are categorized by the size of their particles. Fillers with small particles are used for shallow wrinkles or for under the eyes, while fillers with large particles are used for volumizing purposes. It is more difficult to inject biphasic fillers with large particles using small gauge needles or cannulas. However as there are advantages and disadvantages to using larger gauge cannulas, it is difficult to say which option is better.

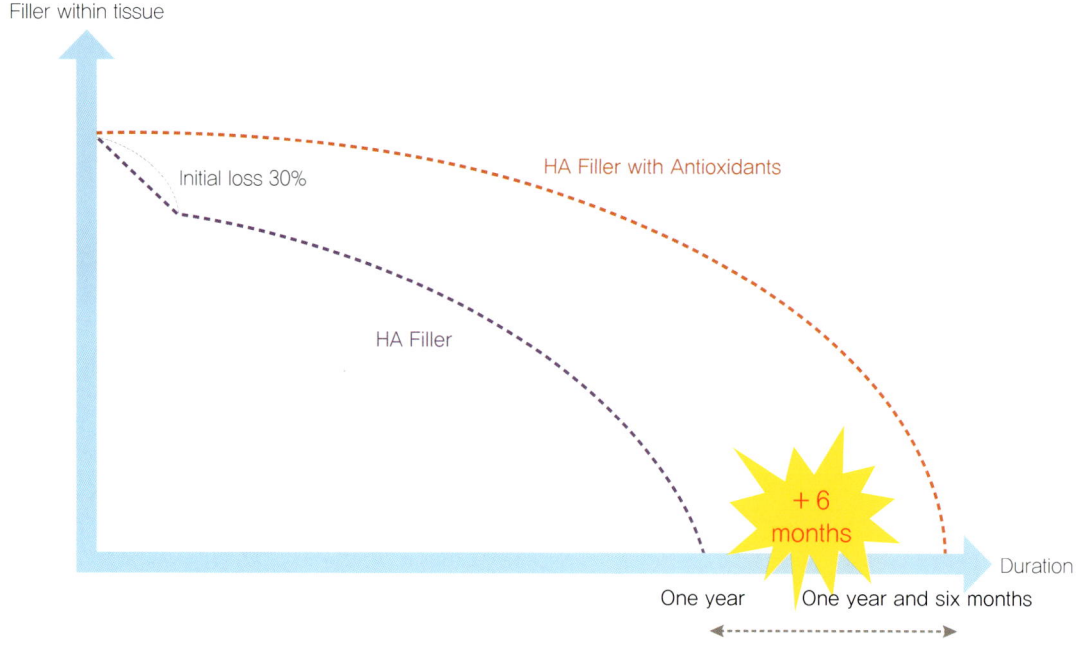

Fig. 1-8 Fillers with antioxidants are protected from initial free radical attack, reducing initial loss. This is the basis for increased the duration.

(Source: Stylage, Chong Keun Dang)

Monophasic fillers are categorized by HA concentration in the filler. The less concentrated fillers are used for shallow wrinkles or under the eyes and the higher concentrated fillers are used for volumizing. The homogenous characteristic, a feature specific to monophasic fillers, does not change as the HA concentration increases. Therefore, injecting monophasic fillers using relatively smaller needles or cannulas is not problematic. This ease of use can be attributed to the homogenous nature of the monophasic fillers.

Tissue damage that may occur when a filler is injected stimulates free radicals. Filler degradation is not only catalyzed by hyaluronidase alone. In fact, free radicals are involved in the initial process of filler degradation. Free radicals, which are very small in size, can freely access pores that exist naturally in between the filler components. Consequently the HA structure that has been compromised by free radicals is more easily degraded by hyaluronidase. Hyaluronidase is an enzyme with a large molecular size so its entry into the pores is restricted by its size. Therefore, hyaluronidase can only break down the outer surface of the injected filler material.

It is predicted that monophasic fillers, composed solely of crosslinked HA, are less vulnerable to degradation by hyaluronidase. Further research is anticipated in this area.

A filler that could suppress the activity of free radicals associated with tissue damage caused by initial injection will be more stable and have longer duration. Currently, fillers with antioxidants with resistance against free radicals are being manufactured and are available in the market. Reducing the initial loss of filler material will result in an increase in filler duration. The authors have been satisfied with fillers containing antioxidants and conservatively predict that this will serve as an important topic for the development of fillers in the future. The authors await further research and development.

(8) Fillers that Harden after Injection

Solid research results on changes in filler material after injection have been very difficult to find. Inevitably, the authors have had to provide information based on their own clinical experiences. However, the authors expect more research to be conducted in this area in the near future and that the breadth of information and recommendations will broaden. The authors await outstanding research findings from researchers and professors.

Since the current trend for filler procedures is volumizing rather than adjusting wrinkles in the dermal layer, there is a lot of interest in the changes in the fillers once they have been injected. The changes in filler material after it has been injected in the dermal layer is determined by whether the filler is monophasic or biphasic. The maintenance of filler shape is dependent on the viscoelasticity and hardness of the filler. Generally, biphasic fillers tend to become harder and stronger after injection while monophasic fillers become smoother and softer. To ensure lasting results and increase patient satisfaction, the initially molded shape of the filler must be maintained to a certain degree. More importantly, the filler must harden into an aesthetically pleasing shape after it has been injected. Especially in the forehead where the subcutaneous soft tissue layer is very thin, injected filler material must harden uniformly to maintain the originally molded shape. In order to perform touch ups, it is important that the previously filler injected has hardened reasonable. This will provide stability during the procedure and allow molding into desired shape. If the filler injected in the previous procedure is not stable and moves around, it will be difficult to design and maintain the intended shape, even with the touch up procedure.

Based on the authors' experiences, monophasic fillers harden and become reasonably stable in three to four weeks. It is important to avoid bleeding during the initial procedure. In the authors' experiences, if there is a lot of bleeding during the procedure, fillers tend not to harden as well. The authors anticipate additional research to be conducted on the rheological changes of fillers after injection.

With biphasic fillers, we can feel that these are harder than monophasic fillers. Accordingly, biphasic fillers procedures are more difficult especially in injection. In the event that hard fillers are injected in a soft tissue layer with insufficient space, internal pressure may increase. Vascular complications associated with fillers can occur from accidental intravascular injection of fillers or from external compression. (Opinions differ in this area. However, considering that necrosis from ischemia occurs even 2~3 days after procedures, extravascular accidents from external pressure exerted on vessels can definitely occur.) The hardness and ability to retain shape are advantages of biphasic fillers. However, disadvantages are that biphasic fillers are associated with difficulty in injections and volume reduction after procedure.

Moreover, it is very important to perform touch up procedures in the appropriate period. If the filler injected during the first procedure has not yet hardened, an unnecessarily large amount of filler may be used during the touch up procedure. Moreover, it is difficult to shape into desired form.

There are rare cases in which the fillers injected do not harden and move around, even at one month after the injection date. In such a case, the fillers do not serve the volumizing function at all, but only causes aesthetic problems. It is recommended that the filler is sufficiently dissolved using hyaluronidase and to re-perform the procedure. It is unclear what causes the injected fillers to maintain their softness and not harden. This causes great discomfort to both the patient and the physician. The authors expect much more research to be conducted in this area as well.

Treated areas need to be assessed at the follow up visit three to four weeks after the procedure. If treated areas have hardened to an acceptable extent, the touch up procedure can be performed. For touch up procedures, cannula is not necessary and a needle is sufficient. The most practical injection method is the perpendicular pulling method. With biphasic fillers, it is important to determine the number of injection points bearing in mind that these fillers do not spread out as much.

(9) Spread of Fillers

Viscoelasticity, an important property of the filler, allows the filler to maintain its shape at the time of injection. This is the strength that maintains the result after the procedures such as volumizing sunken areas or elevating the nasal tip. Fillers that spread well helps in initially creating the desired shape and reduce the risk of exerting external pressure on vessels. However, this quality of low viscoelasticity does not help maintain the shape. As seen in Fig. 1-9, monophasic fillers spread evenly within the dermal layer, whereas biphasic fillers spread unevenly in lumps.

Whether uniform spreading is necessarily an advantage is unclear. Based on the authors' experiences, the hard fillers clearly delivered good results in areas that are subject to a lot of pressure.

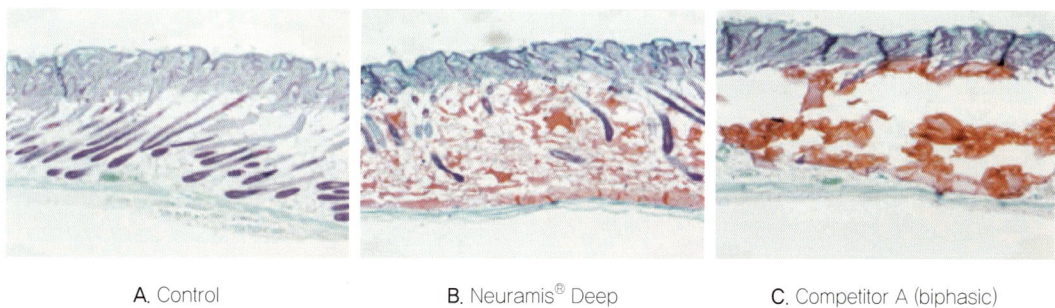

A. Control   B. Neuramis® Deep   C. Competitor A (biphasic)

Contrary to Products of Biphasic penetrate only in the injected part
Neuramis® deep, makes natural volume formation because it spreads evenly between the Skin Tissue

Fig. 1-9 **Changes after administration depending on the filler property.** In case of monophasic HA fillers, they integrated evenly within the skin layer after injection, but biphasic HA fillers did not spread evenly.

(Source: Neuramis, Medytox)

(10) Cohesiveness

Cohesivity is a filler characteristic that may be favorable or unfavorable. When performing filler procedures, products with high cohesivity are ideal in some cases, depending on the area especially in forehead. The difference in cohesiveness can be identified clearly through the following test (compression test).

<High cohesivity = High internal bondage strength that allows filler to maintain its shape = Advantageous in maintaining the shape of volume>

Generally monophasic fillers have higher cohesivity than the biphasic fillers.

Advantage: When external force is applied, the highly cohesive (=monophasic) filler more easily recover its own morphology compared to the less cohesive (=biphasic) filler. The importance of cohesiveness is decreased in patients who have thick skin and abundant subcutaneous fat tissue.

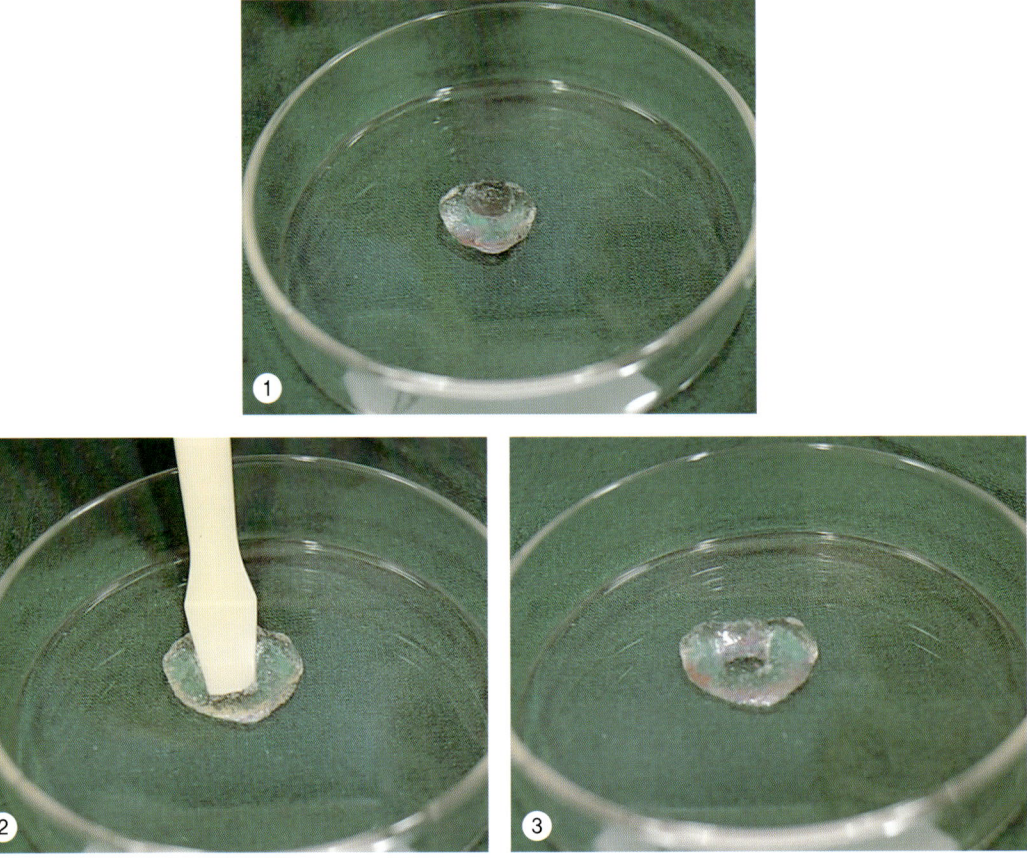

Fig. 1-10 Shows low cohesiveness. When the plastic spoon is pressed against the filler and removed, the separated area in the filler do not combine with each other but remain separate.

(Source: Restylane, GALDERMA)

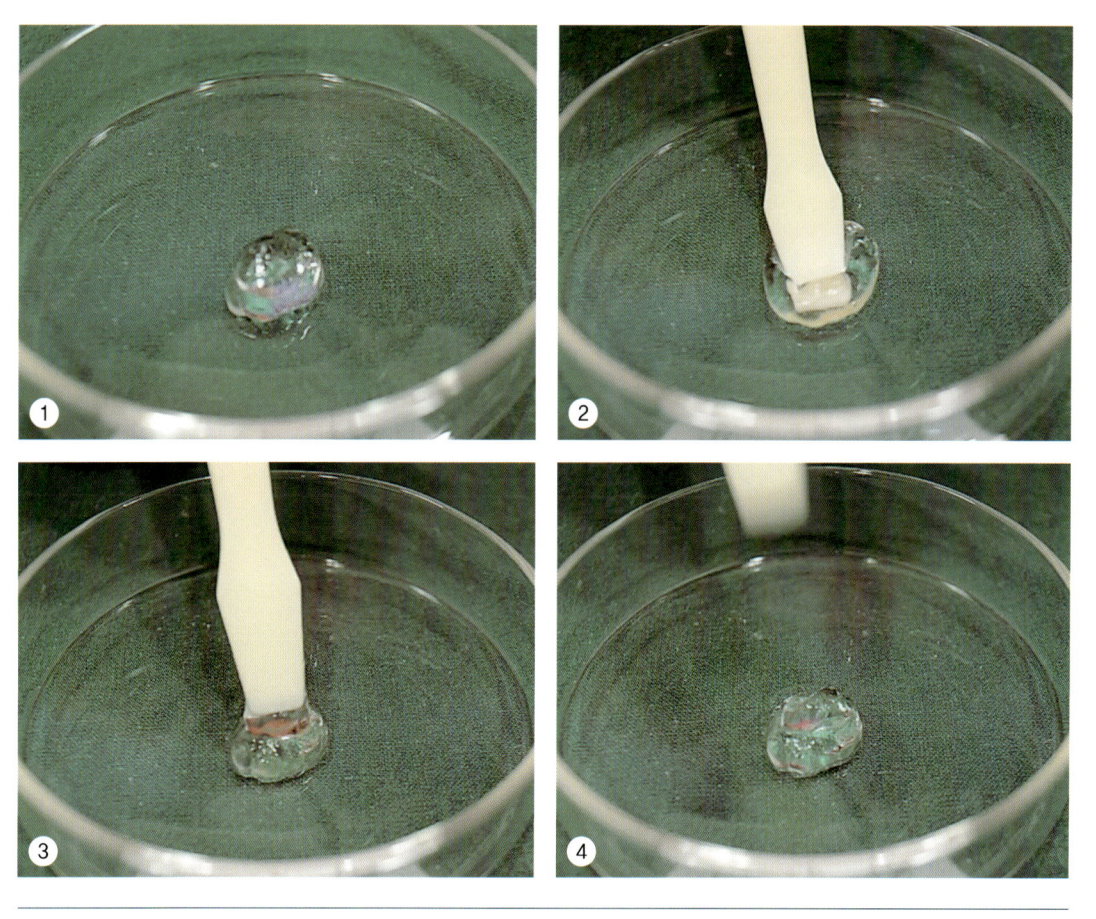

Fig. 1-11 The monophasic filler above shows high cohesiveness. When the plastic spatula is pressed against the filler and removed, the separated areas combine again.

(Monophasic filler: Neuramis, Medytox)

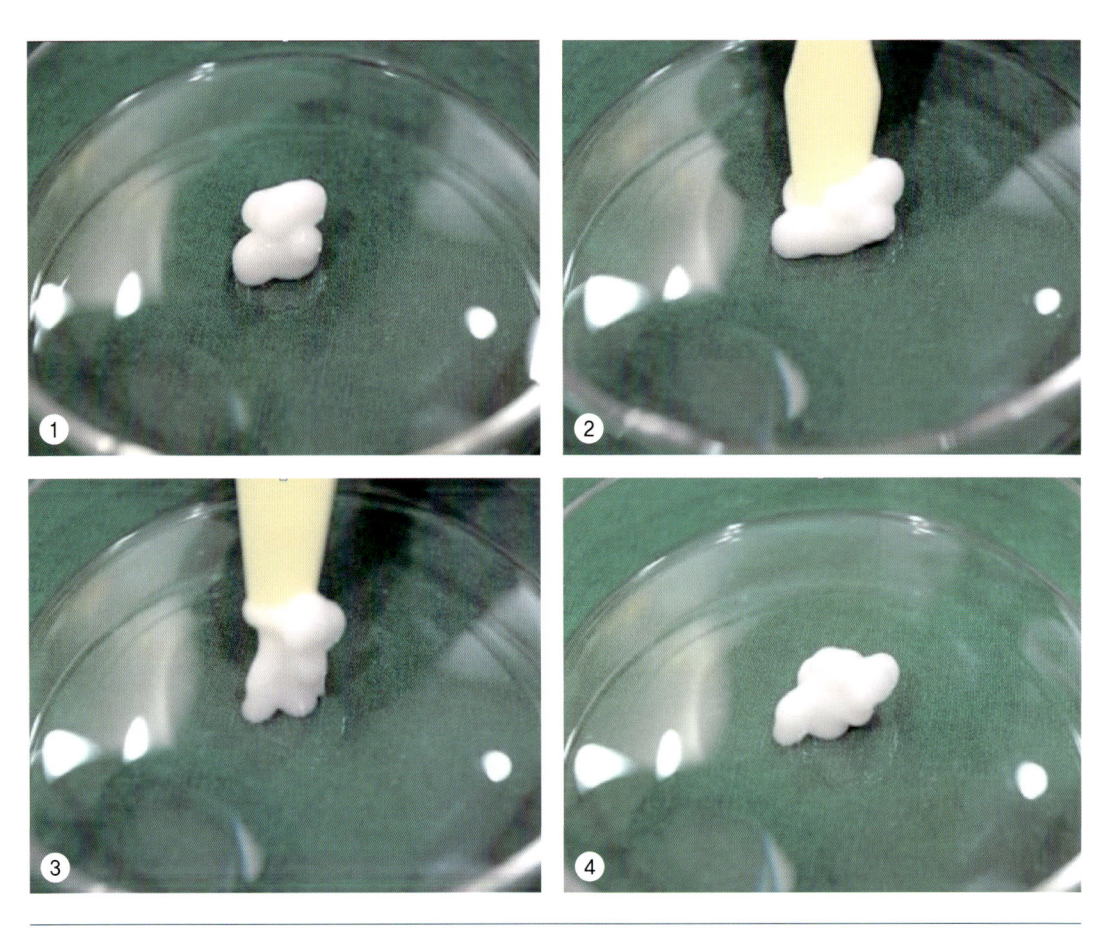

Fig. 1-12 Polycaprolactone filler also shows high cohesiveness.

(Source: Ellansé, JW Pharm)

2) HA Filler from Physician's Perspective

Physicians have limitations in obtaining accurate information about the various physical characteristics of fillers. Physicians have to rely on the manufacturing company for information about the degree of cross-linking, degree of hydration, and consistency.

However, the following physical characteristics of fillers can be evaluated by the physicians.

1. Firstly, ease of injection : in general, the smaller the particle size, the easier it is for the gel to flow through the needle. Also, the addition of free HA, which acts as a lubricant, can improve the ease of injection. It can be said that most of the physical characteristics of fillers explained previously is related to the extrusion force.
2. Secondly, the hardness of the gel : once injected, some fillers are easier to mold and spread well. However some fillers are hard and are more difficult to mold. This characteristic is important from a physician's perspective when selecting a filler. Some physicians prefer hard fillers, whereas some prefer soft fillers. Of course, selection also depends on the area to be injected. For areas with lots of movements, such as the nose, nasolabial fold and forehead or areas with lots of pressure, hard fillers generally bring better results.
3. Thirdly, lifting capacity : lately fillers have been injected in the dermal layer to improve wrinkles but fillers are still largely injected into the subcutaneous layer to restore volume. In the latter case, fillers must be able to hold their position and be able to lift the soft tissues. If the holding strength is too weak, the desired shape cannot be achieved and it may appear as though it has reverted to its original state. Naturally, the satisfaction of the physician and the patient decreases.

Table 1-4 Filler characteristics are related to following items

Ease of injection	• Particle size, needle size and type, viscosity
Gel strength	• Shape maintenance, lifting power
Lifting capacity	• Firmness, hardness, degree of cross-linking
Degree of post-injection swelling	• There is possibility of overcorrection due to post-injection swelling with monophasic fillers • Less bleeding and tissue damage

3-1. Lifting capacity is determined by two rheological properties: G′ value, a measure of the elasticity and cohesiveness, a measure of the viscosity of the gel. It is this viscoelastic property that plays a pivotal role in forming and maintaining the desired shape.

3-2. The ideal filler will have high viscoelasticity and be able to maintain its smoothness. Filler companies are likely to be conducting research with a goal to develop a filler with these properties.

4. Another characteristic is post injection swelling. In general, bruising and swelling after filler procedures are considered inevitable. However, as the physical characteristics of fillers are being researched and fillers with new concepts emerge, new opinions are put forth about post injection swelling. In general, monophasic fillers cause more swelling than biphasic fillers swelling. According to recent research, it can increase up to three times in weight after the procedure. Such a phenomenon is largely a consequence of the filler characteristic and is not related to the degree of tissue damage caused at the time of the procedure. On the other hand, significant tissue damage at the time of the procedure that resulted in a lot bleeding may leading to swelling and bruising. Considering the mechanism of filler degradation, such post injection swelling will have an adverse effect on the filler longevity. Therefore, it is important to conduct the procedure so as to cause the least amount of bruising and swelling and to select fillers that can assist in providing such a result.

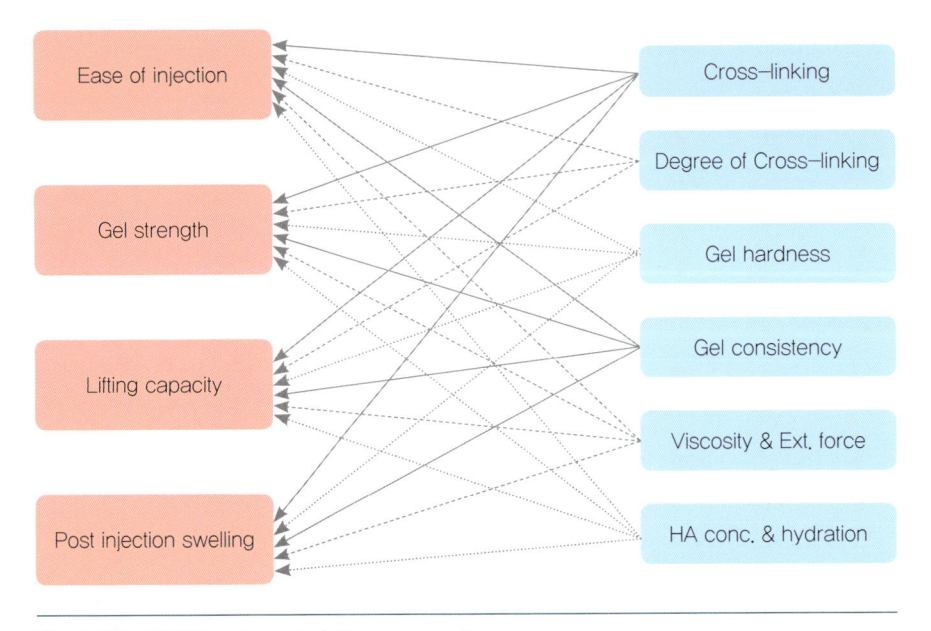

Fig. 1-13   HA filler characteristics - connections

3) Summary of Characteristics of Fillers

- The physical and chemical characteristics of filler products differ at the particle level. However, The important things are the differences which the practitioners feel in their clinical setting.
- The biphasic type has particles and is more difficult to inject, but they maintain a hard shape after being injected by causing an appropriate level of swelling.
- The monophasic type is not composed of particles but forms a homogenous gel mass analogous to whipped cream in cakes or butter. When injected, this type is soft and spreads well, but there is a tendency for swelling. Also, the holding strength, namely viscoelasticity, is weaker than that of biphasic fillers.
- Fillers promoted to have both monophasic and biphasic characteristics have recently emerged. However it is difficult to ascertain if there are actually big differences. These products exhibit both homogenous gel structure and some lump-like properties. It is not clear how these products differ in comparison to monophasic or biphasic fillers.
- In reality the information from test results and description of fillers at the particle level as provided by companies do not aid significantly in the clinical evaluation and selection of fillers.
- From the user's perspective, ease of injection, degree of gel strength, ability to lift soft tissue, and post procedure swelling should be evaluated when selecting the most appropriate filler for him/herself. Evaluation of filler characteristic was done based on actual touching and rubbing.
- Free HA, which acts as a lubricant, is mixed into biphasic fillers. The ratio of free HA differs from product to product but ranges from 10-20%.
- To evaluate the bioequivalence in terms of filler duration, newly developed fillers are usually compared against biphasic fillers manufactured with NASHA technology.
- Results demonstrating equivalence or superiority of the new filler must be interpreted taking into consideration filler type. In the case of comparing a monophasic filler against a biphasic hyaluronic acid filler, it is important to consider that there is early volume loss in biphasic fillers due to the absorption of free HA.
- Results demonstrating longer duration of monophasic filler compared to the biphasic filler may actually not be an indication of product superiority.

(1) Biphasic

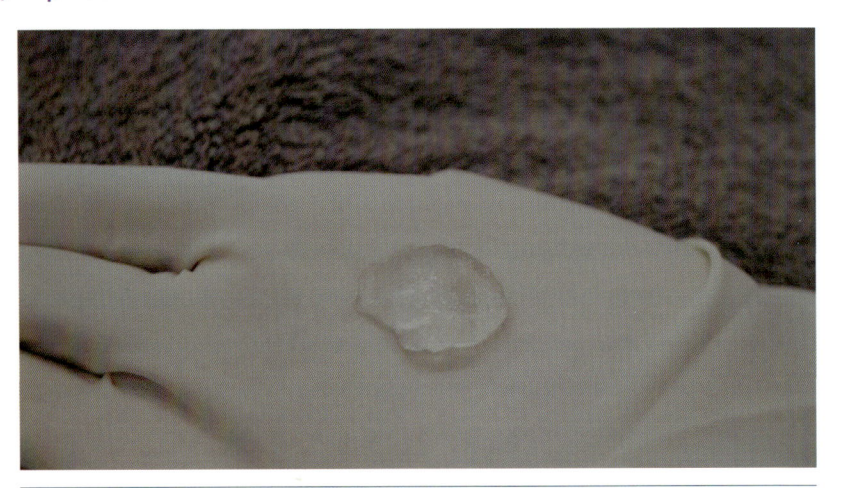

Fig. 1-14 When biphasic fillers are injected on the hand, many small assembled lumps rather than a single mass is observed. Upon examination with the naked eye, the surface is rough and looks like a collection of slightly sticky lumps.

(Source: Restylane, GALDERMA)

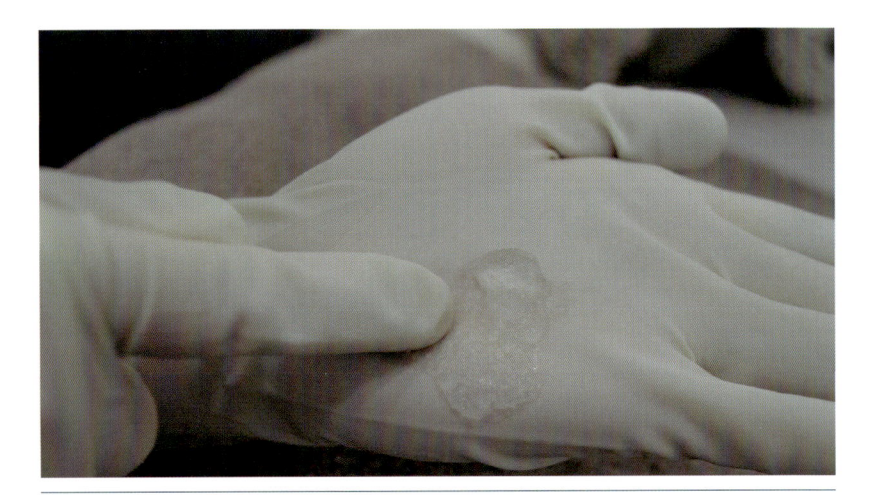

Fig. 1-15 When rubbed with a finger, the mass feels soft but the lumpy particles can be felt. When rubbed, it does not spread evenly and feels as though it breaks down into irregular lumps.

(Source: Restylane, GALDERMA)

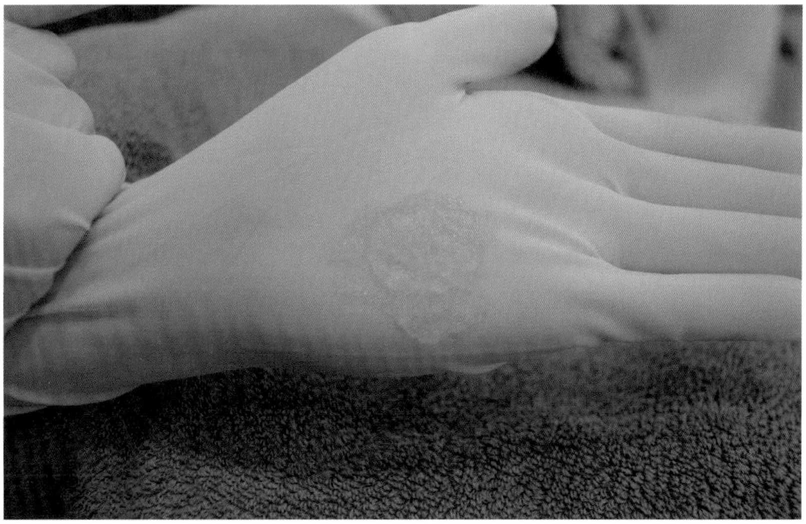

Fig. 1-16 When rubbed with a finger to spread uniformly, it can be see that the mass does not spread to flatten. Due to its relatively high viscosity, particles do not spread evenly and they show tendency to stay in lumps. This factors indicate high viscoelasticity and holding strength.

(Source: Restylane, GALDERMA)

(2) Monophasic

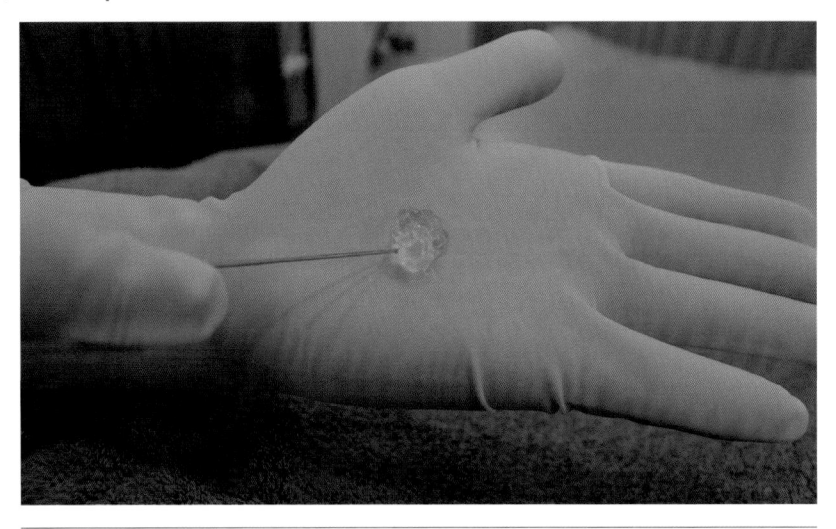

Fig. 1-17 Monophasic filler gel is even and aggregates smoothly to form a single homogenous mass. While the biphasic filler consistency is akin to yeast budding, the monophasic filler does not have this texture.

(Monophasic filler: Neuramis, Medytox)

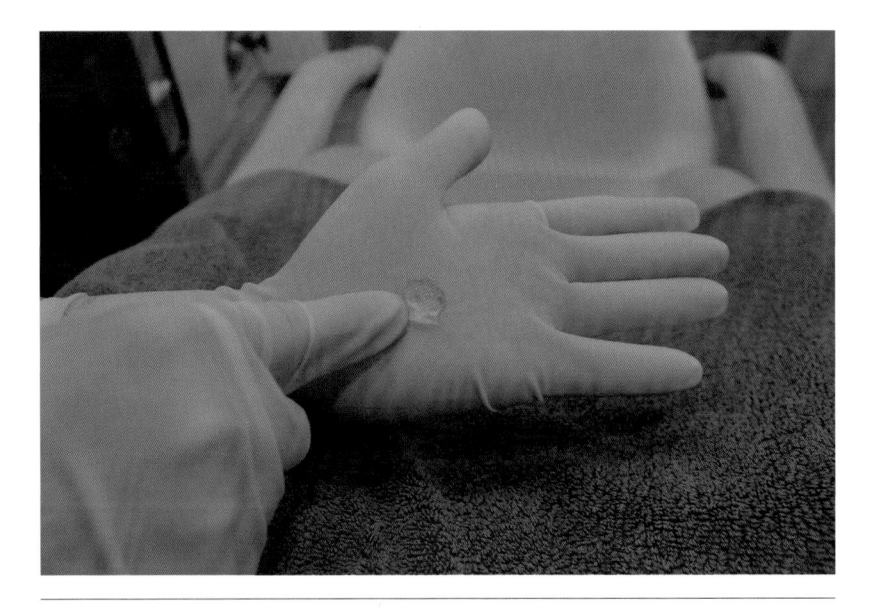

Fig. 1-18 When mass is pressed with the finger, it is soft and the initial volume is maintained to a certain extent.

(Monophasic filler: Neuramis, Medytox)

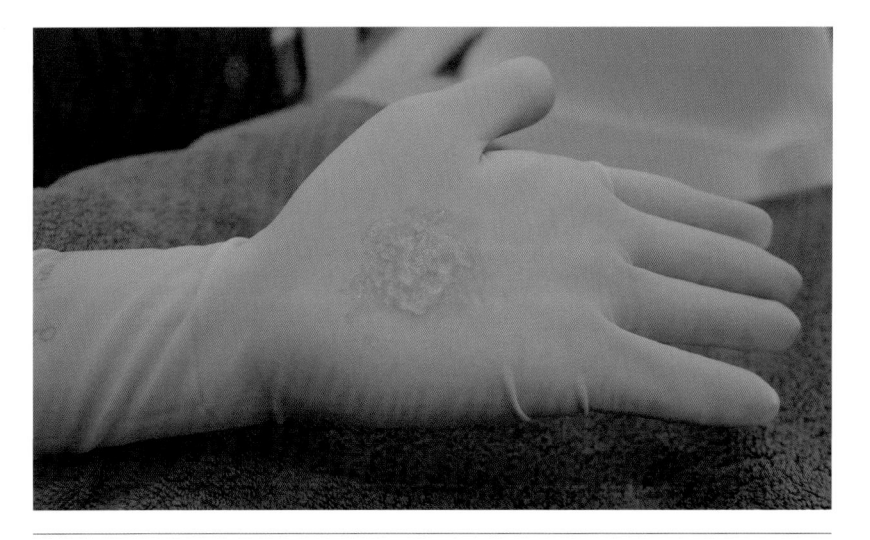

Fig. 1-19 When certain level of force is applied, the initial round form breaks. The mass spreads out smoothly and flattens. The mass is uniform and lumps are not visible.

(Monophasic filler: Neuramis, Medytox)

(3) Monophasic having characteristics of biphasic

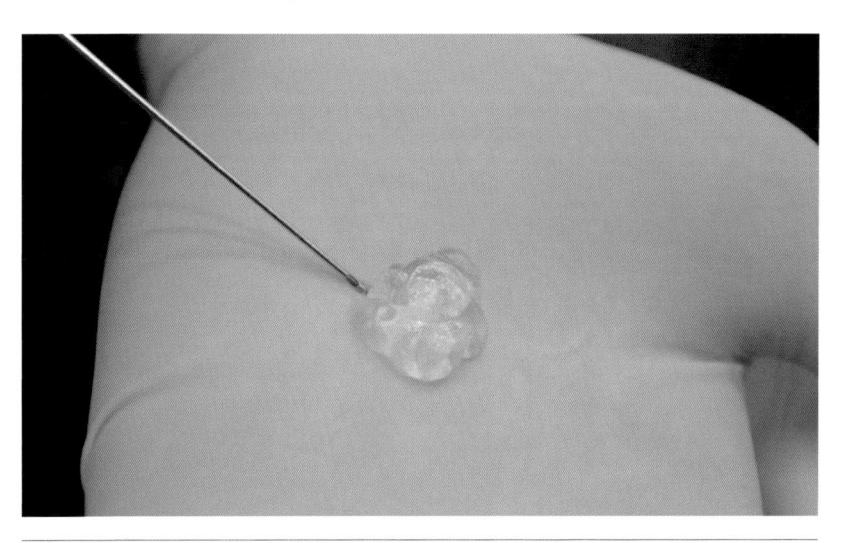

Fig. 1-20 Appearance wise, this filler looks like a monophasic filler. However, unlike purely monophasic filler, slight lumpy areas can be felt.

(Source: The CHAEUM, HUGEL)

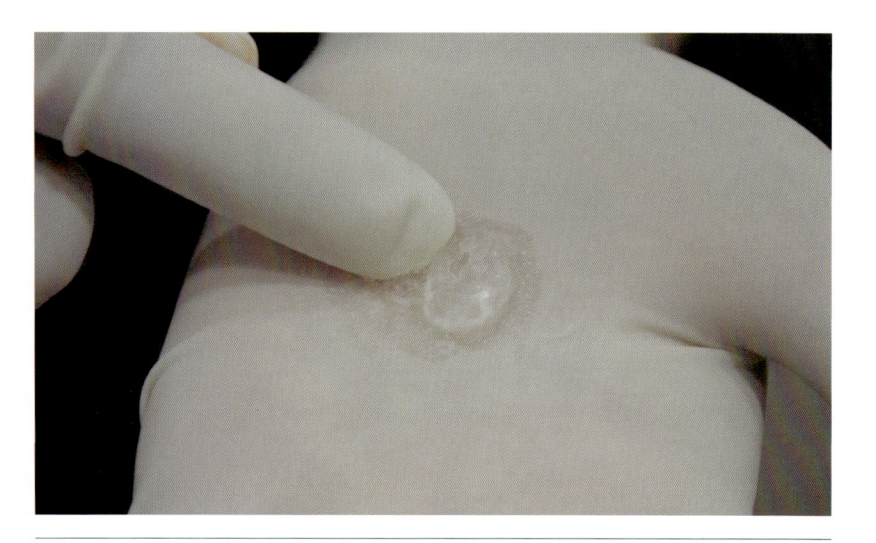

Safe Filler Injection Technique Demonstration – using live imaging tools

Fig. 1-21 When pressed applying light force, viscoelasticity can be felt and likewise, when a certain level of force is applied, the initial shape breaks and spreads.

(Source: The CHAEUM, HUGEL)

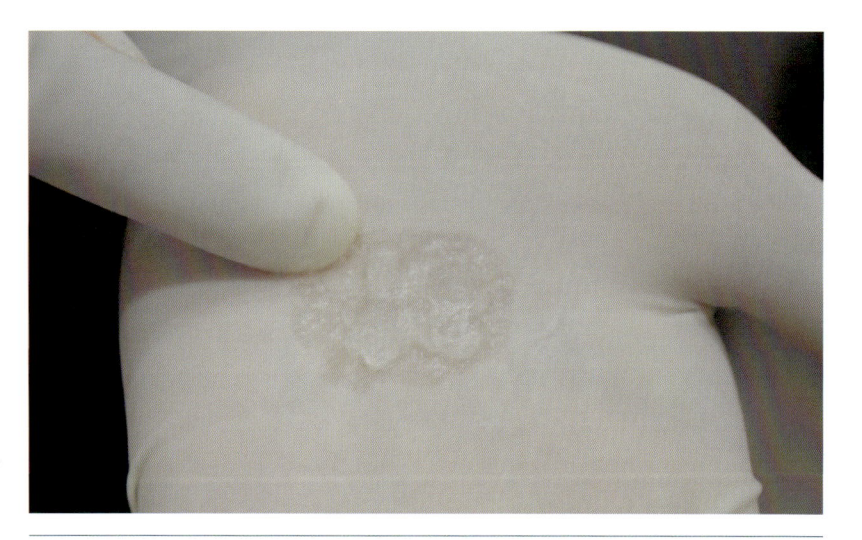

Fig. 1-22 When the mass is broken down by rubbing, the mass does not spread evenly like monophasic filler. Similar to biphasic filler, partially lumpy areas remain. The appearance of the remaining mass does not look identical to a biphasic filler, but the filler's viscoelasticity and ability to aggregate is substantial.

(Source: The CHAEUM, HUGEL)

- Manufacturing process of biphasic fillers involves passing the ground hyaluronic acid through a mesh sieve to produce particles of uniform size. As seen in the figure below, Restylane is composed of uniformly sized particles.
- In the case of monophasic fillers, the cross-linked hyaluronic acid bulk gel is finely ground. The cross-linked units are then left to disperse before use.
- Theoretically, monophasic fillers should consist of one homogenous material. Unlike biphasic fillers, monophasic fillers when touched feel like a single mass.
- Strangely however, when monophasic fillers are observed under microscope it seems that they are also composed of particles.
- As monophasic fillers are not passed through a sieve, the particle size is not uniform.
- Particle consistency can be seen in the figures below.

Restylane Perlane

Restylane

Restylane Vital

Restylane skincare particles

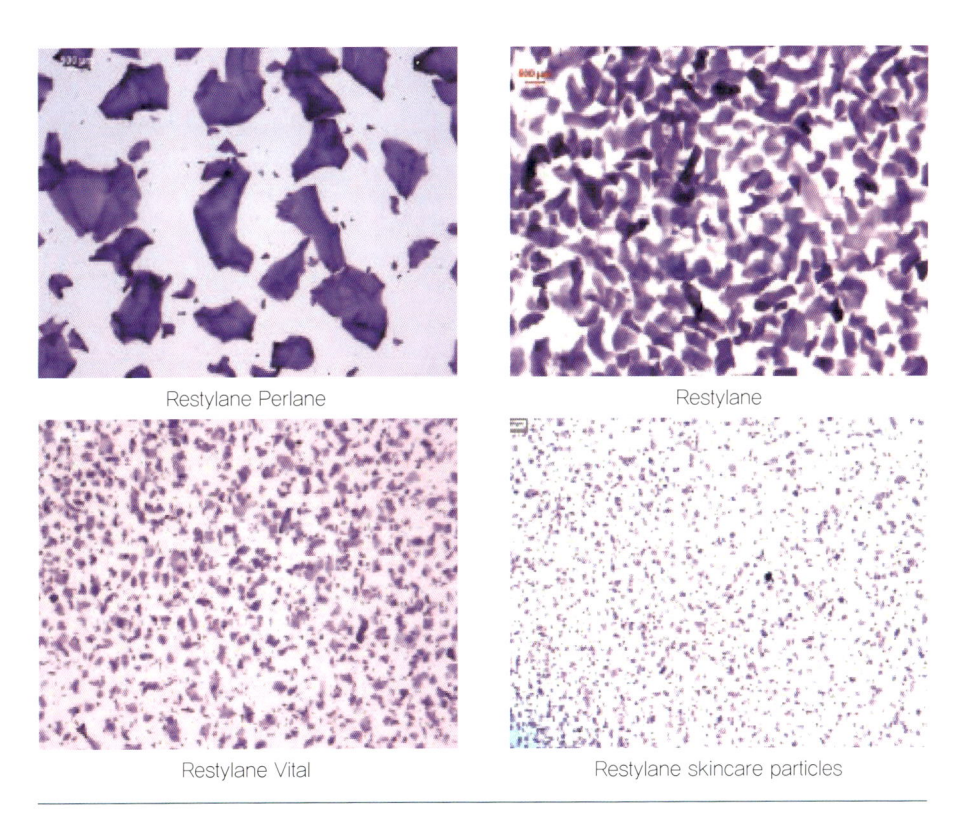

Fig. 1-23   Particle size of Restylane products

- The differences in the monophasic and biphasic filler figures is expected and reflect the effects of the different manufacturing processes.
- When monophasic fillers are felt, they tend to feel smoother and feel as one continuous mass.
- It is important to be aware that laboratory results and clinical study results may differ from results obtained by directly examining the filler products.

2 Characteristics of Calcium Fillers

1) Constituting Components

- **Calcium Hydroxylapatite (CaHA) — $Ca_{10}(PO_4)_6(OH)_2$**
  - 30%
  - A component existing in the human body and made up of beads the size of 20~45 μm.
  - Gradually over time collagen synthesis is promoted and then it is degraded (after degradation, calcium and phosphate ions are metabolized naturally through normal metabolic processes).

- **Gel carrier**
  - 70%
  - Consists of sodium carboxymethylcellulose, glycerin, and sterile water
  - Due to the large amount of particles and good viscoelasticity, augmentation effect is observed instantly.

2) Physical Characteristics

Viscosity and elasticity tend to be better than those of HA fillers.

3) Clinical Advantages

- Volumizing and lifting capacities are excellent, and ease of injection is also good.
- Promotes collagen synthesis.

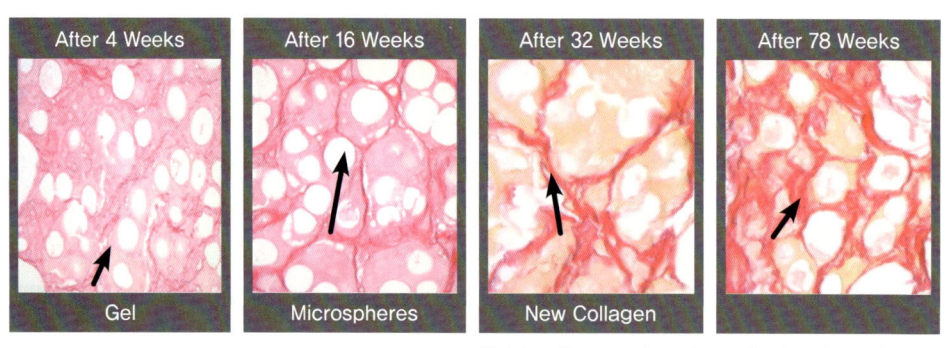

Safe Filler Injection Technique Demonstration – using live imaging tools

Staining: New matrix stains red using picrosirius red

Fig. 1-24 Time course study demonstrating collagen formation after Radiesse® injection
This is a time course study of Radiesse® injected into the subdermis of canine skin. Punch biopsies were taken at 4 weeks, 16 weeks, 32 weeks and 78 weeks.
The white spheres indicate the location of the calcium hydroxylapatite microparticles while the amorphous pink surrounding the particles at 4 and 16 weeks is remaining gel. The fibrillar red structures coursing throughout the images and seen in increasing density are the new collagen fibers being produced in and around the Radiesse® microspheres.

(Source: Radiesse, Merz)

· Rheology Test

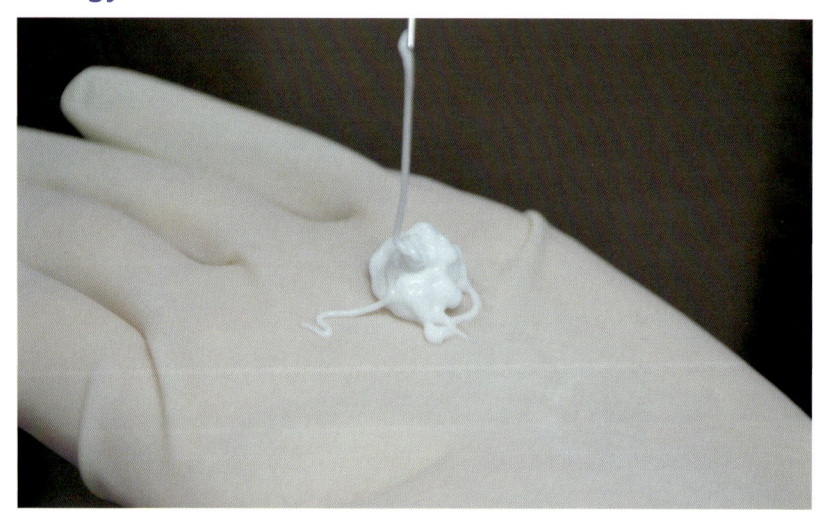

Fig. 1-25 When the calcium fillers are squeezed, a substantial amount of viscoelasticity can be felt. Rather than forming one lump, calcium fillers maintain the shape at the time of injection for a substantial period of time.

(Source: Radiesse, Merz)

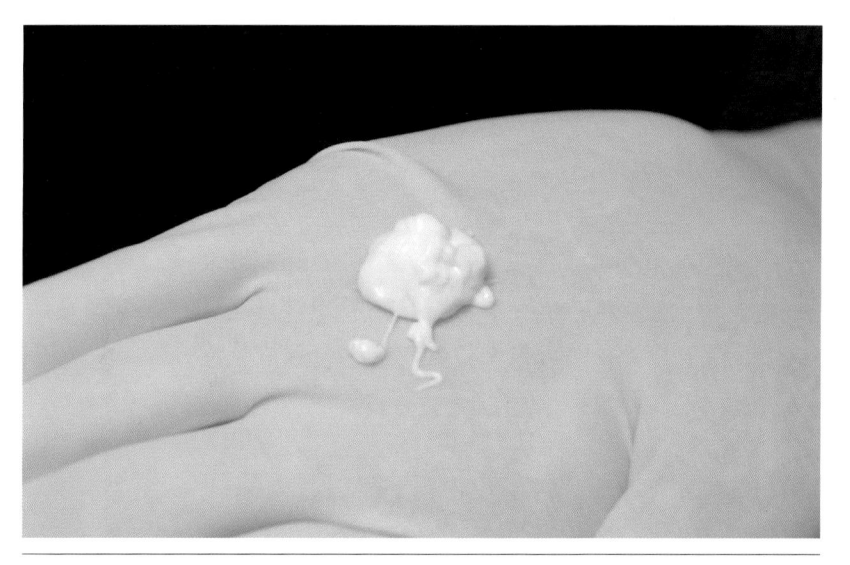

Fig. 1-26 As time passes, it does change to a lump form, but the strength for shape-maintenance is high. This shows that it has much higher lifting capacity than that of HA fillers.

(Source: Radiesse, Merz)

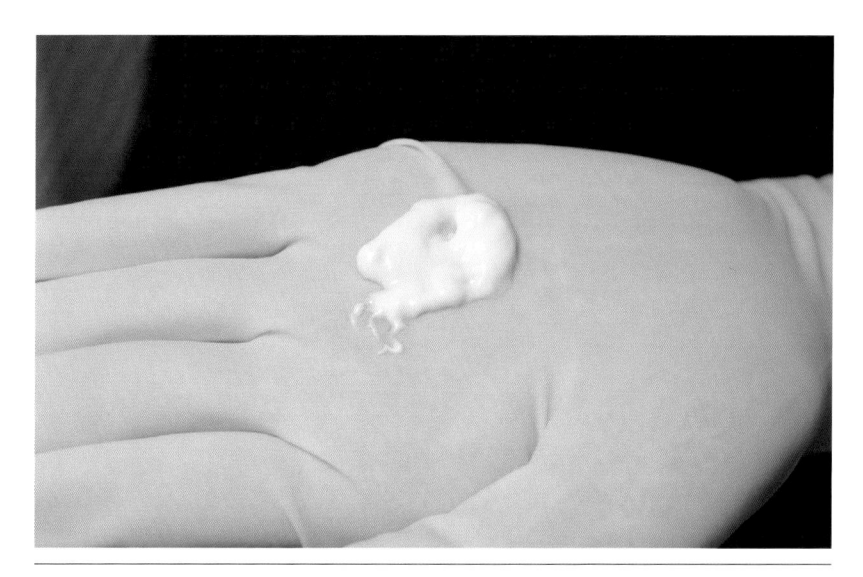

Fig. 1-27 When rubbed, it does not spread out very well. It feels like rubbing a hard form of ointment material. After being injected, it can be learned that the filler maintains its shape stably.

(Source: Radiesse, Merz)

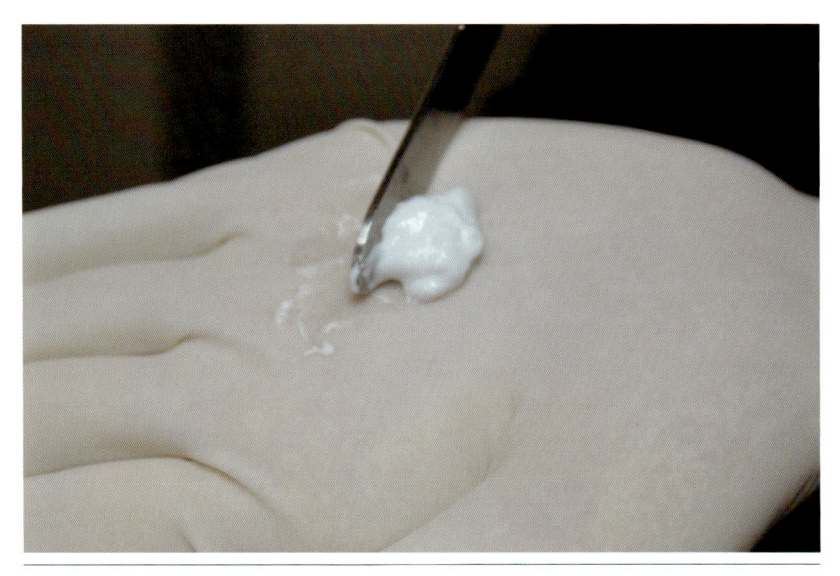

Safe Filler Injection Technique Demonstration – using live imaging tools

Fig. 1-28 When crumpled again, it crumples well.

(Source: Radiesse, Merz)

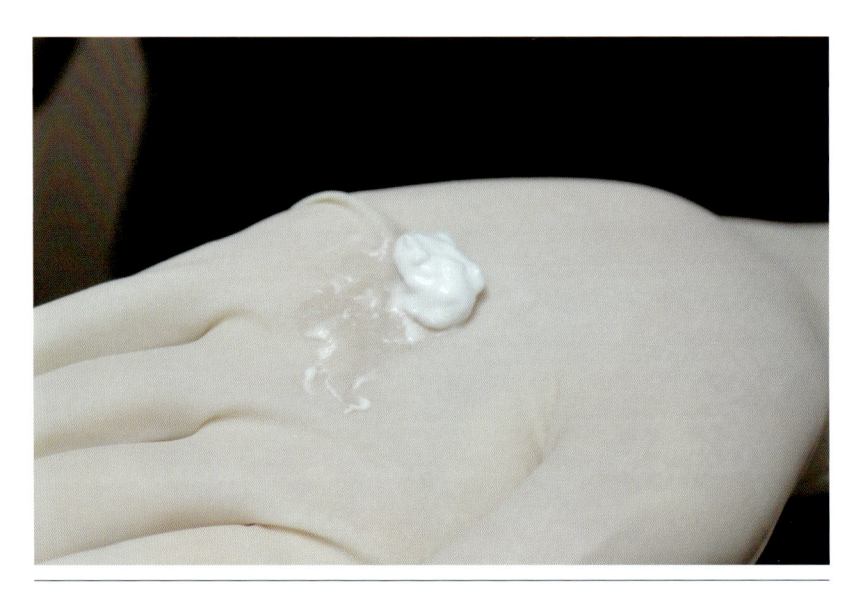

Fig. 1-29 Compared to the time before the initial rubbing, there is not much difference in the amount felt. This demonstrates strong viscoelasticity. However, such an advantage is a factor that causes accidents arising from putting pressure on the blood vessels, also making this a potential disadvantage.

(Source: Radiesse, Merz)

3 Characteristics of Fillers Composed of Polycaprolactone (PCL)

1) PCL Filler - Ellansé

- Hyaluronic acid fillers are easy to use and relatively safe as they can simply be dissociated by hyaluronidase when needed.
- However, they have a weakness that they do not last long, which has led to high demand for fillers with great longevity.
- Consequently, fillers that exhibit longer longevity than HA fillers are being continuously developed.
- Amongst many different polymers, materials that have affirmed safety for medical use are generally being used for manufacturing fillers.
- Fillers comprised of polycaprolactone have been newly developed and currently being used.
- PCL filler consists of 30% of particles with a smooth surface and a spherical shape, and 70% of carboxy methylcellulose (CMC) gel carriers.
- Both PCL and CMC are completely bioresorbable that have been used as medical devices for a long period of time.
- After injection of PCL, CMC gel carrier becomes absorbed immediately by macrophages within a number of weeks. On the other hand, the PCL particles do not become digested by macrophages and form surrounding layers instead, stimulating collagen synthesis attributed to their particular size (25-50 μm) and smooth spherical-shaped surface
- It is important to understand biological mechanisms of a PCL filler.
- As the gel carrier becomes absorbed collagen synthesis replaces the lost volume at the same place.
- Thus, after filler injection, the reduction of swelling due to recovery makes it seem that the treatment volume has been lost. As gel carrier becomes absorbed and then replaced by collagen, the overall volumes looks smaller in general. However, after a while, the lost volume becomes replenished back as collagen synthesis propels for a number of weeks.
- For this reason, some patients have reported that most of the filler has been excreted from the face within the first several weeks.

- This period may be the intermediate stage between the time of gel carrier absorption and the time of collagen synthesis. It is necessary to inform the patient of this biological process and assure them to wait for the following clinical results. Sympathizing with the patient's needs too much may lead to additional treatments and result in an unwanted over correction.

SAFE PRODUCT COMPONENTS WITH A LONG SAFETY HISTORY

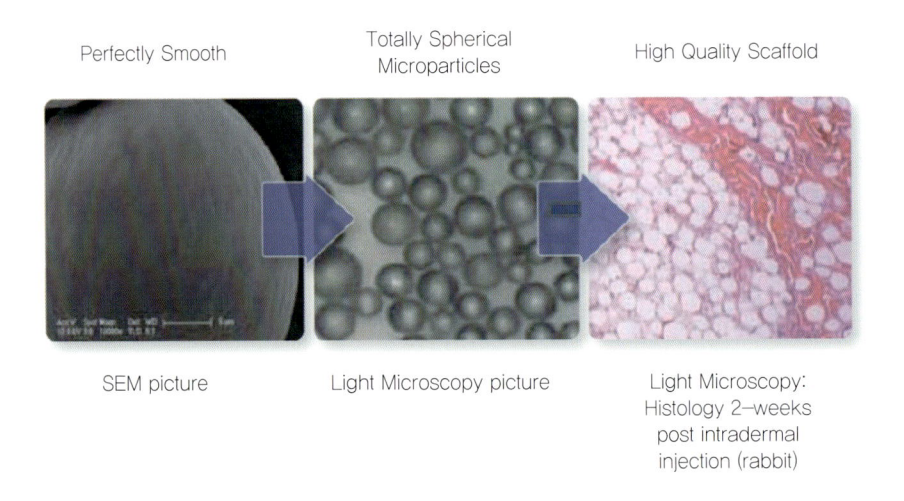

Perfectly Smooth — SEM picture

Totally Spherical Microparticles — Light Microscopy picture

High Quality Scaffold — Light Microscopy: Histology 2–weeks post intradermal injection (rabbit)

Fig. 1-30 Histological changes post injection

(Source: Ellansé JW Pharm, Sinclair)

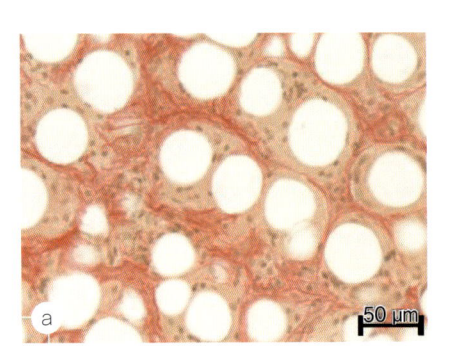

Figure a. Photomicrograph PSR–stained tissue 9 months post–injection with Ellansé™–M using non–polarized light. The figure demonstrates the newly formed collagen scaffold.

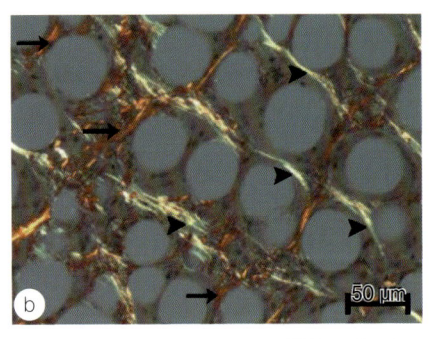

Figure b. Photomicrograph of PSR–stained tissue 9 months post–injection with Ellansé™–M using polarized light. The figure shows a typical orange–red and green birefringence, with red (arrows) collagen Type I and green (arrowheads) collagen Type III.

Fig. 1-31

(Source: Ellansé JW Pharm, Sinclair)

- In general, microspheres that are equal or smaller than 15 μm become phagocytosed, whereas microspheres greater than 15 μm with irregular surfaces likely cause infections and foreign body granuloma.
- One of the most threatening possible complications of using long term fillers would be formation of foreign body granuloma, in which giant cells created by convergence of macrophages encapsulate fillers and cause granulomatous inflammation.
- Therefore, it is highly recommended to double check the potential long-term complications before choosing fillers.
- Until now, PCL fillers have not shown any particular complications in a 2 year-follow up study. Further studies that verify safety for a longer period of time are needed.
- In terms of procedures, PCL filler is not much different from HA fillers.
- However, considering the biochemical characteristics of PCL fillers that stimulate collagen formation, injection into a superficial layer should be avoided.
- It would be better to inject into a deeper dermal layer (subcutaneous layer) for volumization. Since PCL fillers cannot be easily melted unlike the HA fillers, an extreme caution is required at the time of injection. In case of an emergency situation during treatment, a puncture at the injection point should be made and squeeze out the filler.
- However, the homogeneity of the filler components is broken and there is a possibility of particle damage. so the authors think that such an attempt may be dangerous.
- Changes in the filler property after mixing with saline in vitro after 1 minutes and 24 hours are as follows.

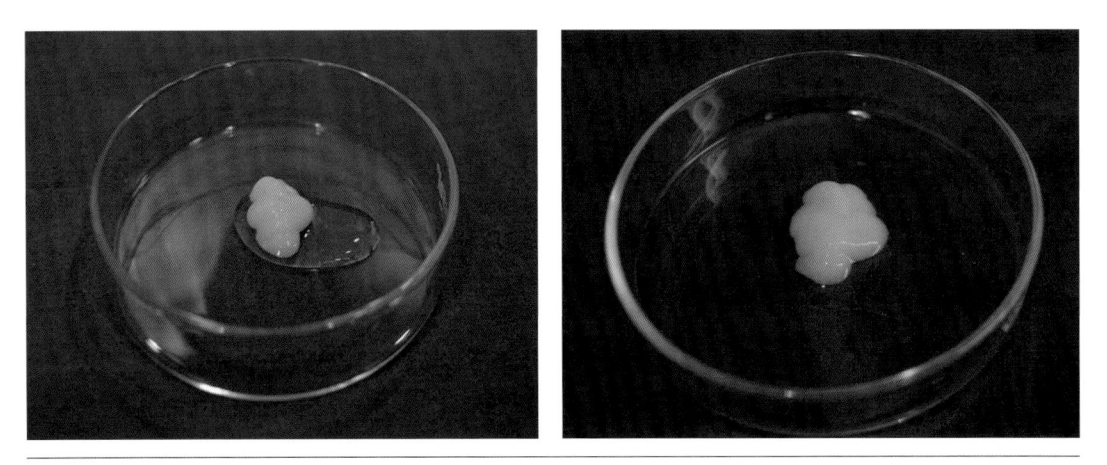

Fig. 1-32　**After 1 min vs. 24 hours.** Polycaprolactone filler is not mixed with saline.

3. Categorization of the Filler Market

••• When selecting fillers with proven safety and efficiency, price has a large effect. Based on the makeup of sales in the Korean filler market, fillers from renowned foreign companies have higher sales, but their high unit cost of import should be taken into consideration. In reality, it is predicted that the most used fillers are the Korean fillers, sold at a relatively low cost.

In selecting fillers, other than mere price and publicity, if other various considerations are evaluated objectively from a physician's perspective, the patient can choose fillers that are most suitable for him/herself.

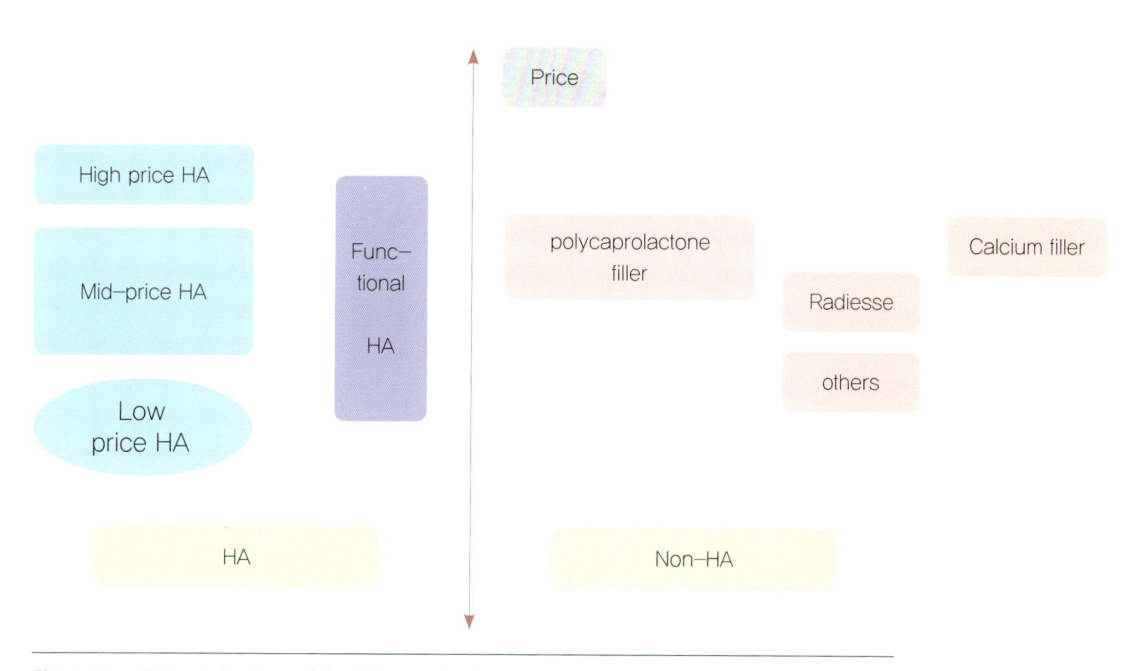

Fig. 1-33 Categorization of the filler market

4. Filler Selection

1 Standards for Filler Selection

Any physician would have deliberated on which filler to use at least once. Those experiencing the filler for the first time tend to use HA fillers that are safe and can be melted. However, with increasing cases and shortcomings with respect to the durability and shape maintenance, interest in non-HA fillers naturally develops. Standards for selecting fillers are affected by property of fillers, physician's experience and confidence, durability, price, etc.

In general, fillers are selected based on the physician's opinion and recommendation. However, one additional consideration ought to be made, which is what fillers should be selected from the patient's perspective. In reality, the standards of selection differ between the physician performing the procedures and the patient receiving the procedures.

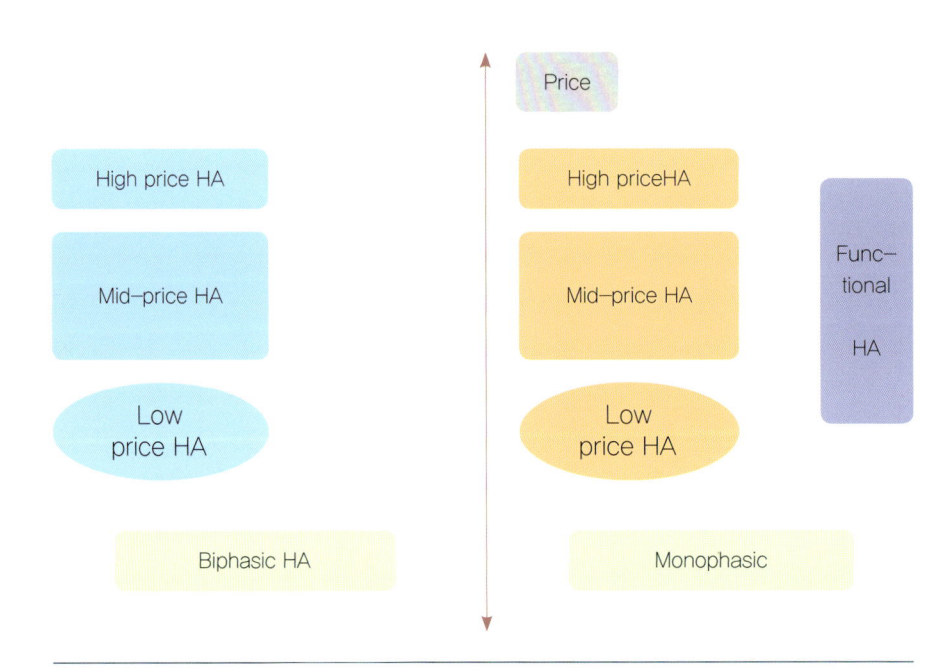

Fig. 1-34 Categorization of HA filler market

| Table 1-5 | Standards for selecting fillers |

Doctor	Patient
• HA or non–HA • Safety • Price • Degree of viscoelasticity: whether the shape is maintained well • Past experience: Experience of side effects cause not to use certain products. • Monophasic vs biphasic • Characteristics of makeup of patients • Appropriate filler for the treatment area • Direction of marketing (High price filler vs. low price filler)	• Filler that has been advertised • Filler experienced by others • Filler recommended by the clinician • Filler with long duration period • Filler with relatively low price • Luxury filler with high price

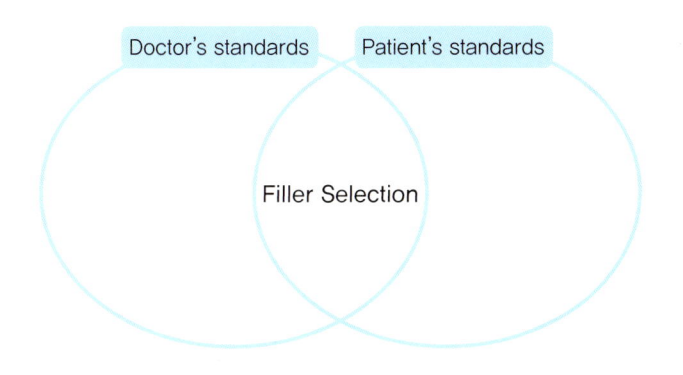

Fig. 1-35   Standards for filler selection

It is helpful to clearly learn the standards for selecting fillers from both sides to make the final decision.

2 Filler Selection and Safety

Filler selection is determined based on various standards but safety must be the top priority.

It is a little more comfortable to use monophasic fillers which put less pressure on the tissue due to the quality which molds and spreads easily. Biphasic fillers, which have large and hard particles, or calcium fillers can be tried for areas with less likelihood of accidents occurring from pressure on the tissue or areas which require high viscoelasticity to maintain the shape. Before getting accustomed with the filler injection, it is recommended to use fillers, which are relatively easy to inject and handle smoothly.

After accumulating much experience using cannula and needles, the hand is able to feel the pressure during the injection and the ability to create space for filler injection through the DPS (deep puncture & separation or subcision) method develops, so it would be considered acceptable to use harder fillers with confidence. It is recommended to avoid using calcium fillers initially on dangerous areas. However, as long as there is solid confidence for conducting safe filler procedures, dangerous treatment areas with high pressures can be targeted with calcium fillers and bring out great results.

Reference

1. S. Y. Park et al. Investigation of the Degradation-Retarding Effect Caused by the Low Swelling Capacity of a Novel Hyaluronic Acid Filler Developed by Solid-Phase Crosslinking Technology. Ann Dermatol. 2014;26(3):357-62.

2. Jean D. A. Carruthers et al. Fillers and Neocollagenesis. Dermatol Surg. 2014;40:S134-6.

3. Laeschke K, Biocompatibility of microparticles into soft tissue fillers. Semin Cutan Med Surg. 2004;23(4):214-7.

4. Anderson JM, Mechanism of inflammation and infection with implanted devices. Cardiovasc. Pathol. 1993;2(3):S33-41.

5. Nicolau PJ, Marijnissen-Hofsté JM. Neocollagenesis after injection of a polycaprolactone based dermal filler in a rabbit. Submitted to EJAMeD 2012.

6. White paper: Neocollagenesis after injection of Ellansé™ in a rabbit. AQTS Medical.

7. Marion Michaela Moers-Carpi, MD. Et al. Polycaprolactone for the Correction of Nasolabial Folds: A 24-Month, Prospective, Randomized, Controlled Clinical Trial. Dermatol Surg. 2013;39:457-63.

8. Jongseo Antonio Kim & Daan Van Abel. Neocollagenesis in human tissue injected with a polycaprolactone-based dermal filler. J Cosmet Laser Ther. 2015;17:99-101.

9. Ahmet Tezel & Glenn H. Fredrickson. The science of hyaluronic acid dermal fillers. J Cosmet Laser Ther. 2008;10:35-42.

10. K. Y. Park, H. K. Kim, B. J. Kim. Comparative study of hyaluronic acid fillers by in vitro and in vivo testing. J Eur Acad Dermatol Venereol. 2014;28(5):565-8.

11. Timothy Corcoran Flynn MD, et al. Comparative Histology of Intradermal Implantation of Mono and Biphasic Hyaluronic Acid Fillers. Dermatol Surg. 2011;37(5):637-43.

12. Coleman K, Voigts R, DeVore DP, Termin P, Coleman WP. Neocollagenesis after Injection of Calcium Hydroxylapatite Composition in a Canine Model, Dermatol Surg. 2008;34(suppl 1):S53-5.

Safe Filler Injection Technique Demonstration
– using live imaging tools

Part
2

Basic Introduction

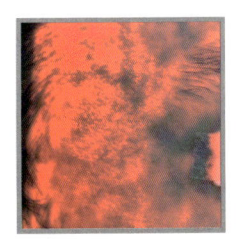

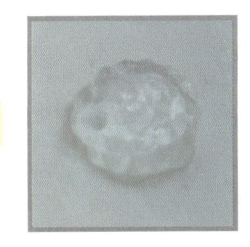

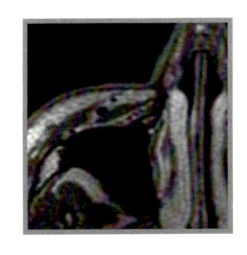

Safe Filler Injection Technique Demonstration
- using live imaging tools

Part 2 — Basic Introduction

1. Design Method

1. Designing the Whole and Parts
2. Design Considering Facial Expressions
3. Tricks for Safe Procedures

2. Filler Administration with Cannulas

1. Puncturing Method for Cannula Insertion
2. Method of Using Cannula Depending on the Depth
3. Cannula Advancement and Separation of Tissue

3. Basic Method of Using a Needle

1. Method of Using a Needle
2. Considerations of Bevel Location in Procedures
3. Post Dermal Subcision Injection Method
4. Perpendicular Pulling Injection Method
5. Perpendicular Injection of a Large Bolus

4. No Bleeding Technique

5. Molding

1. What is Molding?
2. Molding Method for Each Facial Area
   1) Molding Under Eyes (the Smile Line)
   2) Under Eye Guider
   3) Nasolabial Folds and Cheeks
   4) Massage after Injection

6. Dissolution Test

1. How to Use Hyaluronidase
2. An Experiment for Melting HA Fillers

Part 2
Basic Introduction

1. Design Method

1 Designing the Whole and Parts

For perfect results from procedures, the preparation process needs to be strictly adhered to. Filler procedures are not a process of merely injecting and finishing. From the patient's perspective, only after obtaining aesthetic improvement is the satisfaction, making it worth going through the hardship of the procedure.

The design process requires observations to individual sections or parts as well as observations on the whole, in order to create a sense of harmony. Also, there must be harmony between a status when there is no facial expression and a status when there is a smile. Basically, fillers are purported to give a youthful look through strengthening the volume in the subcutaneous layer and improving the appearance of wrinkles through injecting into the dermal layer. If a simple adjustment is made only through injecting filler in sunken areas (based on sectional or partial observations), it is possible to get unsatisfactory outcomes in the future.

Therefore, the harmony between the specific parts and on the whole, as well as changes in facial expressions must be taken into consideration. In order to accurately examine the harmony between the individual parts and the whole, there must be a generally accepted standard for an aesthetically pleasing face, and one must be able to consider which area needs to be changed in order to become prettier.

It is important to learn about the whole facial structure of the patient first. Through conversing with the patient, an accurate understanding should be obtained with respect to the area that the patient is dissatisfied with and based on such understanding, a plan for procedures can be made through comparative analysis with aesthetic standards. Initially, it would be advisable to avoid excessive adjustment affected by trends as beauty standards continuously change depending on the time period

2 Design Considering Facial Expressions

Human's face constantly creates sunken or bulging areas depending on facial expressions. This is especially true for the central area of the forehead where a great amount of dynamic wrinkles occurs.

When considering fillers for the forehead, it is essential to assess the forehead frown lines and glabellar lines prior to the treatment. During physical examination, these lines need to be thoroughly observed while listening to the patient talking. For those who frown a lot while talking, it should be determined whether they have a bad eyesight, which can be fixed simply with vision correction, or the frowning is merely a habit that can be treated with botulinum toxin. Only thereafter, fillers can effectively serve its purpose by stably residing within and maintaining the beautiful shape of the forehead.

In order to treat cheeks or tear troughs, the overall facial expression when smiling must be carefully observed. There are cases where there is a serious difference in the degree of sunkenness between a steady face and a smiling face. In such cases, it is necessary to differently address each sunken area for both facial expressions. Thus, it is advisable to correct the sunken areas that are clearly manifested during both expressions. If a sunken area is manifested more in only one of the two faces, treatment should be planned according to the facial expression that requires less correction. In that way, overcorrection can be avoided and creation of an unnatural face can be prevented. After a sufficient amount of time has passed since the treatment and the fillers stabilize to a certain extent, it is possible to adjust deficient areas through additional treatments.

3 Tricks for Safe Procedures

When designing fillers, regardless of whether a cannula or needle is used, there must be a clear understanding of the dangerous areas. In order to avoid damaging the blood vessels and the nerves, it is very important to have an understanding of not only the organization but also the depth of blood vessels.

For thorough attention to be taken with respect to the dangerous areas, various measures should be taken during the design process. It is helpful to mark the distribution of major blood vessels and nerves prior to performing the procedure. Rather than marking the vasculature, a safety borderline could be drawn, determining not to perform filler injection outside the line. In another method, the origins of major nerves and blood vessels are marked with dots, so that needle or cannula could avoid the dotted regions and pass through the surrounding areas with more caution.

Designing Tricks	Understand the areas the patient would like his or her treatment
	Consider the harmony on the whole
	Consider the variability due to the change in facial expressions
	Be prepared for dangerous areas

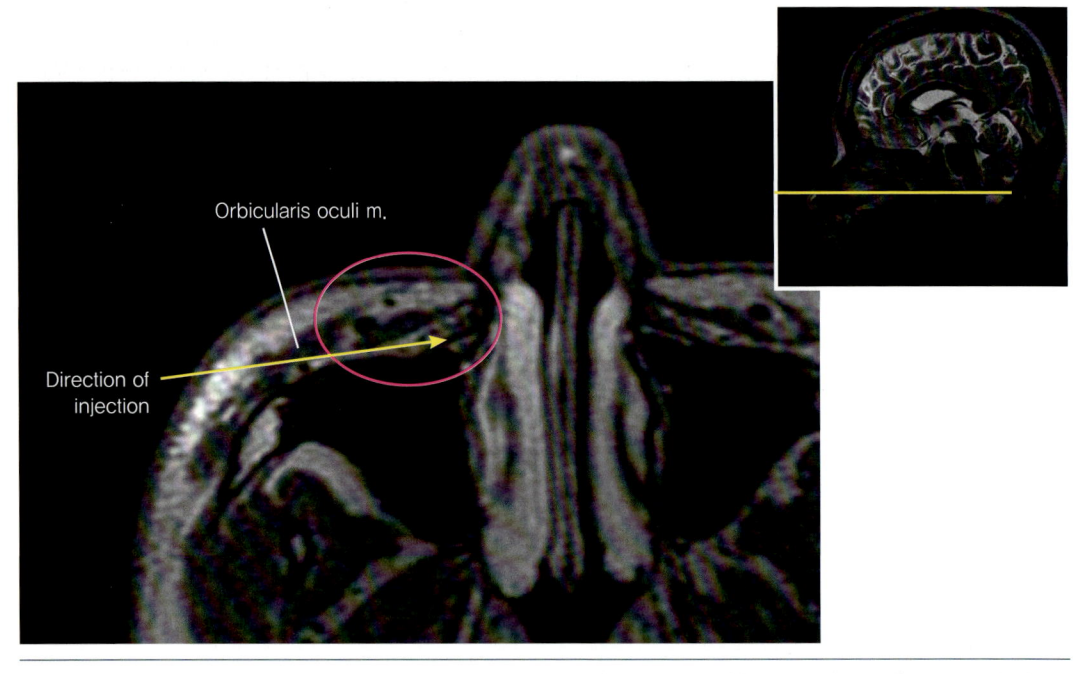

Fig. 2-1 Safe injection depth -Example (1). The safe layer for injecting fillers into the under eye is the layer right above the periosteum. Injection must be made along the layer right below the orbicularis oculi m. In that way accidents rising from angular a & v injection can be avoided.

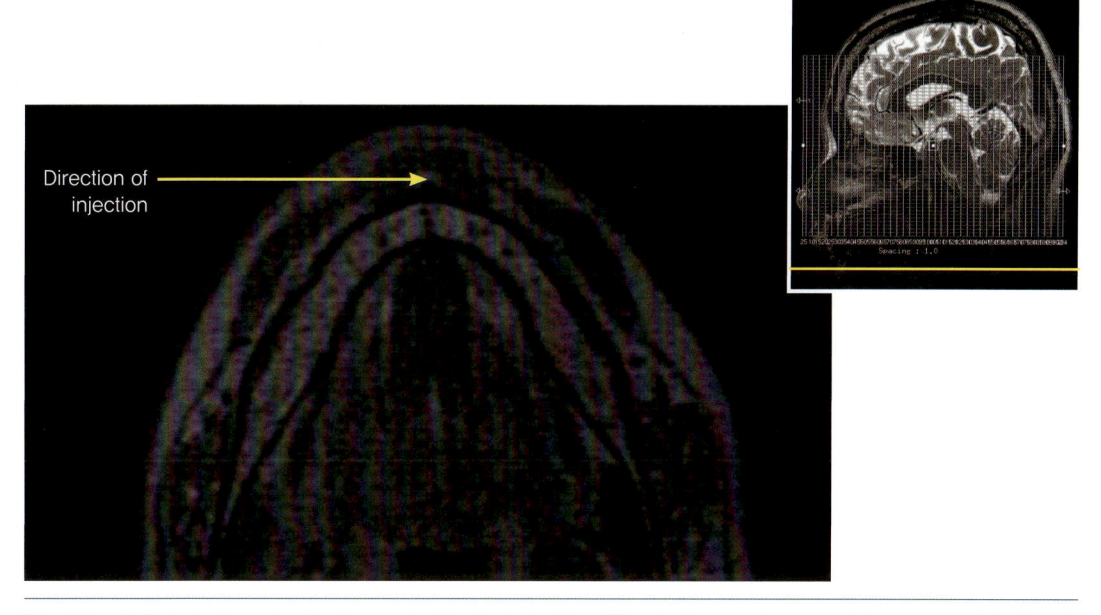

Fig. 2-2 Safe injection depth -Example (2). For injecting fillers in the jaw, in case of the center of the jaw, it is safe to inject in the layer right above the deep layer, periosteum. It is advisable to inject fillers right above the bone by getting to the slightly lateral area.

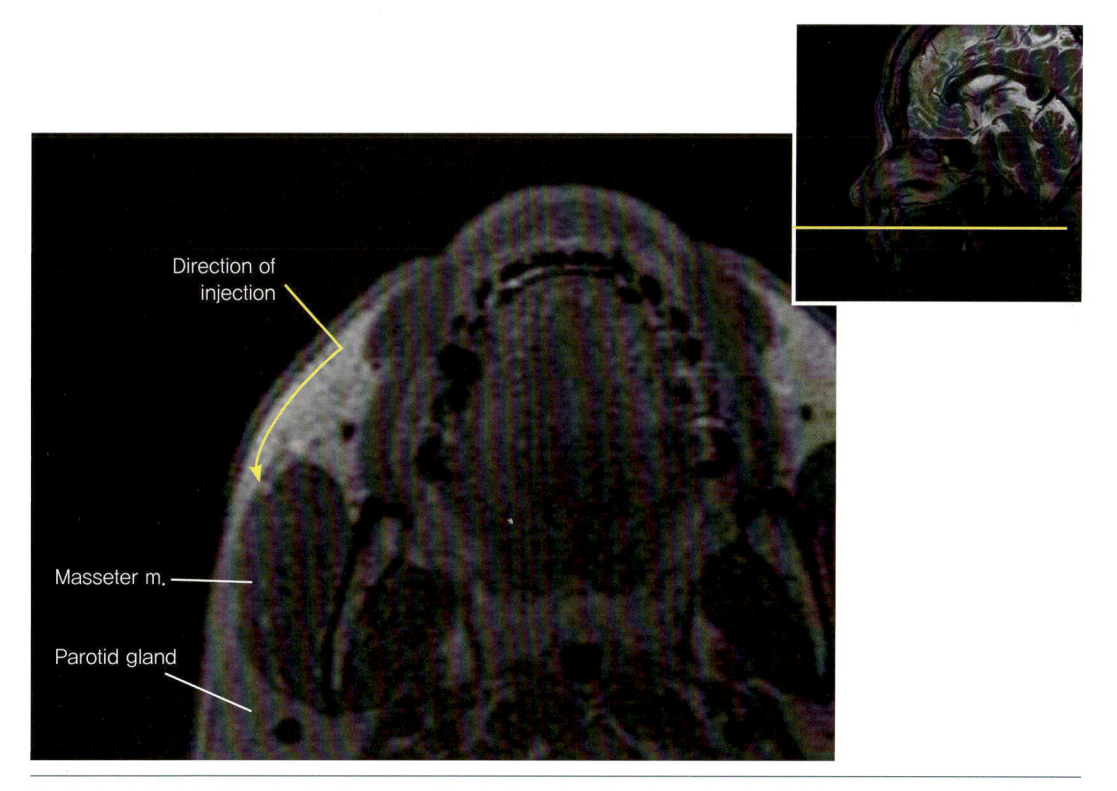

Fig. 2-3 Safe injection depth -Example (3). For injecting fillers into the cheek, it is important not to damage the masseter m. and the parotid gland. It is advisable to proceed along the curve within the subcutaneous layer.

Safe Filler Injection Technique Demonstration – using live imaging tools

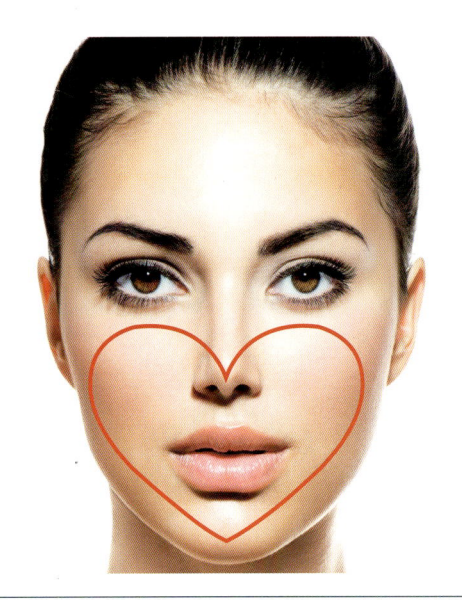

Fig. 2-4 Apple face in complete harmony

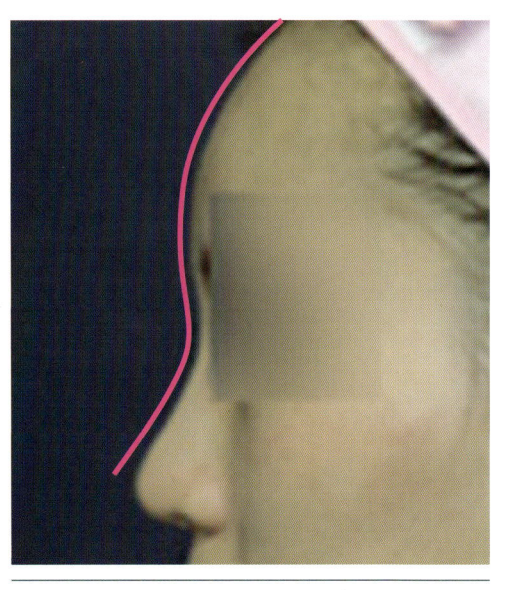

Fig. 2-5 S-line of the forehead and the nose in complete harmony

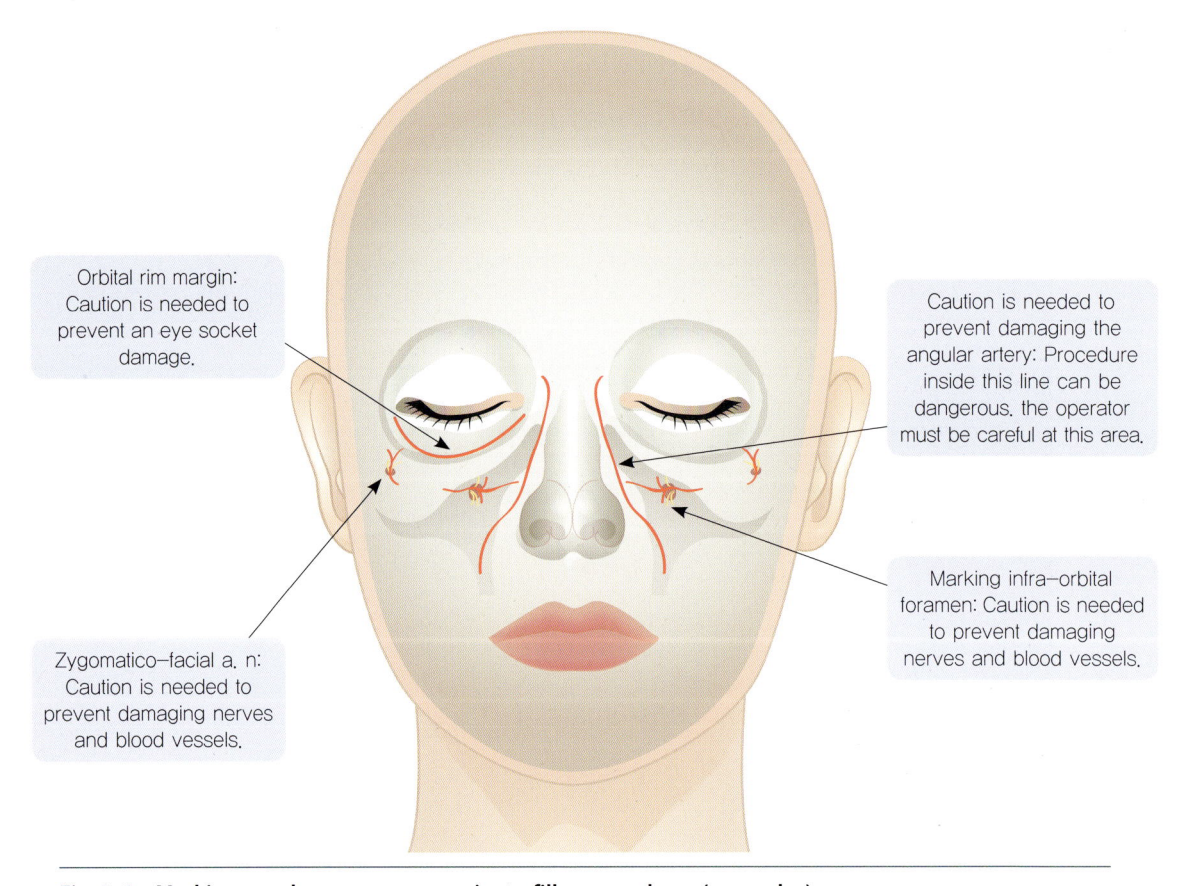

Orbital rim margin: Caution is needed to prevent an eye socket damage.

Zygomatico-facial a. n: Caution is needed to prevent damaging nerves and blood vessels.

Caution is needed to prevent damaging the angular artery: Procedure inside this line can be dangerous, the operator must be careful at this area.

Marking infra-orbital foramen: Caution is needed to prevent damaging nerves and blood vessels.

Fig. 2-6 Markings on dangerous areas prior to filler procedures (examples)

2. Filler Administration with Cannulas

There are no big, fundamental differences between the methods of using a cannula or needle. In general, the linear thread injection method and fan technique can be performed similarly, and yet the perpendicular pulling injection method or perpendicular bulk injection method may not be easily operated using a cannula.

The biggest difference from the needle injection method is that a cannula cannot be injected into the dermal layer and that entry route must be made through a puncture, depending on the insertion areas.

Due to its blunt-end, it is generally expected to cause much less damage to the blood vessels and nerves compared to using a needle. However, based on a number of real case reports, blood vessel accidents have still occurred from using a cannula, alerting that caution must be taken.

It is essential to insert a cannula or a needle after pulling back to release pressure. Namely, the retrograde injection method must be used. Due to the long length of a cannula, it is not necessary to puncture many different places as with a needle. Accordingly, the actual methods being used are mostly the linear retrograde injection method and fan-type linear retrograde injection method.

Here, explanation on the DPS (deep puncture and separation or subcision) method is provided as an additional concept. The DPS method is slightly different from the general injection method, which injects fillers as the needle pulls back after antegrade insertion. It is combined with a method similar to the fan

Table 2-1 Types of injection techniques using Cannula

Linear retrograde technique	General injection method
Fan technique	Injection method for large areas
DPS technique	Safe injection method

Safe Filler Injection Technique Demonstration – using live imaging tools

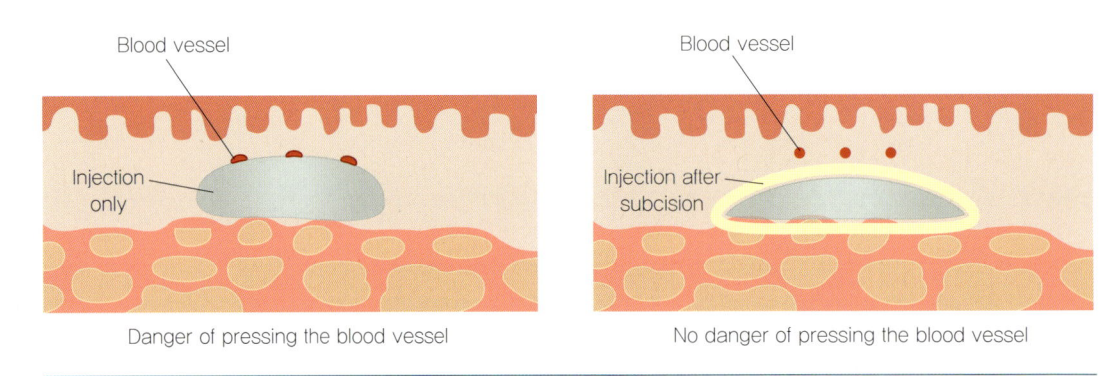

Fig. 2-7 Schematics on the DPS technique

technique, but the purpose of the procedure is different. In case of a fan technique, filler is injected into various areas within a zone created by a minimal puncture area. The DPS method on the other hand repeats forward and backward movements in a fan shape, similarly to the fan technique, but it is performed to create space instead of injecting fillers. It is done with the feeling of making one big space by connecting flat areas made by the fan technique.

After separation of the deep layer using the DPS method, the cannula can be pulled out and the treatment area can be squeezed. If there is any damage to the blood vessels, blood will come out, but if that is not the case, no blood will show. If a small amount of blood comes out, it will be difficult to determine which case it is. In that situation, by pressing the areas the cannula passed on each level, the area of bleeding can be confirmed.

Another method of checking the bleeding area is as follows. If bleeding shows after subcision using the DPS method, the area where the cannula has passed can be pressed and the puncture area can be hemostasized at the same time. Thereafter, if bleeding continues immediately after the pressure is lifted from the puncture area, the bleeding area is considered to be the area between the punctured area and the pressed area. On the other hand, after pressing the area at the time of bleeding, if there is no additional bleeding after the punctured area has been wiped, the bleeding area may be assumed to be near the origin (the area where the cannula proceeded further in) rather than the pressed area.

Opinion differs among groups as to whether blood vessel accidents due to fillers occur from direct injection only or also from the external pressure. Based on the experience of many doctors including ourselves, side effects caused by external pressure acting on the blood vessels seem to be quite possible. Using the DPS method of filler injection, odds of having blood vessel accidents due to external pressures are likely to be reduced.

1 Puncturing Method for Cannula Insertion

Due to the cannula's characteristic of having a blunt end, it is expected to cause less damage to the nerves. With cannulas, the most severe complications, such as accidents arising from vascular occlusion are less expected, yet, procedures must always be performed with caution to minimize any possible side effects. In all processes, the first insertion of the cannula, proceeding into the desired depth, moving to the desired location thereafter, freeing up space and inserting fillers, require detailed handling.

It is difficult to penetrate skin layers with a cannula. After making an entry point using a needle, a cannula can be entered into the layer of interest. In other words, a hole in the top layer of skin can be made using a needle and through this hole, a cannula can proceed to the desired depth and to the desired location. Thereafter, after removing the cannula from the skin, bleeding can be checked.

The areas to take extra caution not to cause bleeding after puncturing are the forehead and the nasolabial folds. Injecting fillers into the nasolabial folds, the angular a. must be taken into consideration.

The forehead is considered as a difficult place to perform procedures without bleeding. Within that area, there is not much soft tissue and there are thick veins passing through the superficial layer. The bone in the forehead is often round and curvy than flat, which makes it easier to hit the blood vessels in the process of freeing up space. Caution must be taken not to cause excessive bleeding even from puncturing, the very first process in the procedure.

If there is only a little amount of blood that can be stopped with hemostasis, the cannula may enter the skin with ease. After proceeding to the periosteum area, it can change its direction to the desired area.

The forehead should be handled differently from other areas. After reaching the desired depth following the puncture, it is advisable to check whether there is bleeding by completely removing the cannula from the skin. As previously mentioned, there are thick veins and arteries residing in the skin layers that contain only a little amount of soft tissues, in which the cannula can cause blood vessel damage as it moves to the desired depth. Therefore, if the physician does not notice the blood vessel damage while proceeding with the cannula, a substantial amount of bleeding can result after the procedure. Consequently, there will be a great deal of bruising after the procedure and the patient will experience discomfort.

2 Method of Using Cannula Depending on the Depth

In performing filler procedures on face, it is very important to determine the depth of the treatment of interest. It is not easy to estimate the injection depth only by palpating with fingers. The areas in which palpation can tell the accurate injection depth is limited to cases where a big difference in sensation is felt due to the change in the tissue density.

When performing procedures on the face, injection depth is generally divided into dermal layer, subdermal fat layer, muscle layer, submuscular layer(supra-periosteal layer). The original function of fillers has been the adjustment of volume deficiency in the dermal layer, but as the recent trend focuses on face augmentation the insertion depth has become significantly deeper. Advancement in the knowledge of facial anatomy has established that filler injection into a deeper layer is safer for augmentation.

There are practically two points for finding out the depth of facial layers. They are a subdermal layer and a layer right above the periosteum, which are felt immediately after puncturing and bone-touching, respectively. Due to the

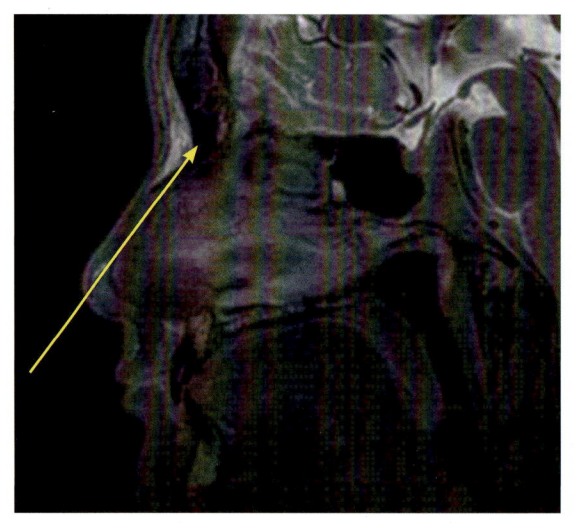

Fig. 2-8 **Proceeding through the same layer**

blunt property of a cannula, it is very difficult to continue proceeding by scraping underneath the periosteum. Thus in many cases, the cannula is steered to enter through the submuscular fat layer, which is right above the periosteum.

In general, for the areas where most procedures are performed, the nose, forehead, under eye, nasolabial folds, jaw, etc., fillers are often injected into the submuscular fat layer. The anatomy has verified that it is safer to go deep for injecting these areas.

- In early days, filler usage was approved only for the purpose of correcting deficiency in the dermis.
- However, the true value of using fillers was found when correcting the loss of facial volume due to aging.
- With time, treatment cases for facial volumization has exceeded those for dermis correction, which ultimately led to Restylane's FDA approval of the clinical indication, called the "cheek volumization".

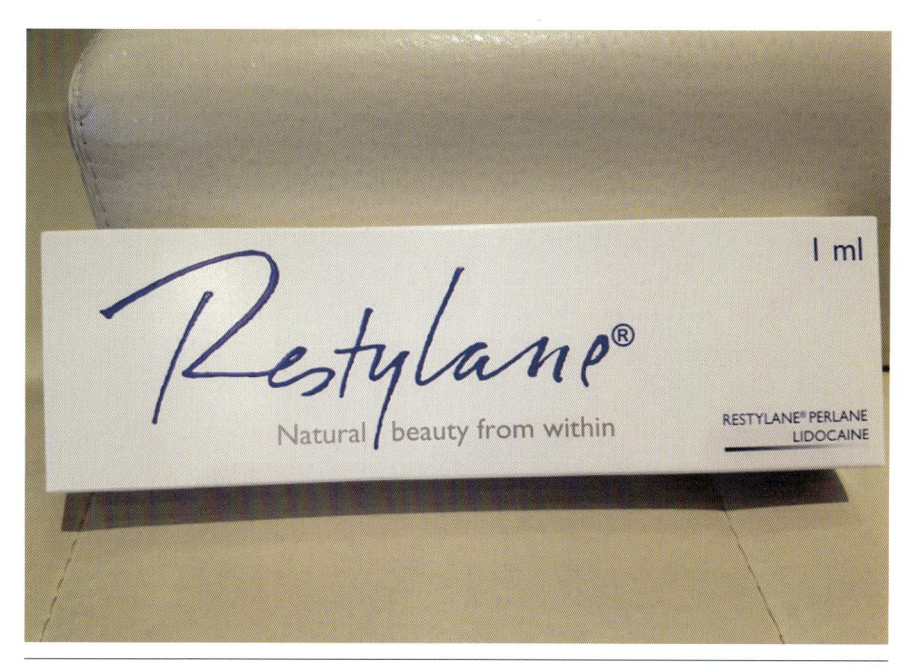

Fig. 2-9　FDA approved Restylane Lyft for volumization

Safe Filler Injection Technique Demonstration – using live imaging tools

The information mentioned above is summarized as follows. For using a cannula, first puncture the skin with a needle, insert the cannula and enter into the area right above the bone. It is recommended to make the puncture in the area without blood vessels, but if bleeding occurs at the puncture and continues beyond the standard point (This point may differ by the physician's judgement: the author proceeds with the cannula as long as the blood is stoppable at the puncture area, not flowing.), it is advisable to make a new puncture elsewhere. When using a cannula, it must be carefully inserted into the skin in a perpendicular direction to the point right on the bone, perform the bone touch, and free up space by moving from the left to right. By moving as softly as possible, bleeding can be avoided while making rooms for treatment.

If the desired region for the procedure is the layer right above the bone, it is easier to predict the depth. However, in regions where there is a possibility of puncturing the mucous membrane, such as the nasolabial fold area, or where injection into the parotid gland must be avoided, such as the cheeks, more caution must be paid.

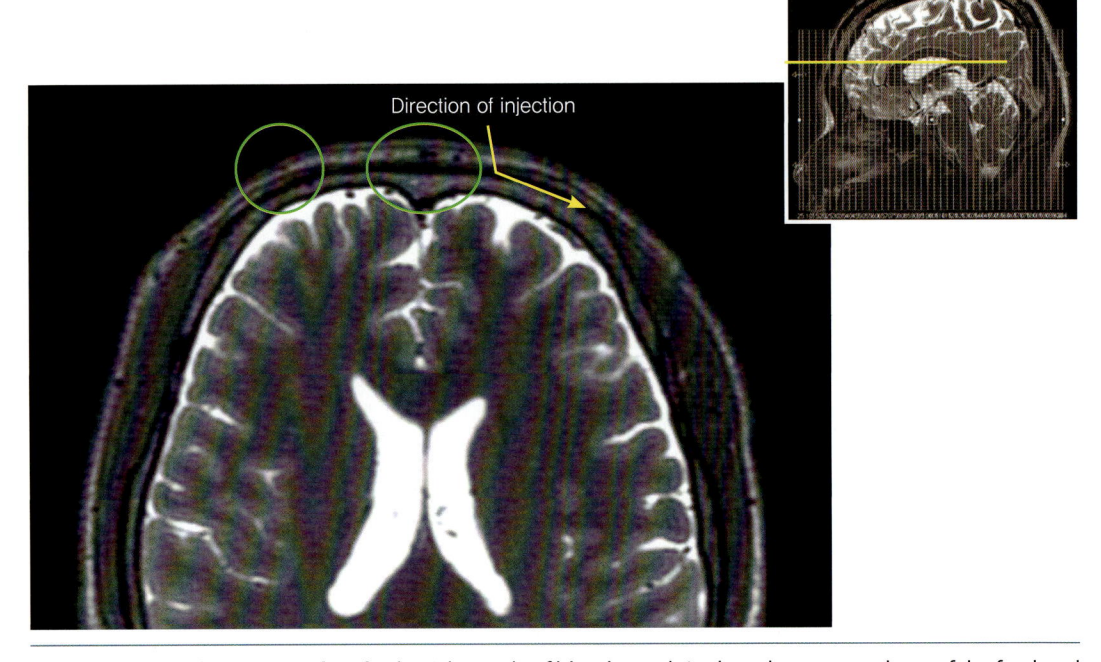

Fig. 2-10 Cannula use – Forehead. The rich supply of blood vessels in the subcutaneous layer of the forehead can be seen. Out of the dermal layer, subcutaneous layer, muscle layer, fat layer below the muscles, periosteum layer, and bone layer, it is recommended that the fat layer below the muscles is suitable space for injections. In the left green circle in the figure, the muscle layer (black) lies below fat layer (white). Another thin layer of fat (white) can be seen below the muscle layer. The black layer below the fat layer is the bone cortex. Cannula should proceed to the fat layer below the muscles.

Consideration of skin thickness, which varies by facial region, will result in better results. The multiple plain dual injection method, which has recently become popular, refers to performing the injection not only into the deep layer, but also simultaneously into the subcutaneous layer and dermal layer. However, as many important blood vessels course through the subcutaneous layer of the face, precise handling is required. It is advisable to perform the procedure after having studied the direction of the blood vessels in the area the procedure is to be performed on.

3 Cannula Advancement and Separation of Tissue

It is advisable to advance the cannula within the same layer and parallel to the surface of the facial bone as much as possible. To avoid vascular accidents, it is important not to advance the cannula too roughly nor use a lot of force in the danger zones. Also, it is important not to inject an excessive volume of filler in the danger zones as this increases the pressure exerted against vessels. Volumizing fillers are generally administered in the fat layer below the muscles and right above the facial bone. From the puncture site, enter perpendicularly into the desired layer, and change the dirction for advancement.

By remaining within the same layer, the advancement of the cannula is very smooth. In order to avoid damage to the blood vessels and nerves, if any resistance is felt during cannula advancement, the route of least resistance should be taken by moving to the cannula slightly to the left and right.

Ligaments that maintain the facial shape exist in certain regions. In order to penetrate the ligaments, slight force must be exerted, in which case, caution must be taken not to damage the blood vessels and the nerves. The regions where the ligaments are attached must be known so that when a slight resistance is felt during the advancement of the cannula, the injector can decide whether to advance with the cannula a little more or whether to take a side step. (Refer to explanation about ligaments in Part 4)

After advancing the cannula and ensuring the tip of the cannula is positioned in desired area of filler placement, space must be procured through tissue sep-

Safe Filler Injection Technique Demonstration – using live imaging tools

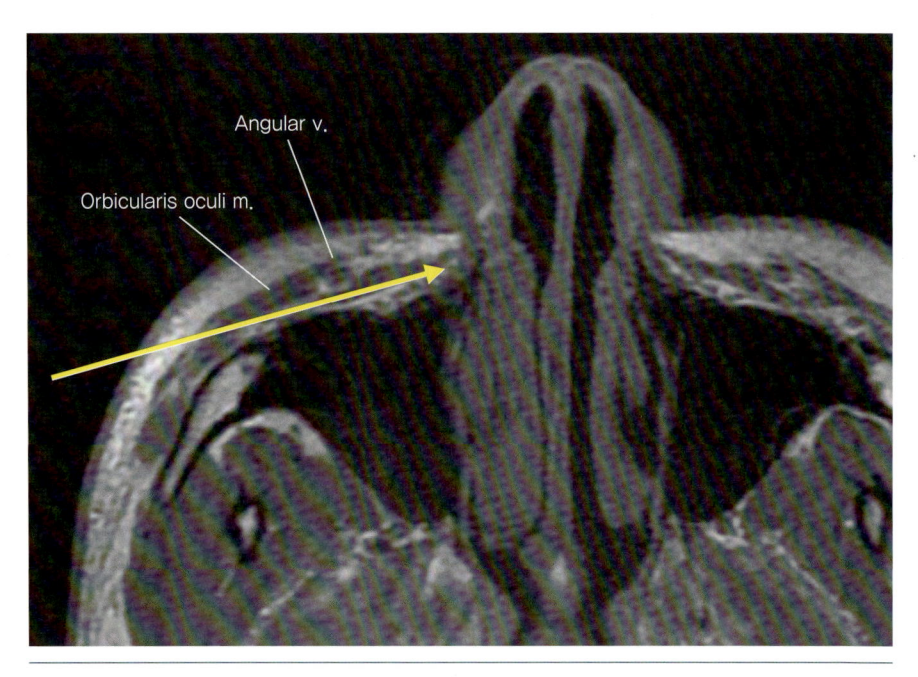

Fig. 2-11 Cannula Advancement. Insert cannula along the fat layer immediately below the orbicularis oculi m. As the muscle is very thin, a small amount of force can puncture the muscle. The only way to prevent vascular accident is to advance smoothly without exerting strength while maintaining a suitable distance from the bone.

aration. Tissue separation is performed within the same layer and is similar to the fan technique in that it involves moving the cannula back and forth. The difference is that unlike the fan technique, this is a process that involves procuring space and no filler administration [DPS (Deep puncture & separation or subcision) method].

After filler administration, the filler may move due to the movement of facial muscles. Space procurement prior to filler administration will reduce the movement of fillers due to facial expression.

Immediately following tissue separation and space procurement, filler can be injected. Or prior to filler injection, the cannula can be withdrawn and pressure can be applied in the direction opposite to the initial direction of cannula advancement to check if any bleeding had occurred. Careful skin puncture, cannula advancement, and tissue separation will ensure minimal to no bleeding.

After completion of the procedure, remove the cannula and re-assess for any signs of bleeding. There tends to be a small amount of bleeding around the punctured area. It is advisable to press lightly on the puncture site for one to two minutes to prevent bruising.

3. Basic Method of Using a Needle

1 Method of Using a Needle

There are various methods for using a needle, but by and large, these methods can be categorized into one of two major groups. One is the traditional four injection method and the other is the widely used perpendicular pulling injection method. With the perpendicular pulling injection method, the needle tip is positioned at a safe depth. In general, the safe depth is the layer right above the periosteum. Negative pressure is created by pinching the skin slightly and the filler is injected as the needle is withdrawn. The various injection methods have similarities. The tower injection technique explained in the Fig. below (Fig. 2-12) is a variation of the perpendicular pulling method and involves injecting the filler into different layers in a non-continuous manner.

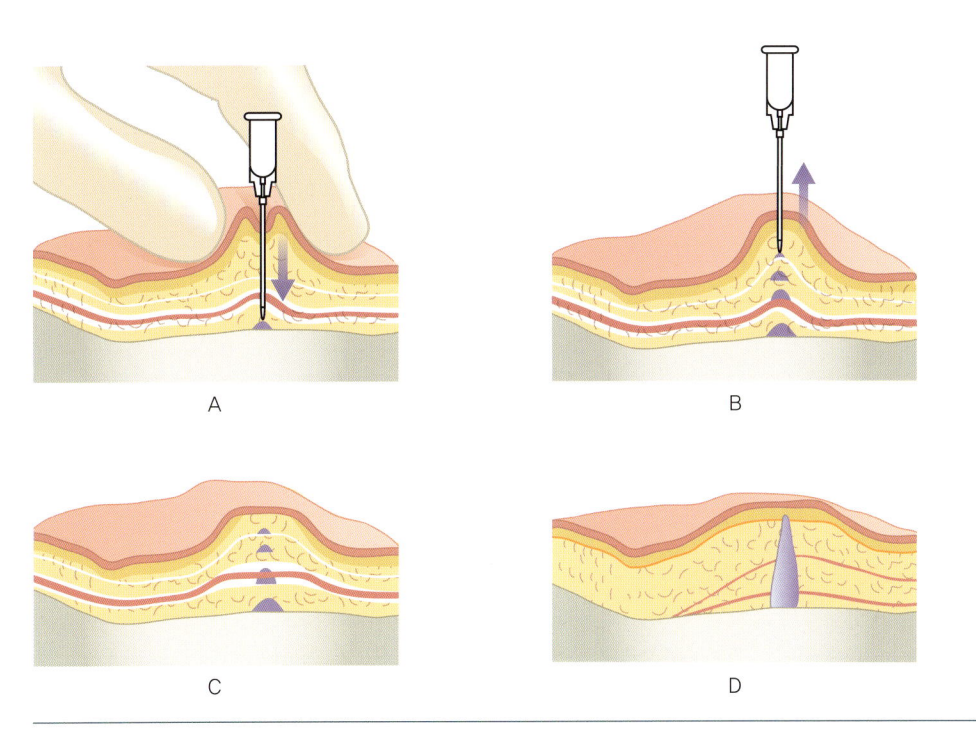

Fig. 2-12 Tower injection technique

Safe Filler Injection Technique Demonstration – using live imaging tools

Among the traditional methods of injection, three methods are used most frequently. The first one is the linear threading technique, which injects the needle into the dermal or the subcutaneous layer in the direction of the purple arrow. Then as the needle is withdrawn in the direction of the red arrow, a consistent pressure is applied on the plunger to inject the filler material. In order to reduce vascular accidents, the filler is injected in this retrograde manner. Anterograde injections may increase the risk of puncturing a vessel and direct intravascular filler injection.

The second is the serial puncture technique, which refers to small bolus injections into the desired layer from multiple injection points. This method minimizes movement of the needle in the facial tissue and can be used for injecting small quantities in multiple areas.

The third technique is the fan technique which is used for injecting filler evenly into a wide area while minimizing the number of puncture sites. Basically, the fan technique is a very useful skill, not only for needles, but also for cannulas. This is a skill which serves as foundation for the DPS (deep puncture & separation or subcision) method, which is highlighted as the most important procedural skill in this book.

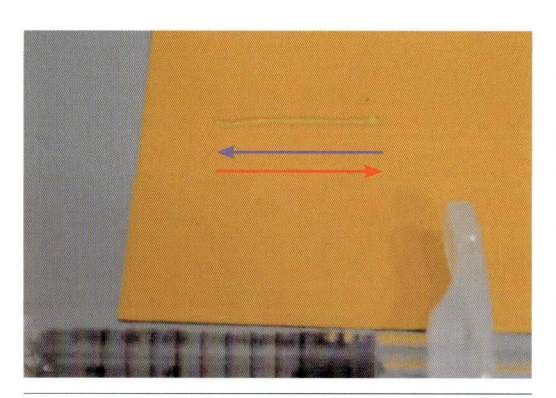

Fig. 2-13 Linear threading technique

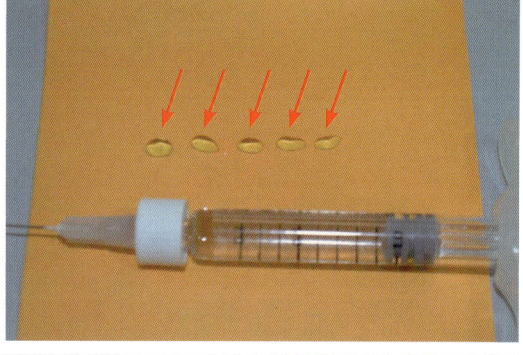

Fig. 2-14 Serial puncture technique

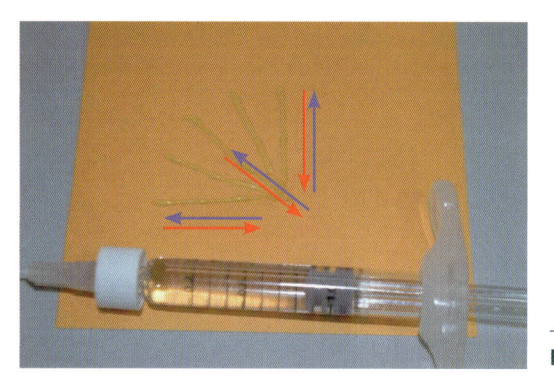

Fig. 2-15 Fan technique

2 Considerations of Bevel Location in Procedures

1) Bevel Down, Up, and Sideways

Whether a needle or cannula is used, material is injected from the syringe in one direction. Especially for procedures involving the superficial layers of the skin, injecting the filler with the bevel up (increased proximity to skin surface) may increase the risk of uneven linear formation of bumps. This is because it is not easy to inject a completely uniform amount across the linear region. In this case, positioning the bevel downwards or sideways will ensure a more even administration resulting in fewer bumps.

2) Bevel Direction

In general, the fillers are injected most frequently into the dermal layer and right above the periosteum. Considering the original purpose of fillers, the dermal layer may be thought of as the layer that is most frequently injected. However, considering the recent volumizing trend, filler are actually injected the most right above the periosteum. It is advisable for the physician to consider the anatomy of the layer to be injected and position the bevel away from regions in which blood vessels are expected to pass.

It is important to learn the skill of selecting the appropriate bevel direction, withdrawing the needle, and injecting evenly. This skill is especially important when injecting into the dermis layer or into the dermal subcutaneous junction. The bevel sideways injection method is useful in these cases.

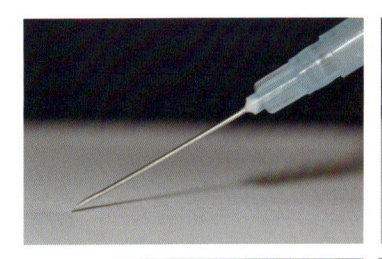

Fig. 2-16 Bevel up

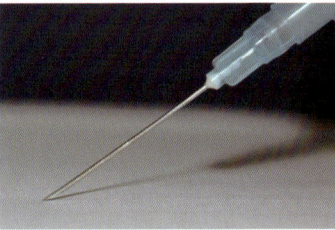

Fig. 2-17 Bevel down

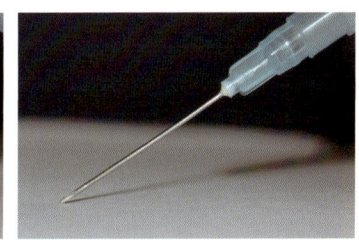

Fig. 2-18 Bevel sideways

3 Post Dermal Subcision Injection Method

Post dermal subcision injection method is a very useful procedure method. This method changes the paradigm of filler administration. The conventional method includes positioning the needle in the dermal layer and injecting the filler in a retrograde manner. Thus, the sunken or depressed areas are lifted. However, in the post dermal subcision injection method, tissue separation to procure space for filler material is performed in advance. The filler is then administered into the space that has been already prepared. After administration, fillers are not spread out through massaging, but inserted into the space that has been already made so the concept is to have the fillers spread naturally.

The advantage of the post dermal subcision injection method is that it allows not only the safe injection of the fillers into the desired shape, but also the diverse application of this technique.

Direction of needle movement (tissue separation while moving sideways

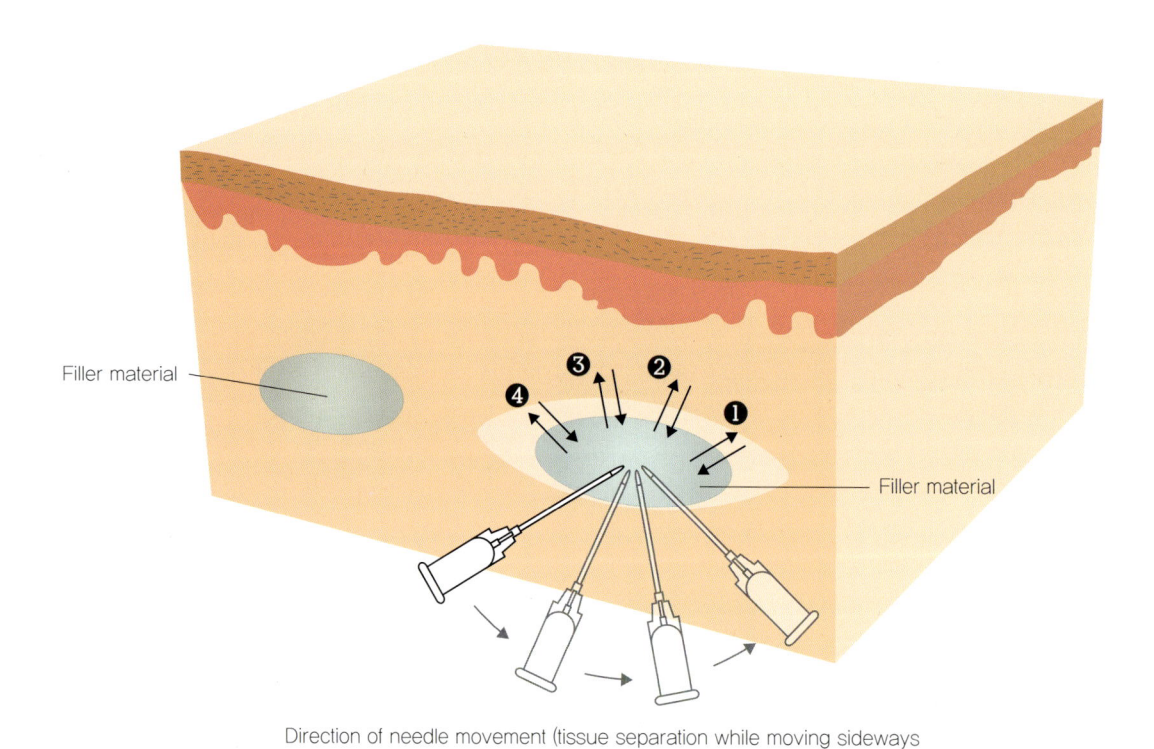

Fig. 2-19 The left shows when fillers are injected into the dermal layer. The right shows tissue separation across a wide area in the dermis using a needle prior to filler administration. The needle is removed after carefully injecting the filler into the procured space.

One such application is in dermal proliferation treatment. Collagen depletion due to infections and damage lead to depressions and furrows. In these areas, dermal subcision is performed to procure space and allowed to fill with blood. Then powerful fractional type laser treatments are performed over these areas to cause additional skin damage. In general, the stronger the energy of the fractional type laser, the greater the magnitude of cellular proliferation. In the treatment of sunken areas or scars, the performance of dermal subcision to procure space and loosen tissue in conjunction with fractional type lasers will have a synergistic effect on tissue proliferation.

4 Perpendicular Pulling Injection Method

This is a method that is frequently used with needles. With the increasing emphasis on safety with filler procedures, the issue with respect to selecting the depth of the injection has been raised. Rather than inserting the needle at a slanted angle or making routes by tunneling, the needle enters perpendicularly and filler is injected only after the needle tip has been positioned precisely in a safe layer. The filler injection is made after loosening the target tissue area by slightly pulling backwards and it is this step that distinguishes this method from the perpendicular puncture injection method.

Based on filler characteristics, filler placement via bolus injection is more advantageous in terms of duration and maintenance of shape.

But this technique can be dangerous when the physician doesn't know the location of vessel and the depth of it.

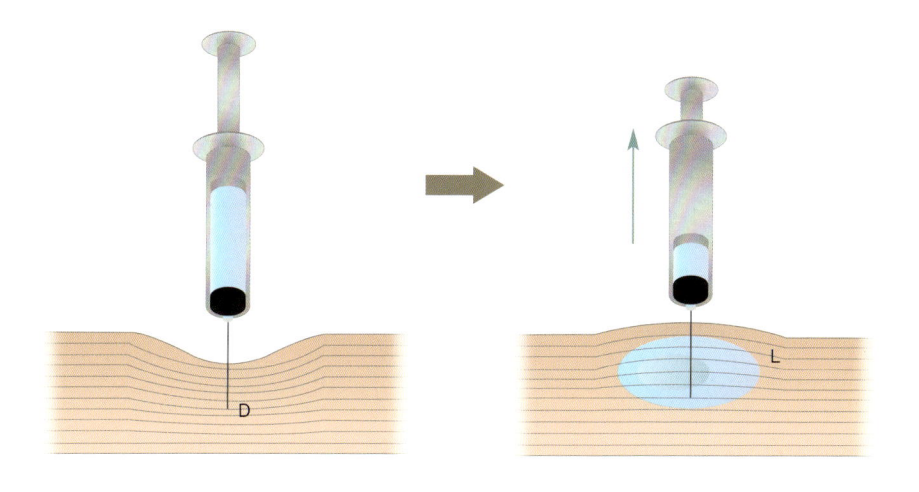

Fig. 2-20 Perpendicular Pulling Injection Method

5 Perpendicular Injection of a Large Bolus

Instead of using multiple puncture sites, this method creates the desired shape by pressing after injecting a large amount of filler. This method requires spreading of the filler lump after injection. However, even after spreading it out, due to its viscoelastic property, there is a possibility that the filler body will form a mass leading to lump formation. Nonetheless, because the filler is injected in one large bolus, even if the filler moves due to pressure, the filler is maintained as one body. In this case, the area of contact with external tissue is relatively small so it has an advantage of better fixation and increased duration is expected.

The desired shape is formed by sufficient massage after initial filler placement. This is a useful method with monophasic fillers, as they have better spreadability. Biphasic fillers on the other hand tend to be more difficult to spread out. With this procedure it is very important not to cause any bleeding. Bleeding increases the risk of intravascular injection of filler and significant complications. This method is for those who have thorough knowledge of safe injection depth and vascular anatomy.

In performing the perpendicular injection of a large bolus, the objective of the filler procedure needs to be clearly defined. If the objective is augmentation, biphasic fillers, which have high viscoelasticity, should be injected as a large bolus in one area and shaped into desired form. On the other hand, if filler needs to be spread over a large area, monophasic fillers can be injected followed by flattening. Even with monophasic fillers, the filler mass may not spread out if an excessive amount has been placed. Accordingly, determination of filler volume required and consideration of the rheological properties in filler selection are essential for this method.

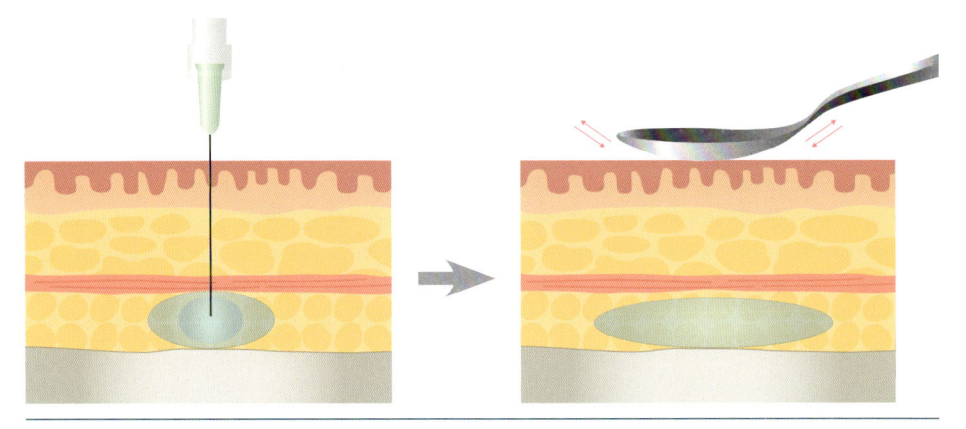

Fig. 2-21 Perpendicular injection of a large bolus involves injection of a large bolus in one injection site. After injection, it is necessary to spread out the filler using pressure.

4. No Bleeding Technique

●●● Whenever the authors provide filler training, certain key points are always emphasized. That is, to be humble, respectful, calm, and cautious. When procedures are performed when the mind is rushed, handling tends to become fast and rough. If the patient happens to have thin blood vessels or have anatomical variations that could not be avoided with the conventional techniques and safety precautions, problems may occur. Therefore, it is necessary to remain focused, aim for minimal bleeding, and always proceed with caution.

The less bleeding there is during the filler procedure, the better. In general, skin necrosis or visual problems resulting from injecting into the artery and pulmonary embolism resulting from directly injecting into the vein are severe complications. Even if it is not a directly injected into the blood vessels, it is very important to reduce bleeding during filler procedures. If blood comes out due to any damage to the blood vessels, this is accompanied by swelling and bruising, causing extended downtime. Moreover, due to the swelling and bruising at the time of the procedure, it makes it difficult to evaluate the final result.

In order to prevent puncturing an artery (intra-arterial emboli are associated with more severe complications), a comprehensive knowledge of facial anatomy is necessary. The most important factors are courses of the arterial branches and the depth at which they course. Moreover, due to individual variations in facial vasculature, cautious and gentle handling is crucial at all times. In order to prevent the complications that arise from arterial damage, cautious handling is required for cannulas and an accurate awareness of depth for filler injection is required for needles. The blunt tips of cannulas do make them safer than needles but they do not guarantee complete safety. Forceful handling and injecting excessive amounts of filler into the danger zones with cannulas will increase the risk of complications. With respect to treating the danger zones, the upmost safety standards must be followed with respect to the injection site and depth.

Venous walls tend to be weaker. In particular, the veins in the temporal and forehead regions are more susceptible to damage. Cautious approach is important but it is also just as important to incorporate the practice of avoiding the visible veins in the superficial layer while injecting. It should also be noted that cannulas can easily puncture veins.

Accordingly, understanding the anatomy, handling with caution, using a cannula, and restricting treatments in the danger zones will help minimize bleeding.

Safe Filler Injection Technique Demonstration – using live imaging tools

Final point to be discussed in this section is minimizing bleeding at the entry site when using a cannula. Prior to filler administration using cannulas, a puncture must be made in the skin. If there is damage to blood vessels at the entry site, the injected filler will mix with blood resulting in significant bruising. Therefore, the puncture must be made as superficially as possible, just sufficient enough to pass the dermal layer. Thereafter it is advisable to proceed into the deeper layers using a cannula.

The following device may reduce the risk of bleeding. This device digitally displays a map of the superficial veins on the surface of the skin. It is used in hospitals to establish IV lines in patients in whom catheter insertion is difficult. Bleeding in the forehead region can cause severe bruising and this device may help minimize the risk of bleeding at the puncture site.

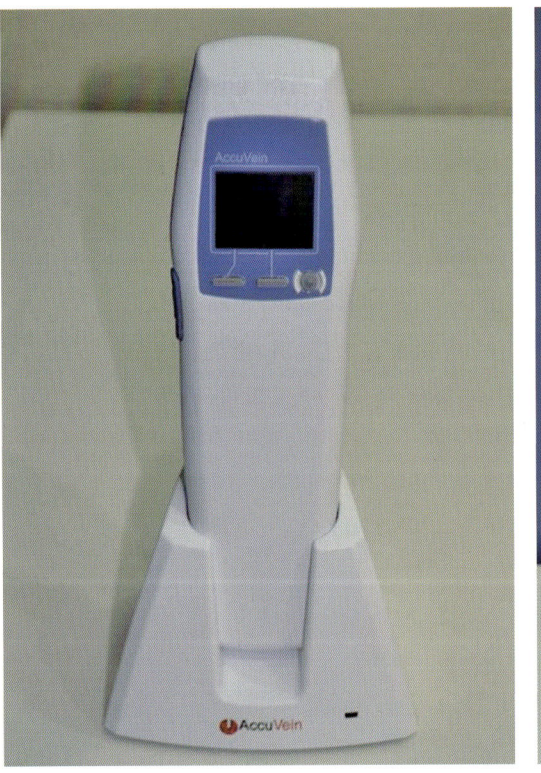

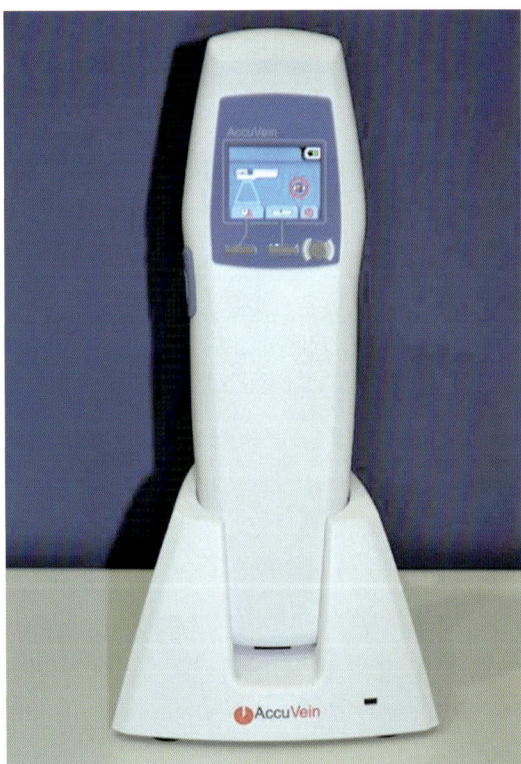

Fig. 2-22 Accuvein is a device that displays blood vessels in the subcutaneous layer.

(Source: Mediana Accuvein)

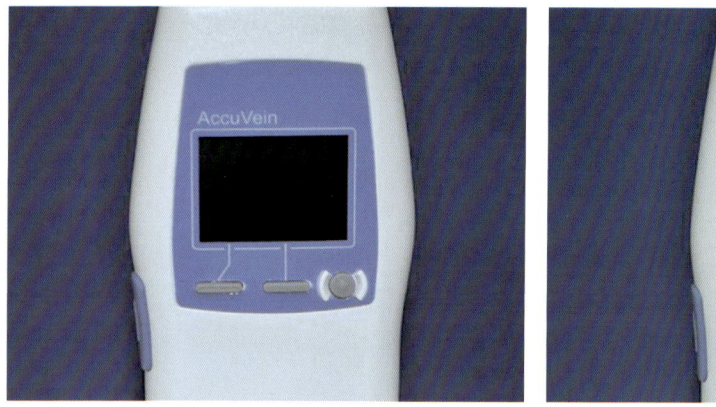

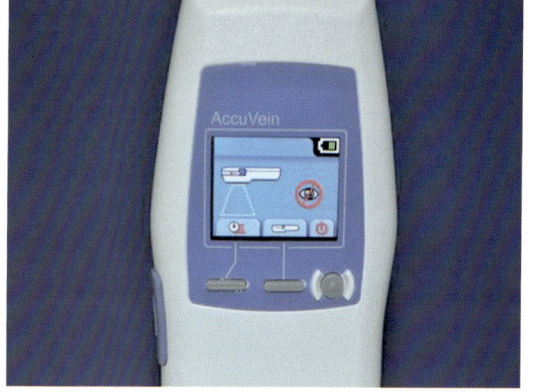

Fig. 2-23   A closer shot of Accuvein

(Source: Mediana Accuvein)

After switching it on, the device is held over the surface of the skin. The veins are displayed in black. This device only displays the veins in the subcutaneous layer and does not display arteries. This device cannot completely prevent arterial accidents but it helps minimize the risk of bleeding at the puncture site.

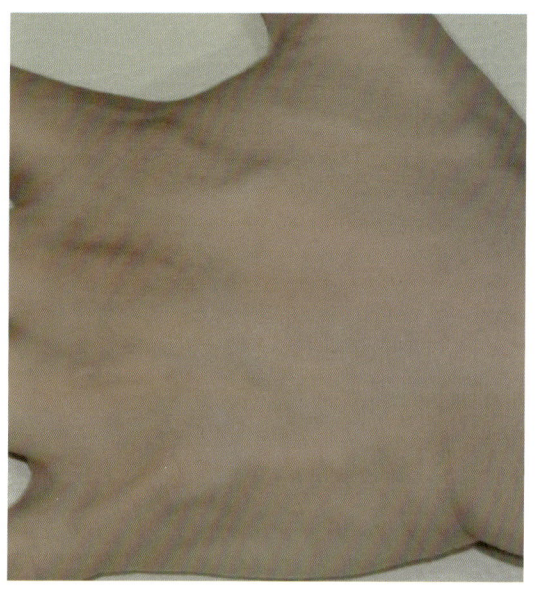

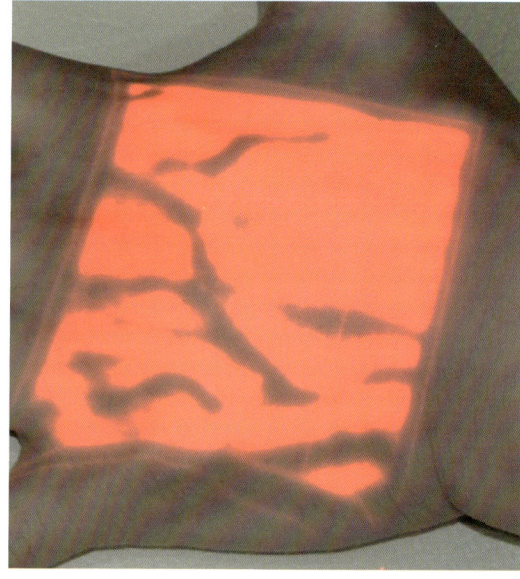

Fig. 2-24   Hand dorsum

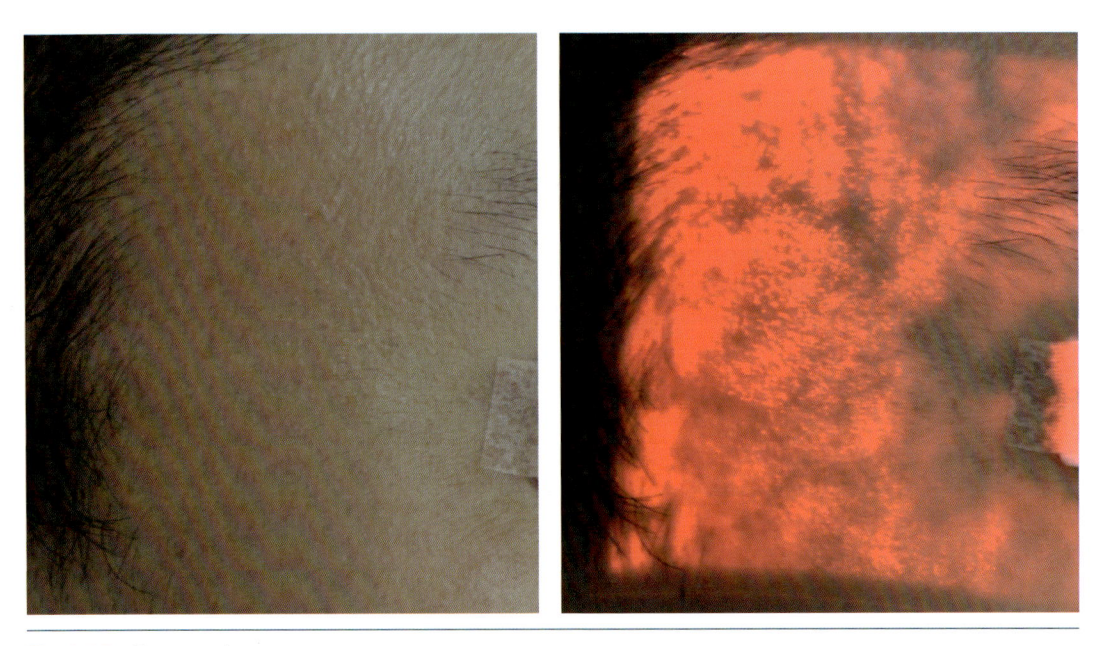

Safe Filler Injection Technique Demonstration – using live imaging tools

Fig. 2-25　Temporal area

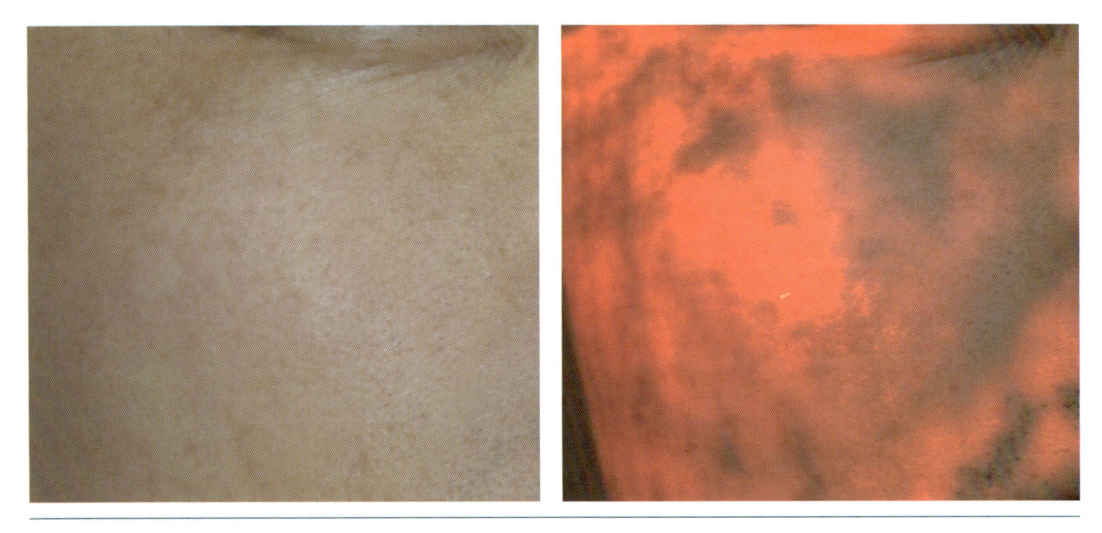

Fig. 2-26　Zygomatic area

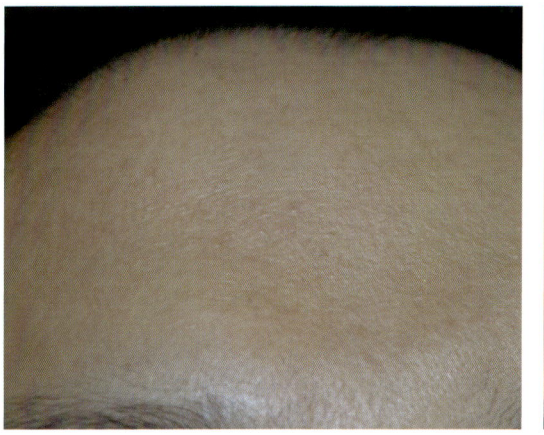

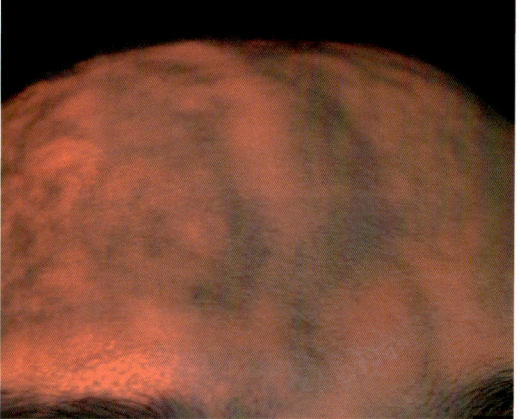

Fig. 2-27　Forehead

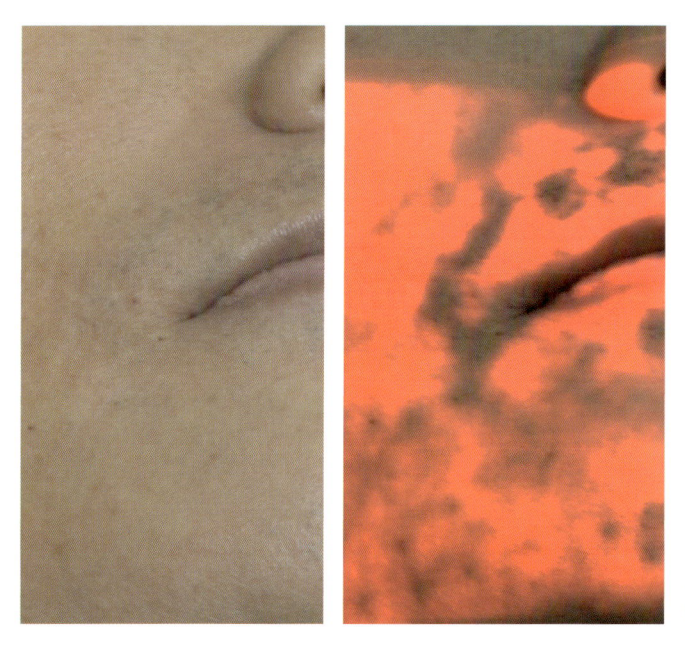

Fig. 2-28　Nasolabial fold

5. Molding

1 What is Molding?

What types of changes are observed when injected filler is rubbed? Immediately after filler administration, the filler rarely is in the form of the desired or intended shape. The viscoelastic property of the filler ensures that the filler body does not lose its original shape. However, as the shape immediately after injection is not the final look, the process of minor alteration of shape, namely molding, is necessary. Fillers with lower elasticity, smaller particles, or lower HA concentration spread out better at the time of molding. On the other hand, fillers with higher elasticity, larger particles, or higher HA concentration tend not to spread out as well.

The filler moving with changes in facial expression or its inability to maintain molded shape may have been observed in clinical practice. The question that arises is if the filler can revert to the initially molded shape by rubbing. Can fillers which have been spread out by shear force be once again molded into the intended shape by subsequent shaping? The answer to this question can be seen in the following figures.

1) Monophasic Filler Molding

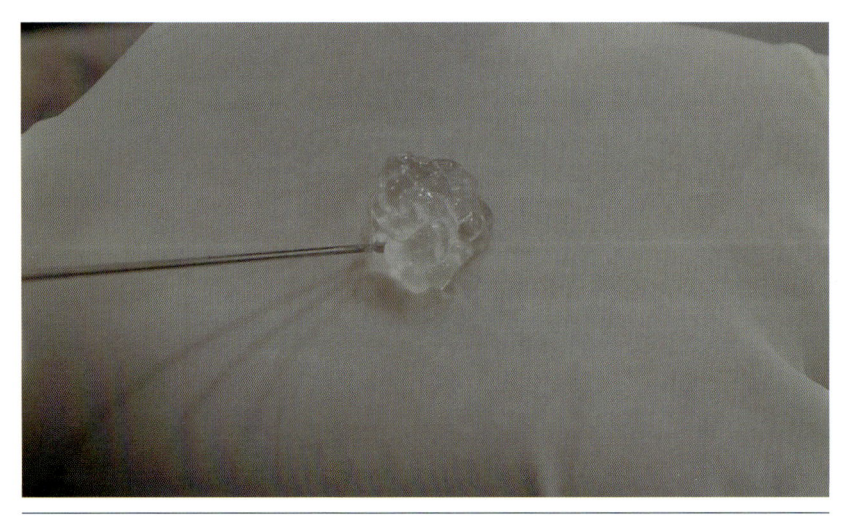

Fig. 2-29 When monophasic filler is injected onto the palm. Viscoelasticity as evidenced by smooth surface and aggregation into a round shape can be observed.

(Monophasic filler: Neuramis, Medytox)

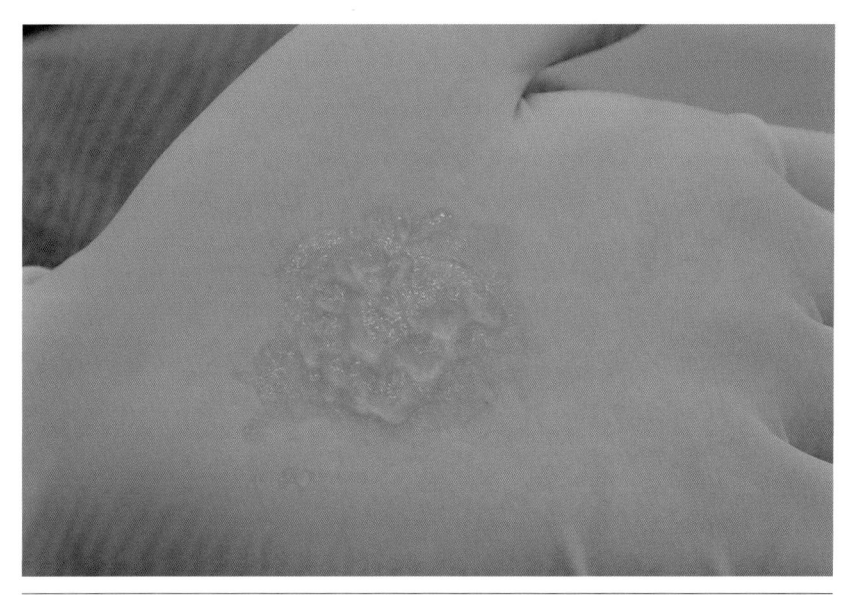

Fig. 2-30 Resistance against external pressure is not high. It spreads well when pressed and rubbed and spreads out evenly.

(Monophasic filler: Neuramis, Medytox)

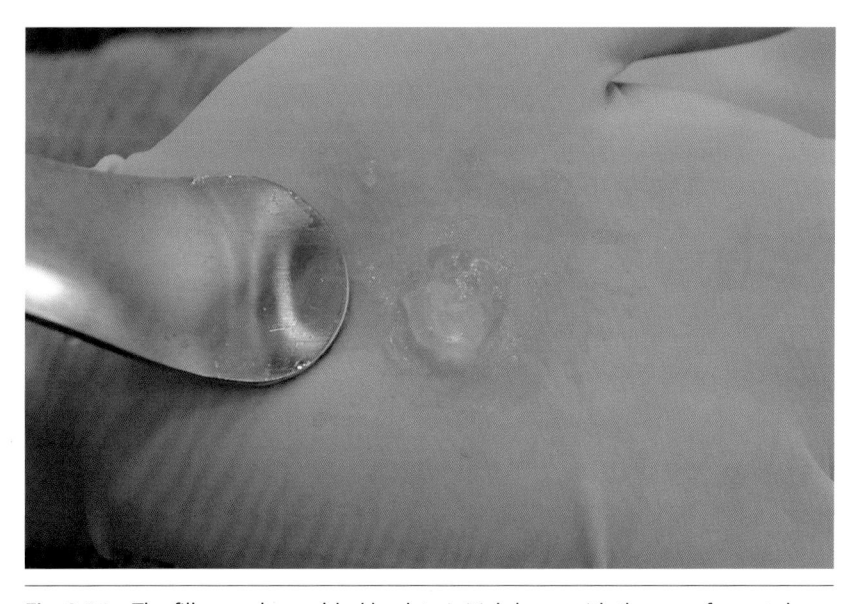

Fig. 2-31 The filler can be molded back to initial shape with the use of a spatula.

(Monophasic filler: Neuramis, Medytox)

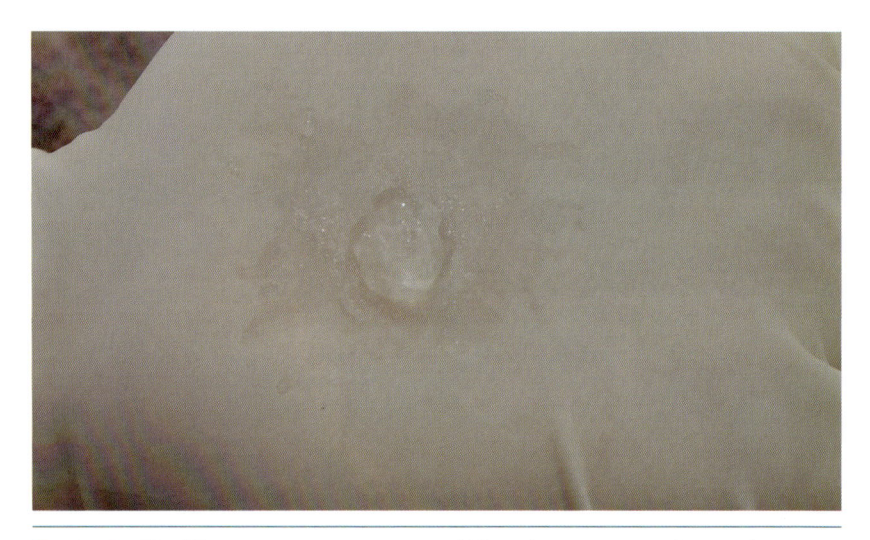

Safe Filler Injection Technique Demonstration – using live imaging tools

Fig. 2-32 The filler seems to aggregate well, but there seems to be a reduction in volume. This process of spreading and aggregating demonstrates that it does not return to its original shape but demonstrates that cohesivity is maintained to a certain extent.

(Monophasic filler: Neuramis, Medytox)

2) Biphasic Filler Molding

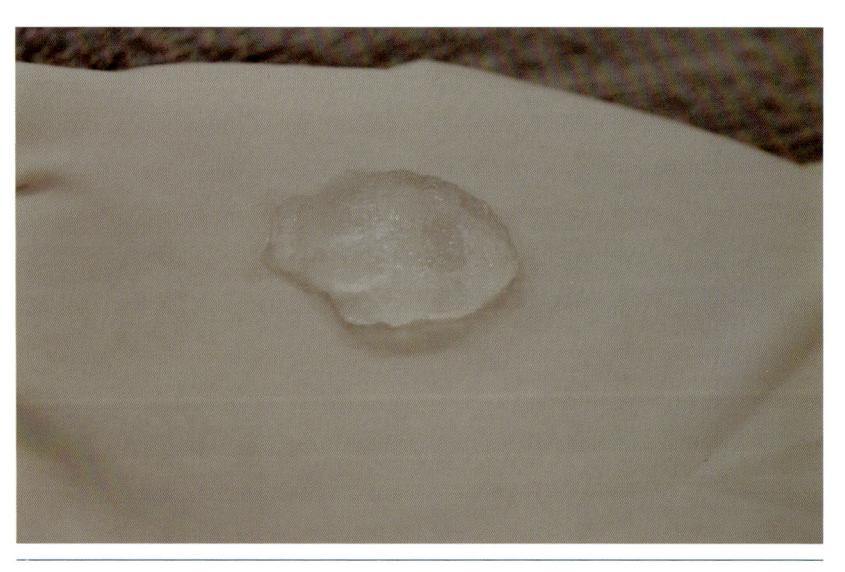

Fig. 2-33 This is how biphasic filler appears when injected on the palm of hand. Irregular surface and highly viscous characteristic can be observed.

(Source: Restylane, GALDERMA)

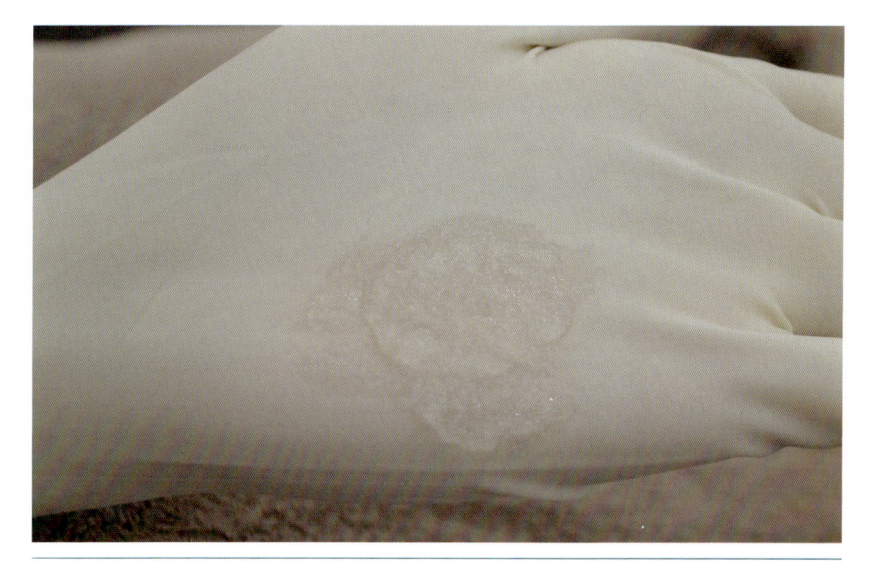

Fig. 2-34 Resistance against external pressure is high. When rubbed by pressing, rather than spreading out evenly it feels more as though the lumps are moving.
(Source: Restylane, GALDERMA)

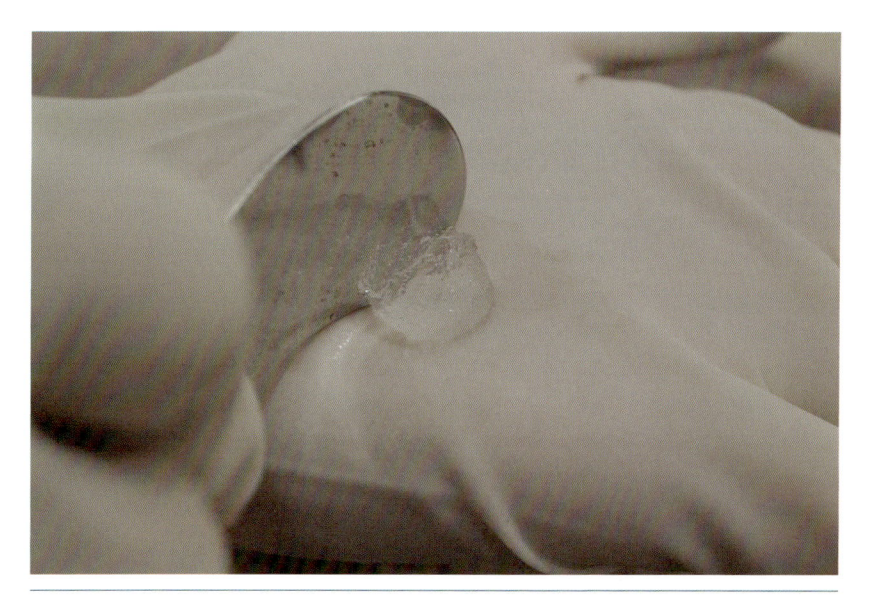

Fig. 2-35 The filler can be molded back to initial shape with the use of a spatula.
(Source: Restylane, GALDERMA)

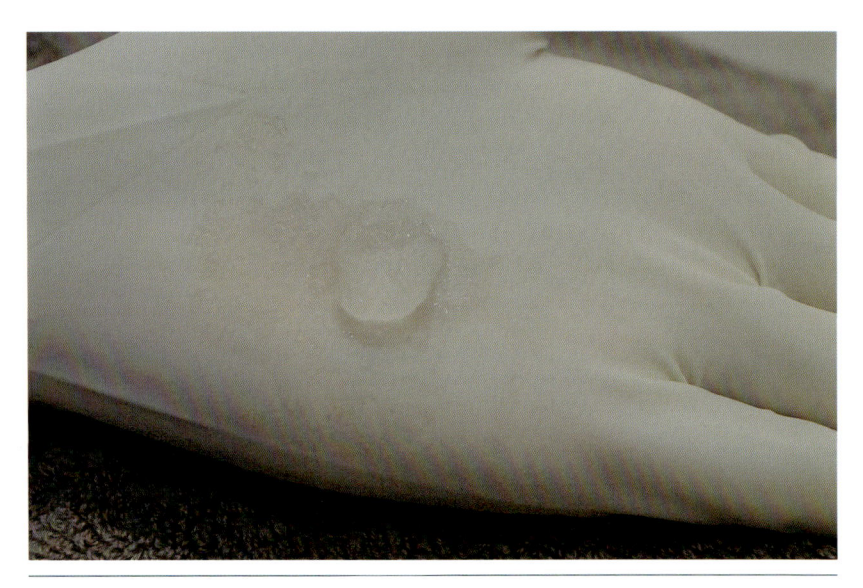

Fig. 2-36 When aggregated again, the volume did not decrease in comparison to the initial shape and almost complete restoration of original shape can be observed. This process of spreading and aggregating shows that it reverts to its original state.

(Source: Restylane, GALDERMA)

3) Molding Monophasic Filler Having the Characteristics of Biphasic

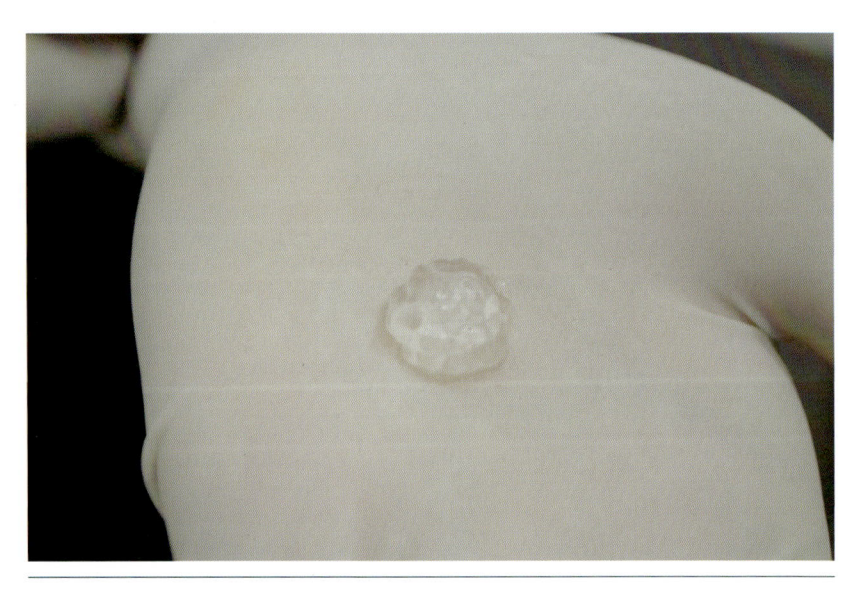

Fig. 2-37 When monophasic filler with characteristics of biphasic is injected on the palm, bumps that are slightly similar to biphasic filler are felt but the entire shape appears closer to monophasic filler.

(Source: The CHAEUM, HUGEL)

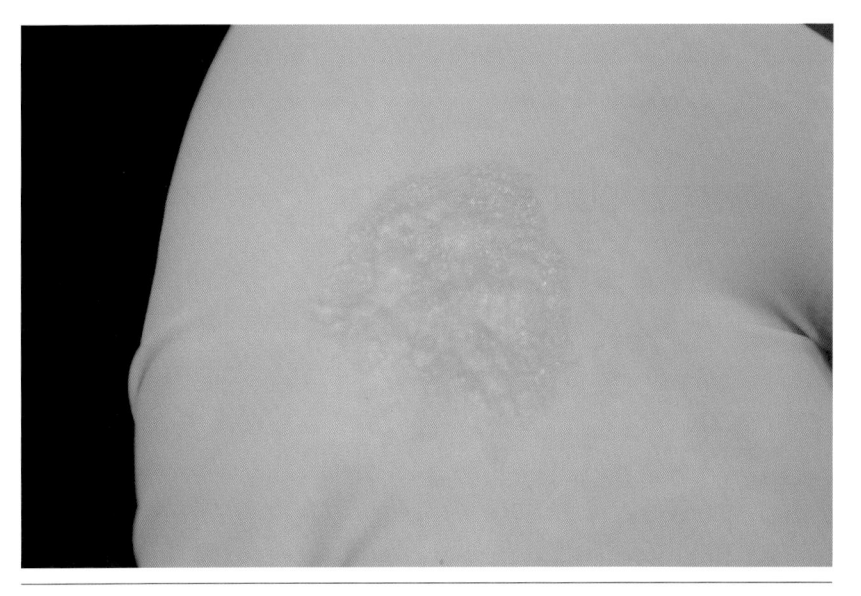

Fig. 2-38 When spread out by pressing against the palm, viscoelasticity can be felt and it spreads evenly. After injecting the filler, it shows that it spreads evenly during molding.

(Source: The CHAEUM, HUGEL)

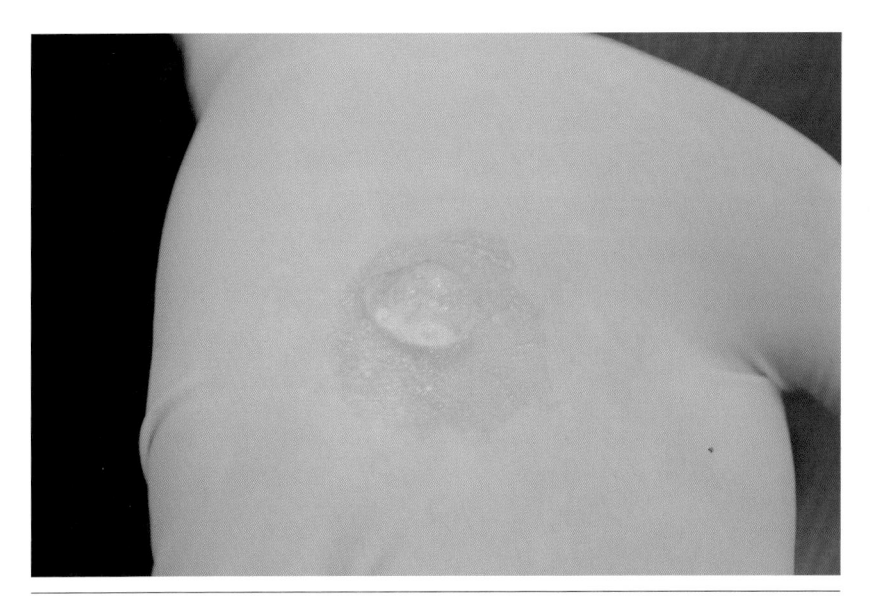

Fig. 2-39 When aggregated again, viscoelasticity is restored showing that not much has been lost. After the initial injection, it can be predicted that through molding, the desired shape can be achieved.

(Source: The CHAEUM, HUGEL)

4) Calcium Filler Molding

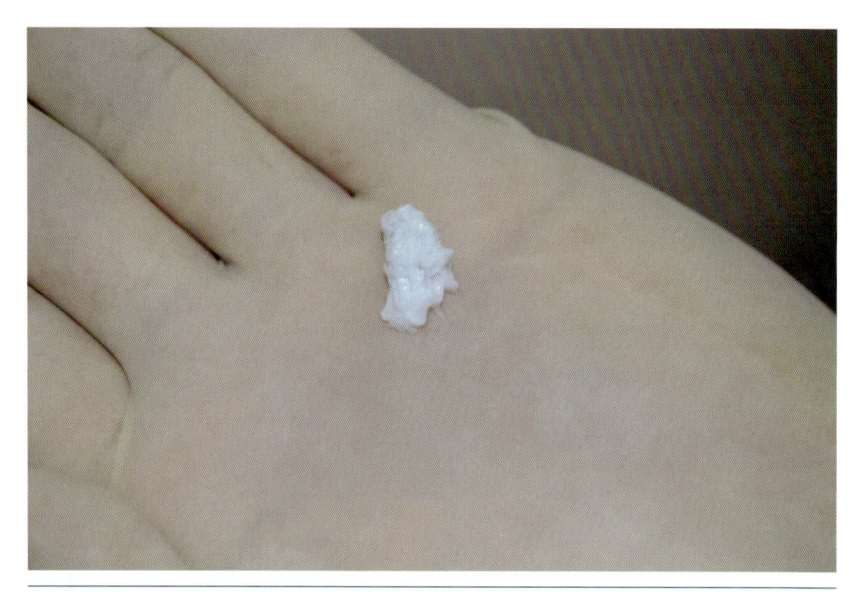

Fig. 2-40 Calcium filler molding (1). As time passes its form changes to a lump and the strength for maintaining the shape is great. This shows that it has much higher lifting capacity than HA filler.

(Source: Facetem, Daewoong)

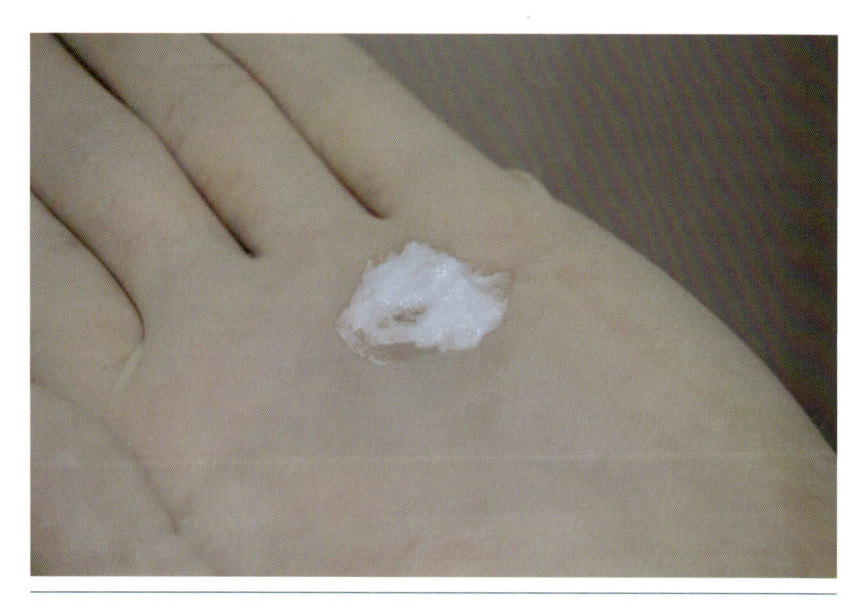

Fig. 2-41 Calcium filler molding (2). It does not spread out very well when rubbed. It feels similar to rubbing hard form ointment. This suggests that the filler will maintain its shape stably after being injected.

(Source: Facetem, Daewoong)

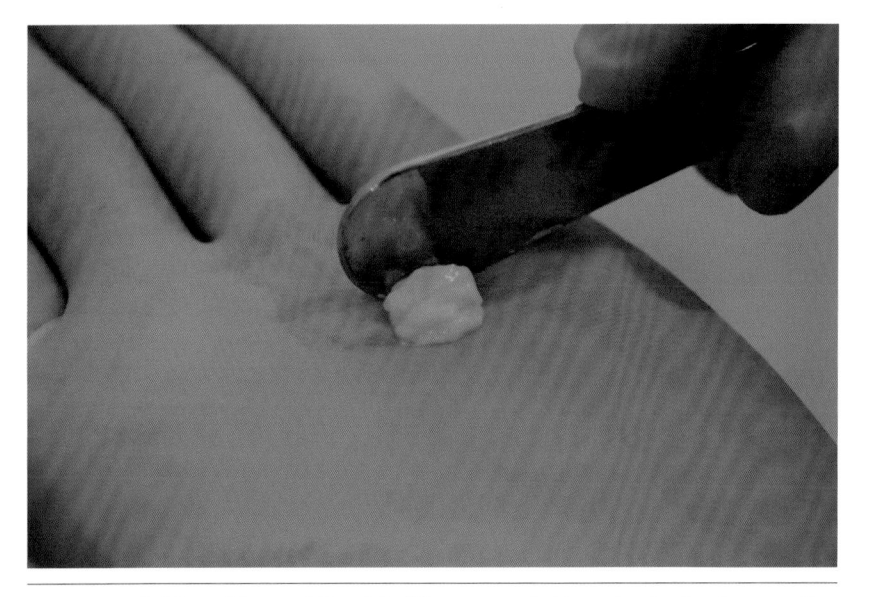

Fig. 2-42 Calcium filler molding (3). When crumpled it maintains its shape well.

(Source: Facetem, Daewoong)

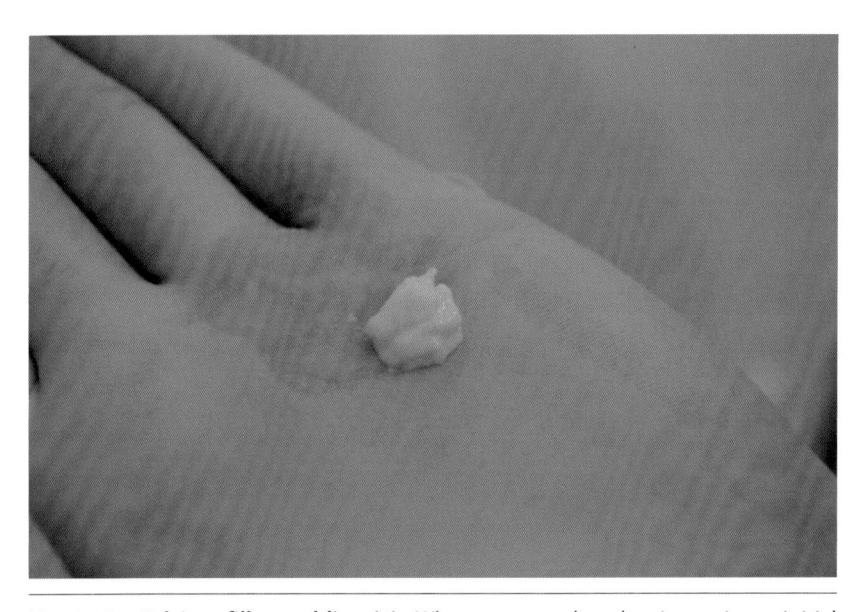

Fig. 2-43 Calcium filler molding (4). When compared to the time prior to initial rubbing, there is not much difference in the total amount of the filler. This demonstrates strong viscoelasticity. However, such advantage could also cause vascular complications resulting from pressuring the blood vessels, suggesting that high viscoelasticity is a double-edged sword.

(Source: Facetem, Daewoong)

When molding, it is easier to make the desired shape on a hard base. It is difficult to perform molding in areas made up of soft tissues, such as the cheek and tear trough. In such case, it is advisable to inject fillers with caution in order to avoid overcorrection. Besides, using tongue depressors or other special equipment can help mold in the soft regions. The following figures are examples of equipment that are used for molding.

2 Molding Method for Each Facial Area

1) Molding Under Eyes (the Smile Line)

Performing procedures along the smile line under eyes is relatively difficult and tricky. It is due to the high likelihood of getting bruises as well as the curvy characteristic of the lower eyelid, which makes it difficult to perform molding. Using a needle, the procedures can be completed in about three injections. However, this may result in bruises more easily, and if injections were performed at different injection depths, the treatment area can appear to be layered. As such, when performing a procedure under the eyes, under eye guider comes in handy. The equipment allows you to forecast the smile line shape of the under eye and to insert stably at injection. Moreover, it prevents fillers from moving downward, so the under eyes does not become saggy after the procedure. In general, when the soft tissue and skin in the lower eyelid area have low strength and elasticity, the fillers injected are likely to move downward. Thus, after the procedure, it is strongly advised to fix the under eye by taping and prevent forming any tracts that could possibly send fillers downwards under eyes. The under eye guider can be helpful for such tasks.

2) Under Eye Guider

The enlarged photograph of a guider on the right in Fig. 2-45 demonstrates that creation of a smile line under eye is dependent on the adjustment of the glider. For making the smile line, a cannula or needle should enter from the lateral area, make routes by penetrating the center of under eye shape made, inject evenly while pulling backward, and then exit. Fillers that are highly moldable with weak viscoelasticity are recommended to be used.

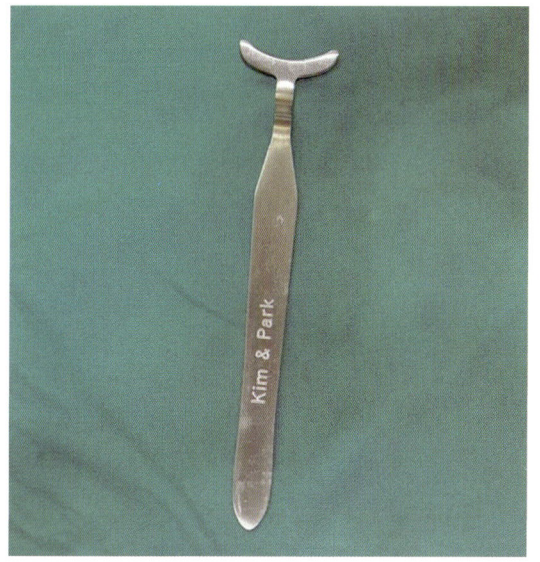

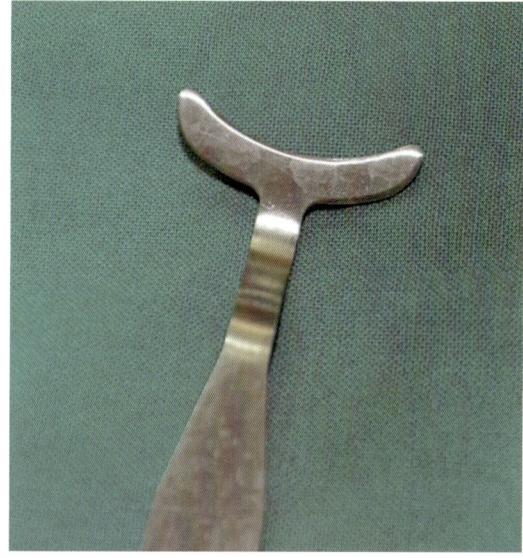

Fig. 2-44 **Under eye guider**

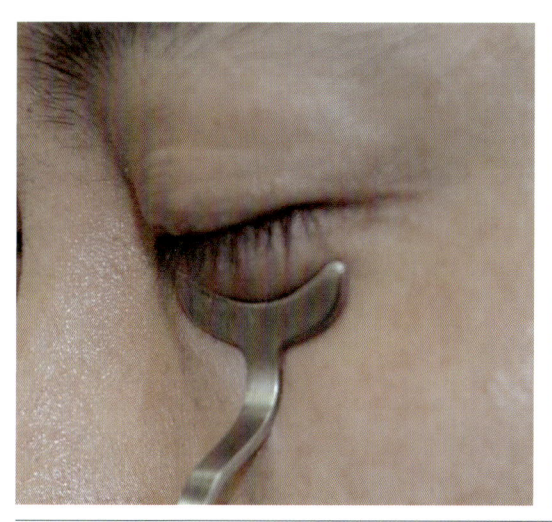

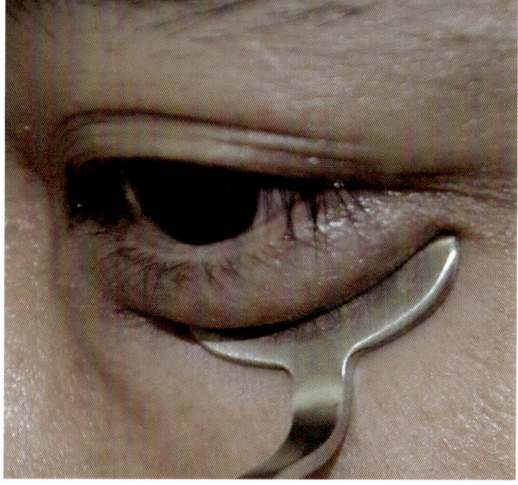

Fig. 2-45 **Under eye guider molding**

85

3) Nasolabial Folds and Cheeks

Since the cheeks and nasolabial folds do not have hard bottoms, it is quite difficult to make shapes in these areas. But if fillers with weak viscoelasticity are used, shape cannot be maintained due to recurrent small movements.

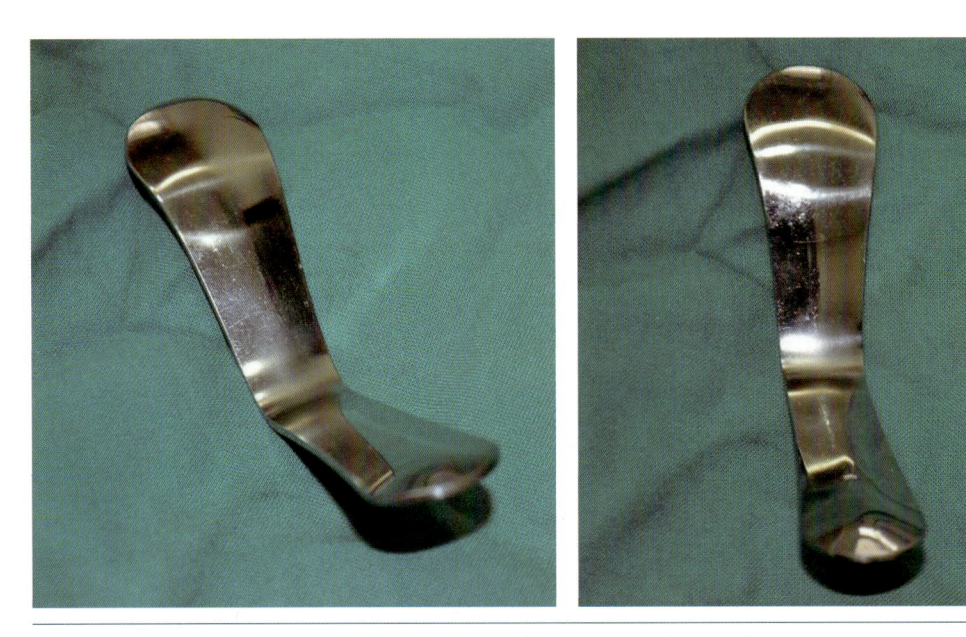

Fig. 2-46 Molding equipment for the nasolabial folds and cheeks (product name: Nurumee)

4) Massage after Injection

It may not be possible to make the desired shape immediately after injecting fillers. At that time, the desired shape may be obtained through various handlings. This is through pressing, gathering or massaging. Due to the viscoelasticity of fillers, it does not change its shape unless a certain level of pressure is applied. Massaging the nasolabial folds and the cheeks is especially tricky as the pressure cannot be delivered entirely as it is due to the soft tissue located right below the skin. Also, it is difficult to deliver the pressure evenly. Therefore, good results can be obtained by using various equipment properly.

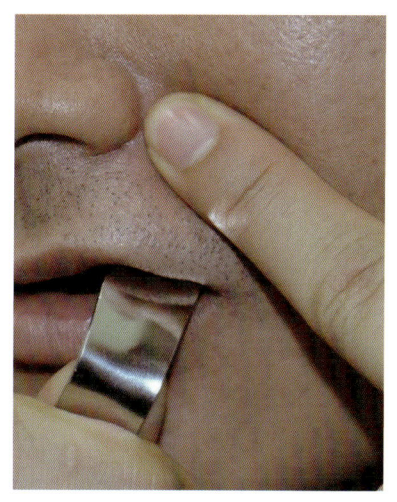

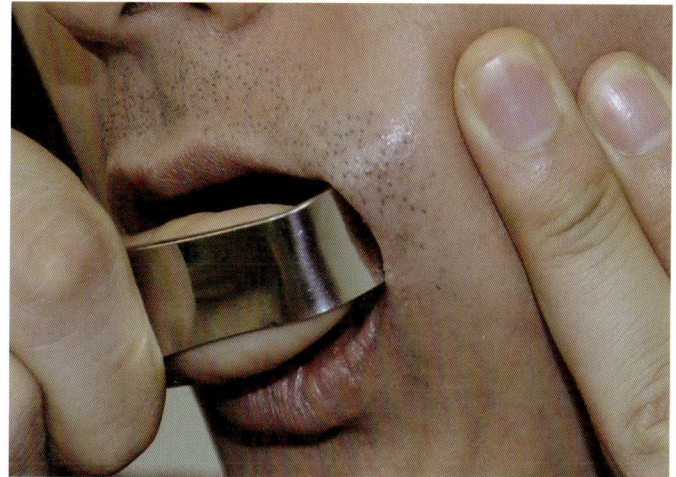

Fig. 2-47 Molding nasolabial folds and cheeks

6. Dissolution Test

1 How to Use Hyaluronidase

Amongst many different types of fillers being used today, hyaluronic acid fillers are the most common type of all. Hyaluronic acid has the disadvantage of having a short longevity; conversely, its ability to dissolve readily in the skin is an advantage when compared to other kinds of fillers. Research shows that fillers may cause side effects to blood vessels at a frequency of about 0.001%. As these side effects could be serious, the characteristics of HA fillers are appreciated, specifically for their ability to dissolve. In recent studies, treatments using hyaluronidase have been explored as well.

In general, complications such as vascular occlusion or vascular compromise occur when fillers block blood supply. They happen because fillers have been injected directly into a blood vessel, or fillers that have been already injected install external pressure to nearby blood vessels. We define these phenomena as intravascular injection vs extravascular compression, respectively. From intravascular injections, complications generated by embolism are commonly found.

In reality, no questions are concerned with the use of hyaluronidase for diminishing the side effects.

Based on experimental results from a 2011 study by Kim, et al., hyaluronidase use at 4 hours and 24 hours showed significant differences in results.

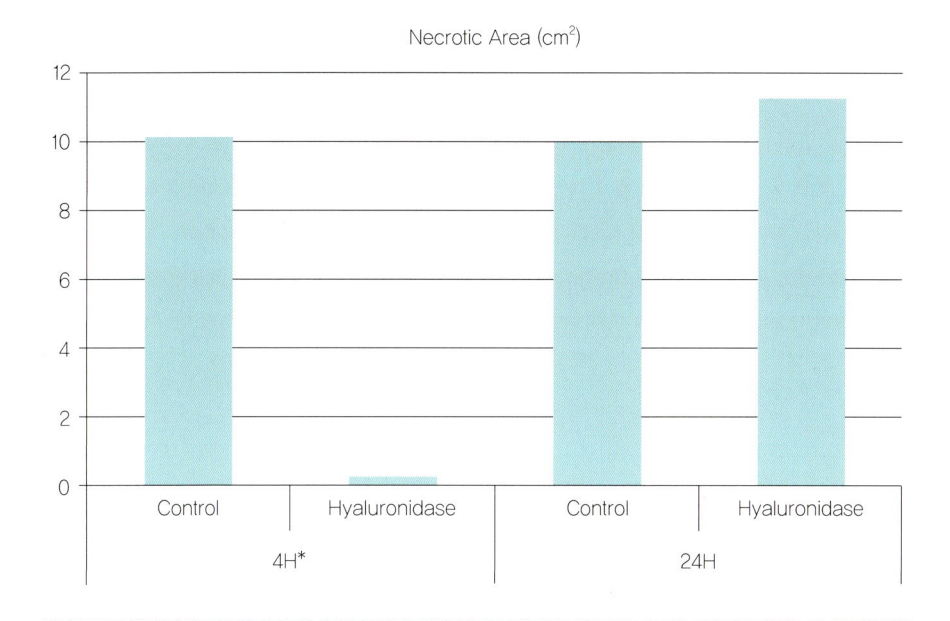

Fig. 2-48 The necrotic area was significantly smaller in the hyaluronidase-injected ears in the 4-h intervention group. In the 24-h intervention group, the difference in the necrotic area between control and hyaluronidase-injected ears was not significant.
*Significant difference for p <0.05.

In light of these research results, it has been clearly demonstrated that hyaluronidase must be used as early as possible. However, there are no clear standards for how to use it and how much of it is necessary.

Many studies have been conducted based on the recommendations of experts. Most of these theses have stated the recommended amount of hyaluronidase smaller than the amount actually being used in clinics.

However, in 2015, Cohen JL, et al. recommended using a sufficient amount of hyaluronidase, 200 units at a minimum. The authors also agree with this study regarding the amount of hyaluronidase that must be used.

For further clarification, the authors have performed filler dissolution experiments. Consequently, additional comments have been included based on the test results.

In order to melt hyaluronic acid filler effectively, we must consider not only hyaluronidase capacity, but also the amount of saline solution.

In other words, changes can occur only when sufficient amount of saline solution is mixed with hyaluronic acid filler. Thus, it is crucial to add a significant amount of saline solution. This will likely be helpful to understand treatments for resolving filler complications.

2 An Experiment for Melting HA Fillers

Types of fillers
a. biphasic HA filler
b. monophasic HA filler
c. polycaprolactone filler

Experimental conditions
- Most hyaluronidase consists of 1,500-units of capacity per vial.
- Make a hyaluronidase solution with a concentration of 5 unit/0.1 cc by mixing in 2 cc of saline solution.
- Afterwards, add 1 cc of hyaluronic acid filler into a beaker, and then pour the solution of hyaluronidase mixed with saline. After mixing them together, observe the appearance of the solution over time.

a. Biphasic Filler

Experiment contents
1. Hyaluronic acid filler 1 cc + hyaluronidase 0.1 cc (75 unit)
2. Hyaluronic acid filler 1 cc + hyaluronidase 1 cc (750 unit)
3. Hyaluronic acid filler 1 cc + normal saline 1 cc

a-1 Hyaluronic acid filler 1cc + hyaluronidase 0.1 cc (75 unit)

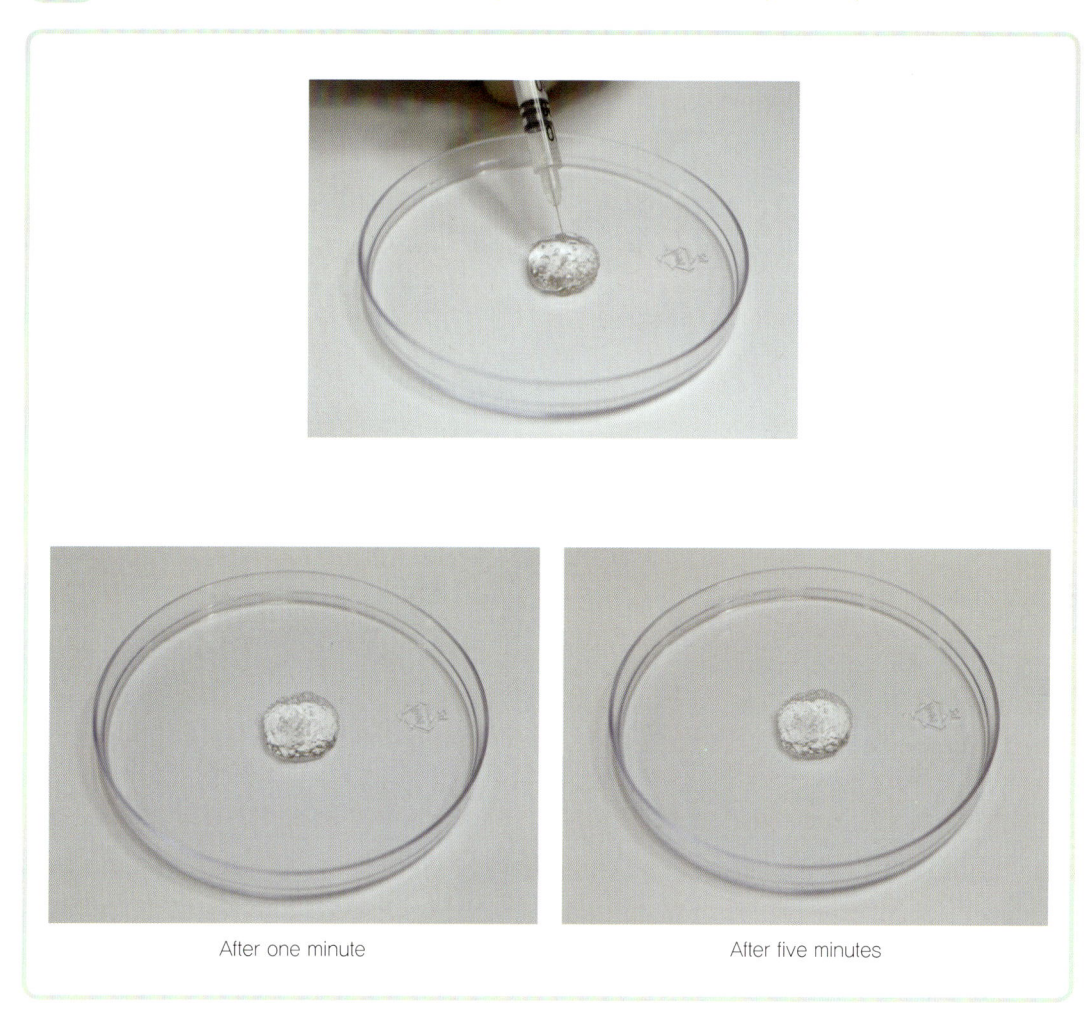

After one minute

After five minutes

As seen in the figure a-1, 0.1 cc of hyaluronidase was insufficient to dissolve 1 cc of hyaluronic acid filler. It can be seen that the amount of hyaluronidase that has been stated in many previous theses does not have a significant effect in reality.

Safe Filler Injection Technique Demonstration – using live imaging tools

a-2 Hyaluronic acid filler 1 cc + hyaluronidase 1 cc (750 unit)

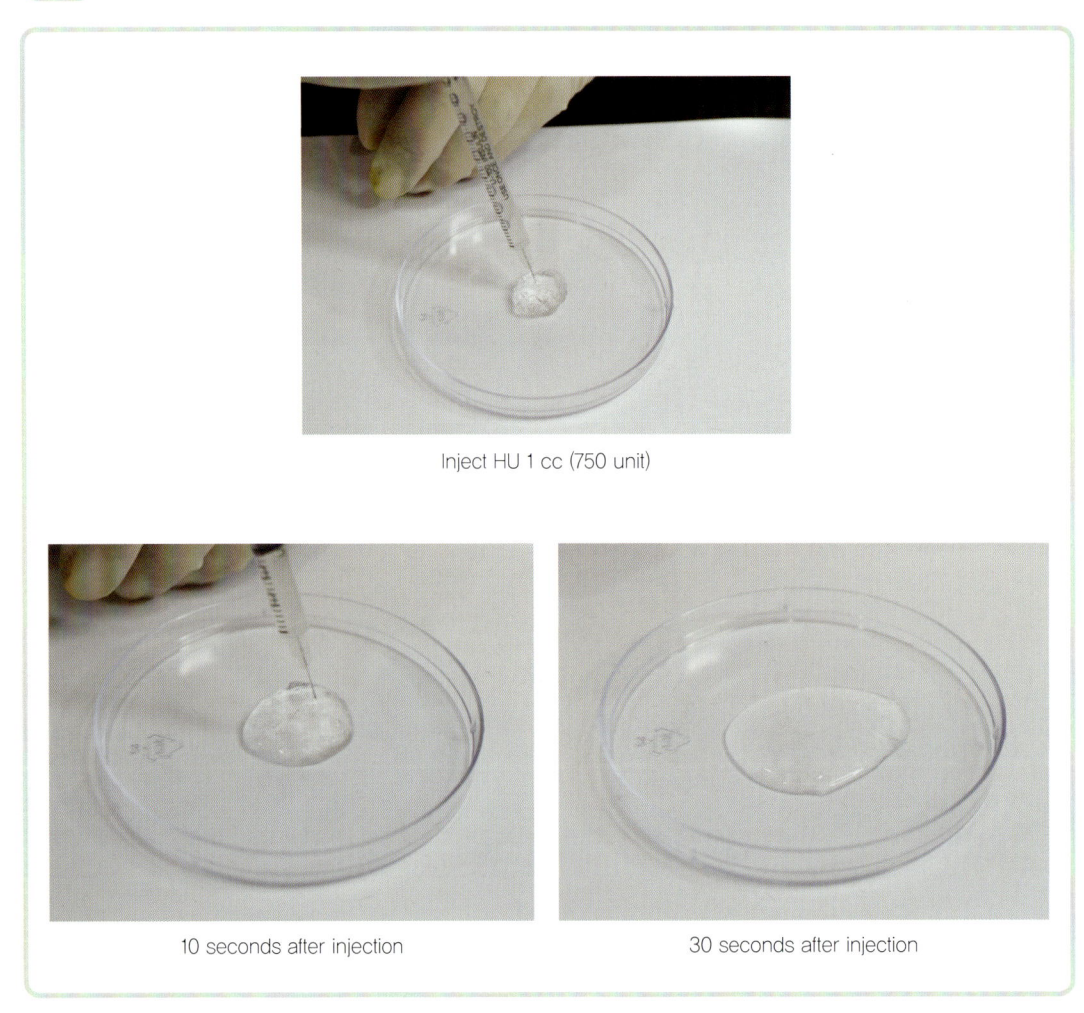

Inject HU 1 cc (750 unit)

10 seconds after injection

30 seconds after injection

    When a sufficient amount of hyaluronidase is added, fillers become dissolved right away. In the case of impending necrosis, hyaluronidase must be used as an urgent emergency treatment. Accordingly, it is important to use a sufficient amount of hyaluronidase to quickly dissolve the filler.

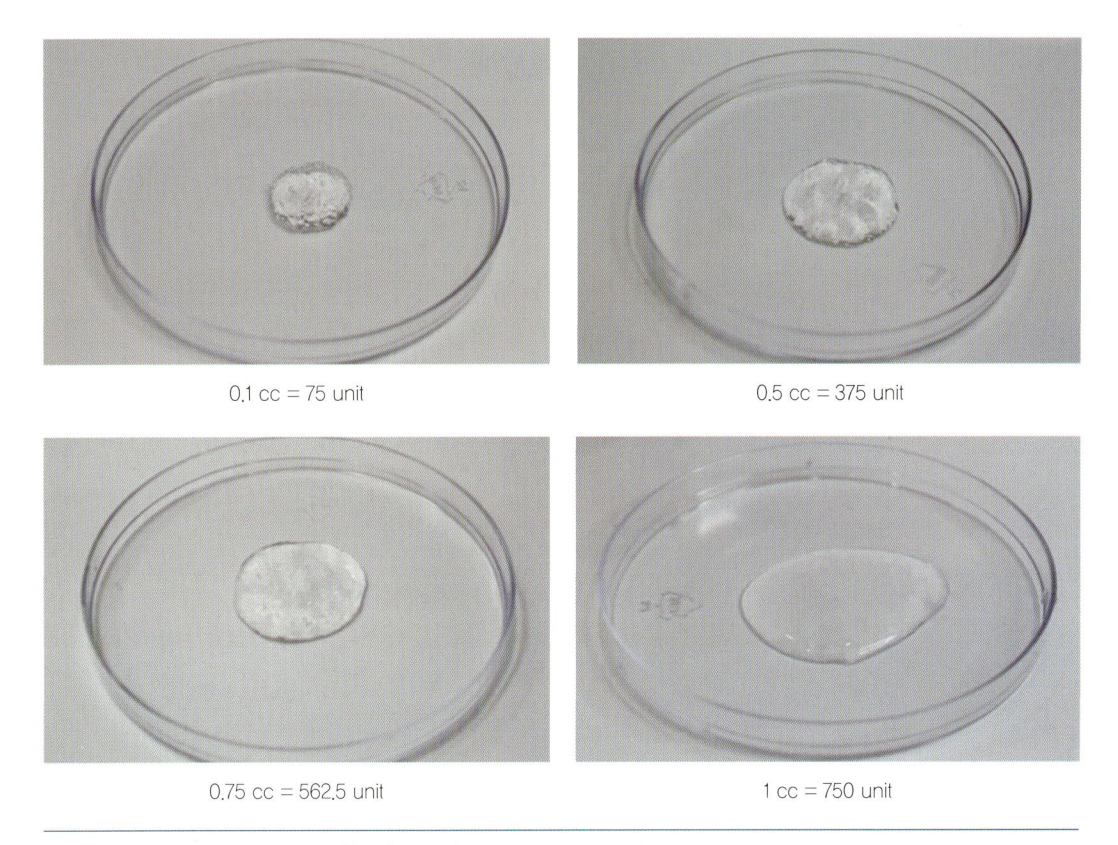

0.1 cc = 75 unit	0.5 cc = 375 unit
0.75 cc = 562.5 unit	1 cc = 750 unit

Fig. 2-49   For each amount of hyaluronidase (75 unit/0.1 cc)

Fig. 2-49 shows the degree of filler dissolution proportional to the amount of hyaluronidase added.

It demonstrates that the more hyaluronidase is used, the more hyaluronic acid dissolves completely.

This finding significantly supports the idea of the previous discussion that a sufficient amount of hyaluronidase is necessary for dissolving hyaluronic acid filler.

a-3 Hyaluronic acid filler 1 cc + normal saline 1 cc

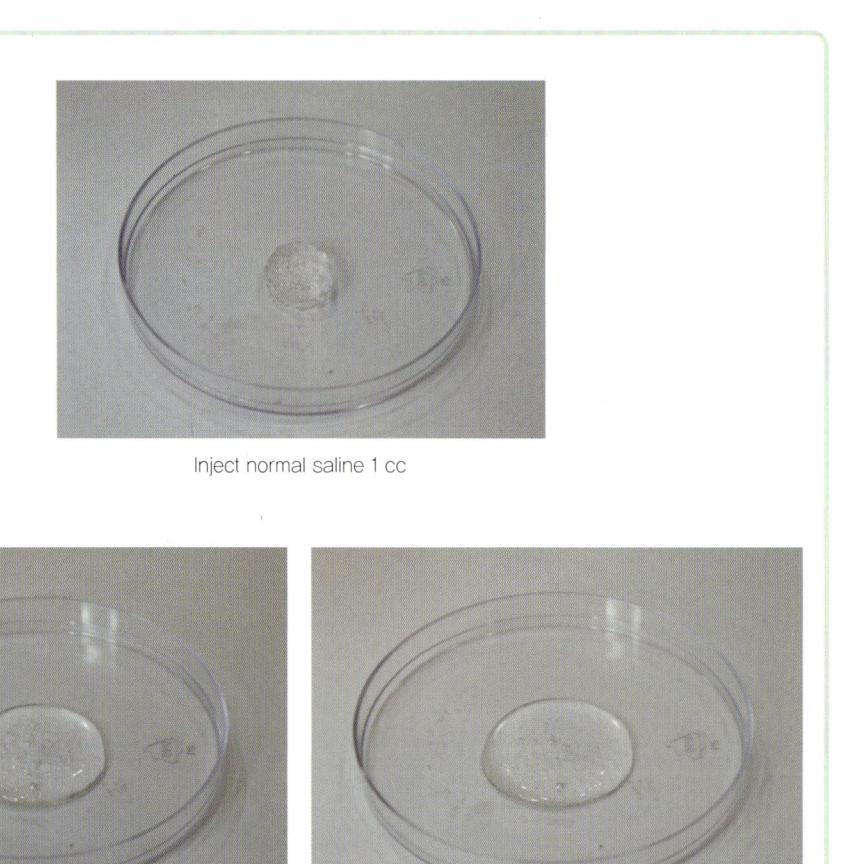

Inject normal saline 1 cc

After one minute

After 5 minutes

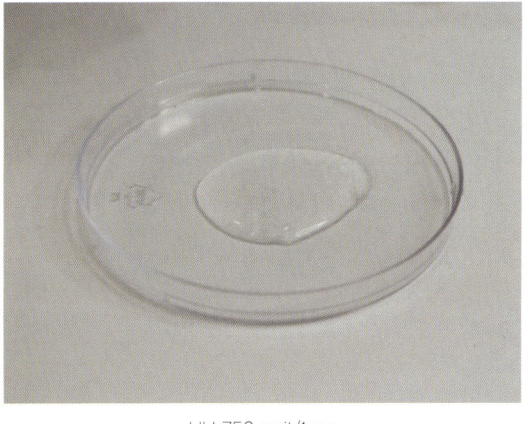

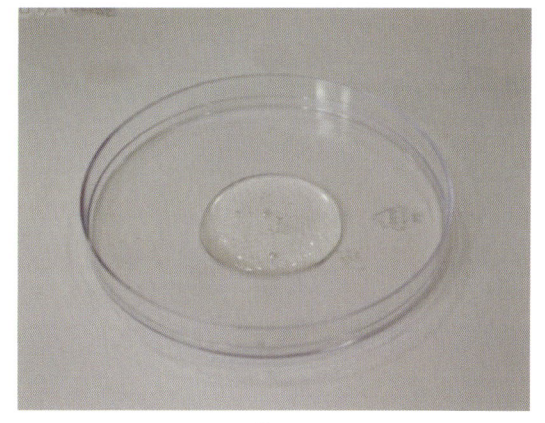

| HU 750 unit/1 cc | N/S 1 cc |

Fig. 2-50 This shows that using a sufficient amount of saline solution is as important as using a sufficient amount of hyaluronidase.

The figures above demonstrate that it is necessary to use sufficient amount of saline as much as using sufficient amount of hyaluronidase. They also suggest to use a large volume of hyaluronidase rather than a small volume.

Vascular complications may arise from direct intravascular injection; they may also occur from ischemia caused by pressuring the blood vessels externally. Accordingly, by eliminating the viscoelasticity of hyaluronic acid, which is the source of pressure, the internal or external pressure caused by filler can be released. It can be seen that when filler is mixed with saline, it absorbs the saline and make a new saturated form of physical state.

In reality, hyaluronic acid fillers are not completely saturated, but are manufactured so that they can absorb only a small amount of water. Therefore, in treating filler complications, it is absolutely essential to reduce the strength of the filler. This step can be accomplished by inducing crumpling by adding a sufficient amount of saline solution.

The impact of strength reduction is more clearly seen in biphasic fillers than in monophasic fillers.

b. Monophasic Filler

Experiment contents

1. Hyaluronic acid filler 1 cc + hyaluronidase 0.1 cc (75 unit)
2. Hyaluronic acid filler 1 cc + hyaluronidase 1 cc (750 unit)
3. Hyaluronic acid filler 1 cc + normal saline 1 cc

b-1 Hyaluronic acid filler 1 cc + hyaluronidase 0.1 cc (75 unit)

0.1 cc

After one minute

After 5 minutes

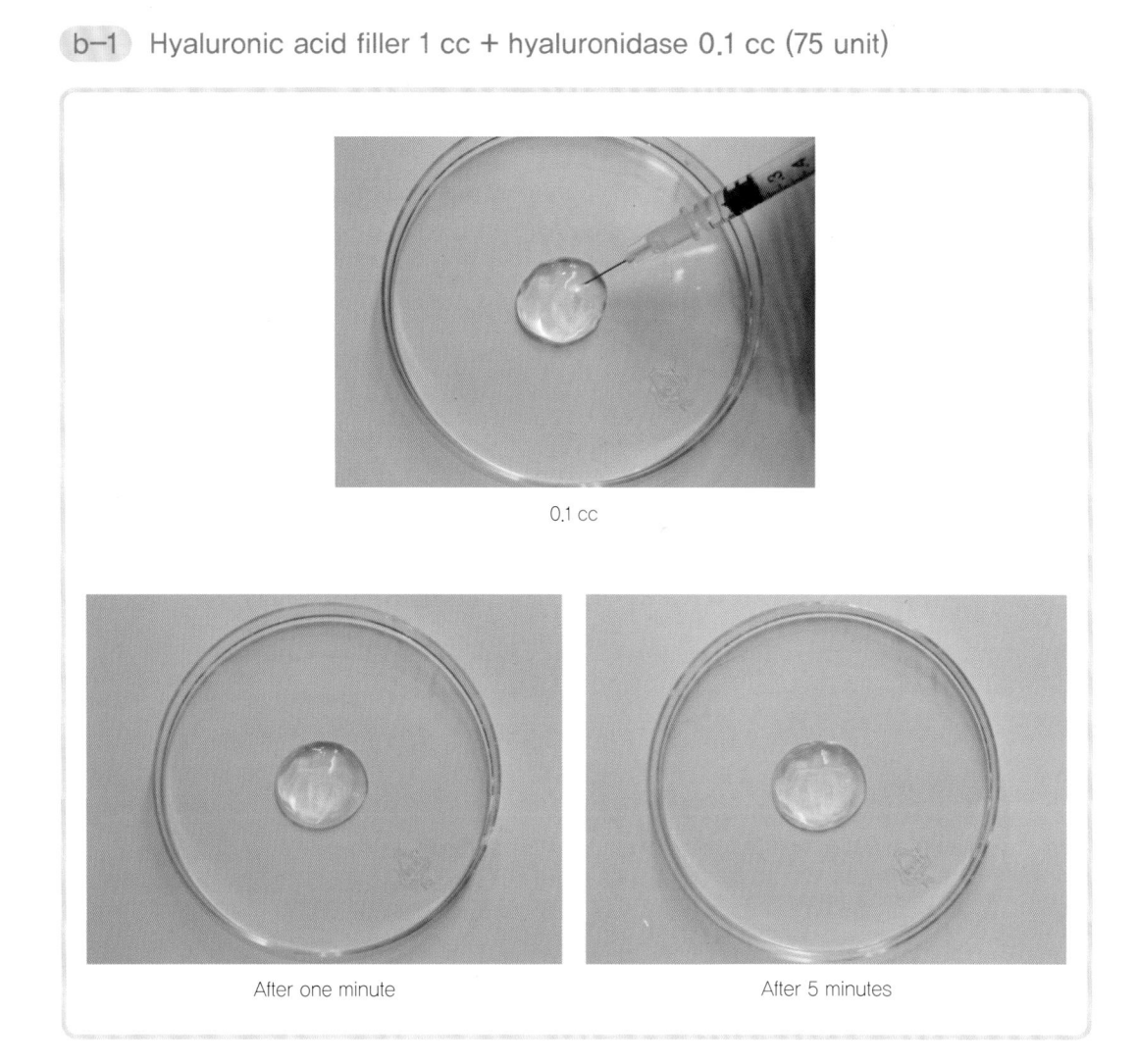

    As seen in figure b-1, monophasic fillers could not be dissolved with 0.1 cc/ 75 units, which was used in the previous theses. Additionally, the monophasic fillers were relatively weak with respect to the degree of mixing between the saline and hyaluronidase. Some fillers have relatively little effect in attracting liquid and maintaining stable characteristics. When such types of fillers need to be dissolved, a slightly larger amount of hyaluronidase and massaging the filler are necessary.

b-2 Hyaluronic acid filler 1 cc + hyaluronidase 1 cc (750 unit)

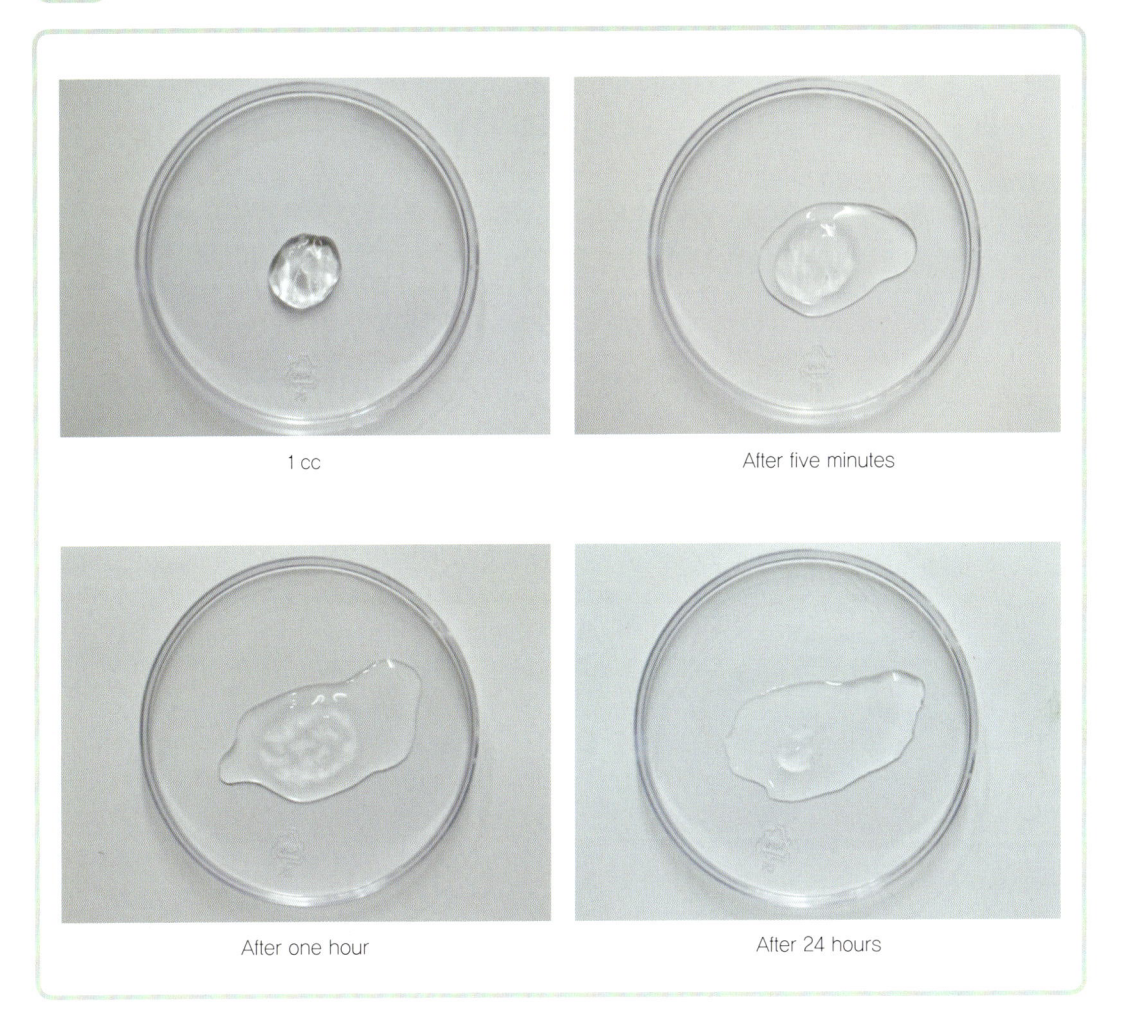

1 cc

After five minutes

After one hour

After 24 hours

In figure b-2, it can be seen that the fillers did not dissolve completely even after 24 hours. The effect of hyaluronidase, which innately exists within our body, is expected to be greater in the body, and therefore, the fillers would probably dissolve faster in a clinical setting than they do during in vitro tests.

It must be noted that the melting procedure should be repeated if fillers do not become dissolved completely.

b-3 Hyaluronic acid filler 1 cc + normal saline 1 cc

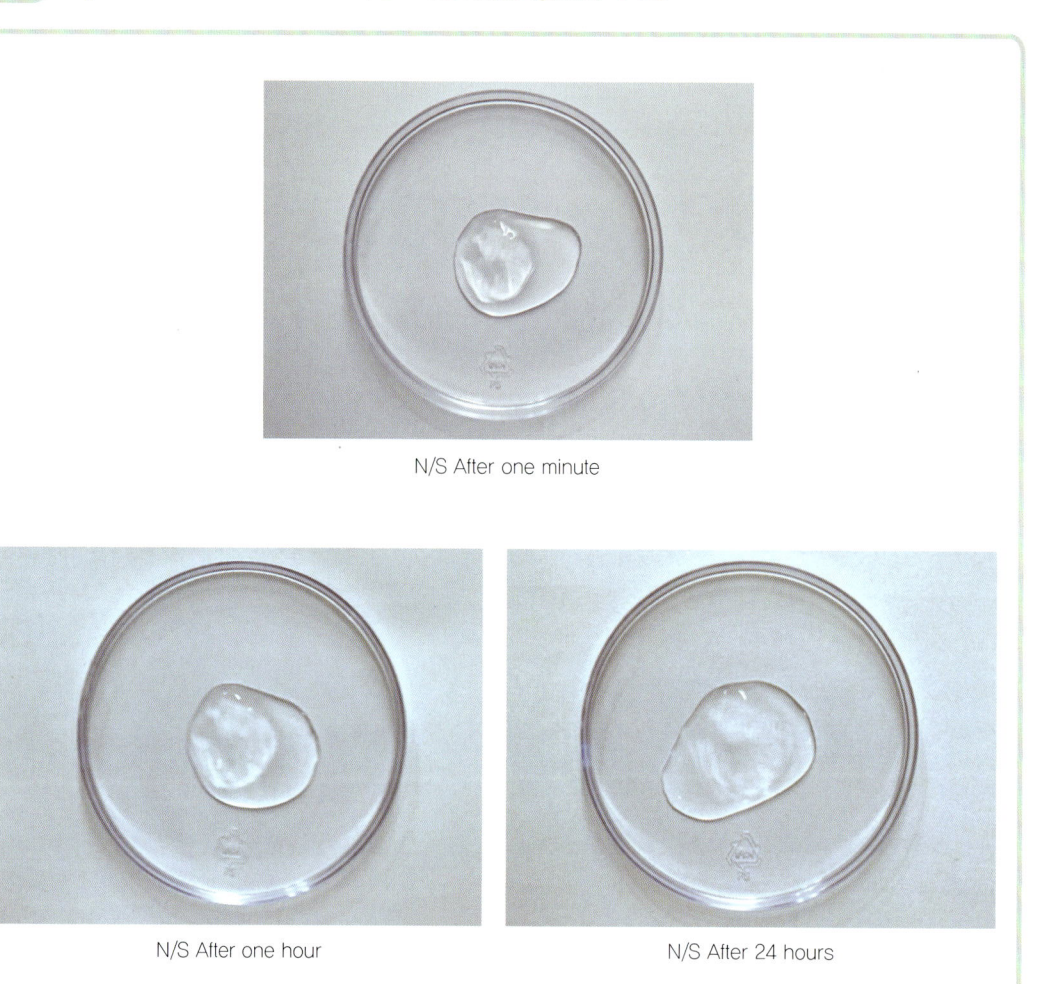

N/S After one minute

N/S After one hour

N/S After 24 hours

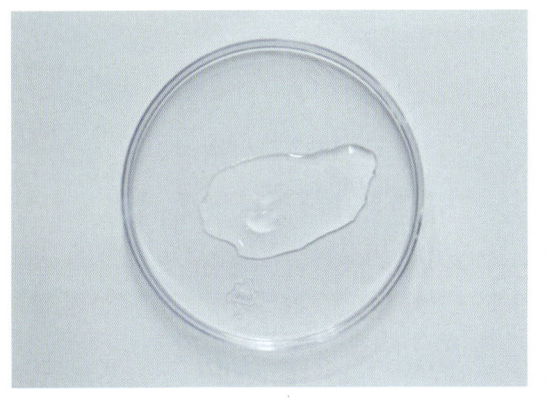

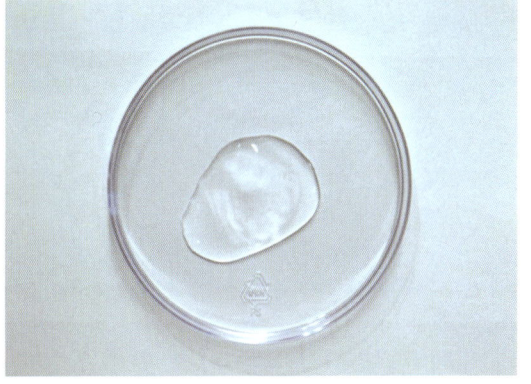

Fig. 2-51　Comparison - hyaluronidase 750 unit 1 cc vs. normal saline 1 cc

Fig. 2-51 shows the results when saline is mixed with monophasic filler. It can be observed that although the fillers do not melt entirely, combination with saline leads to change in their physical form different from their initial shape. From the result, it can be speculated that the fundamental, physical characteristic of viscoelasticity has been changed. Still, the filler is completely separable from the liquid on its own. It can be also predicted that less swelling will occur after procedures, but this requires additional research.

It should be noted that this observation does not apply to all monophasic fillers, as each product has different characteristics.

c. Polycaprolactone Filler

Experiment Contents

1. Polycaprolactone filler 1 cc + hyaluronidase 1 cc (750 unit)
2. Polycaprolactone filler 1 cc + normal saline 1 cc

c-1 Polycaprolactone filler 1 cc + hyaluronidase 1 cc (750 unit)

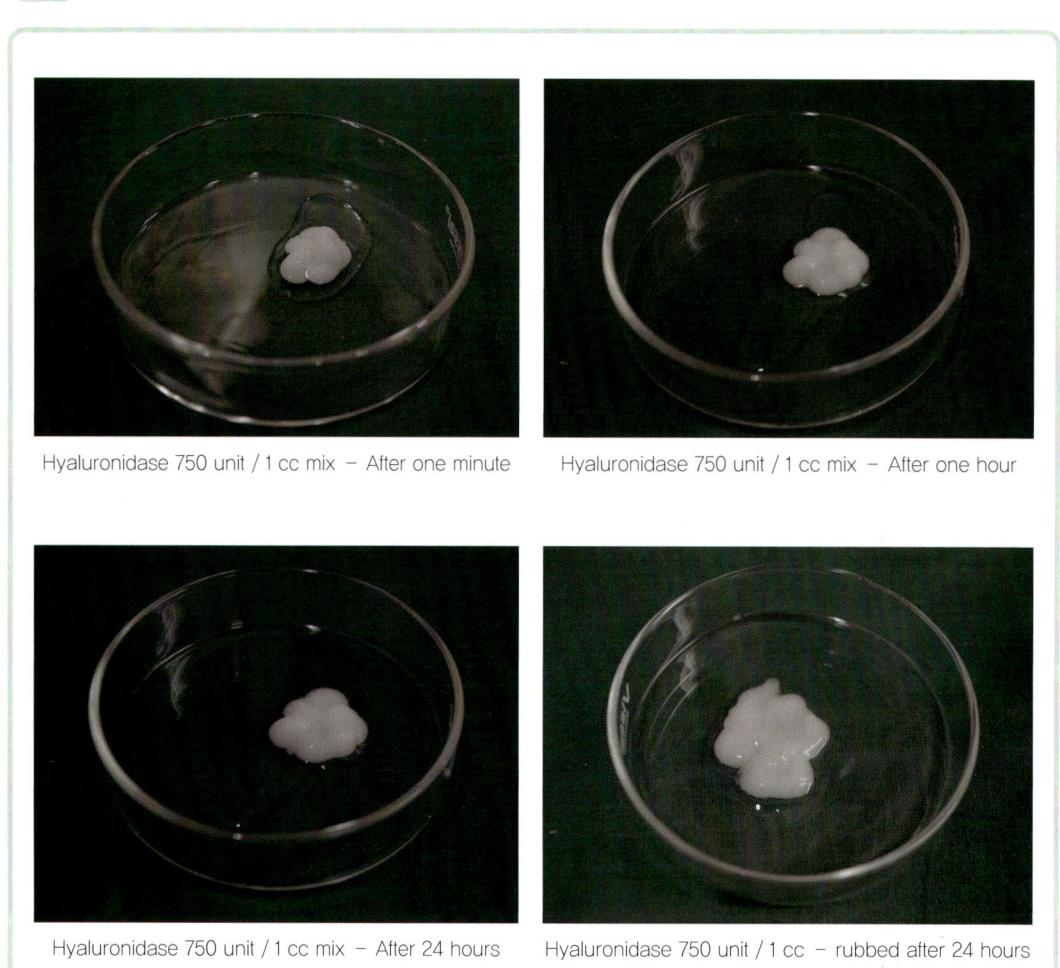

Hyaluronidase 750 unit / 1 cc mix – After one minute

Hyaluronidase 750 unit / 1 cc mix – After one hour

Hyaluronidase 750 unit / 1 cc mix – After 24 hours

Hyaluronidase 750 unit / 1 cc – rubbed after 24 hours

c-2 Polycaprolactone filler 1 cc + normal saline 1 cc

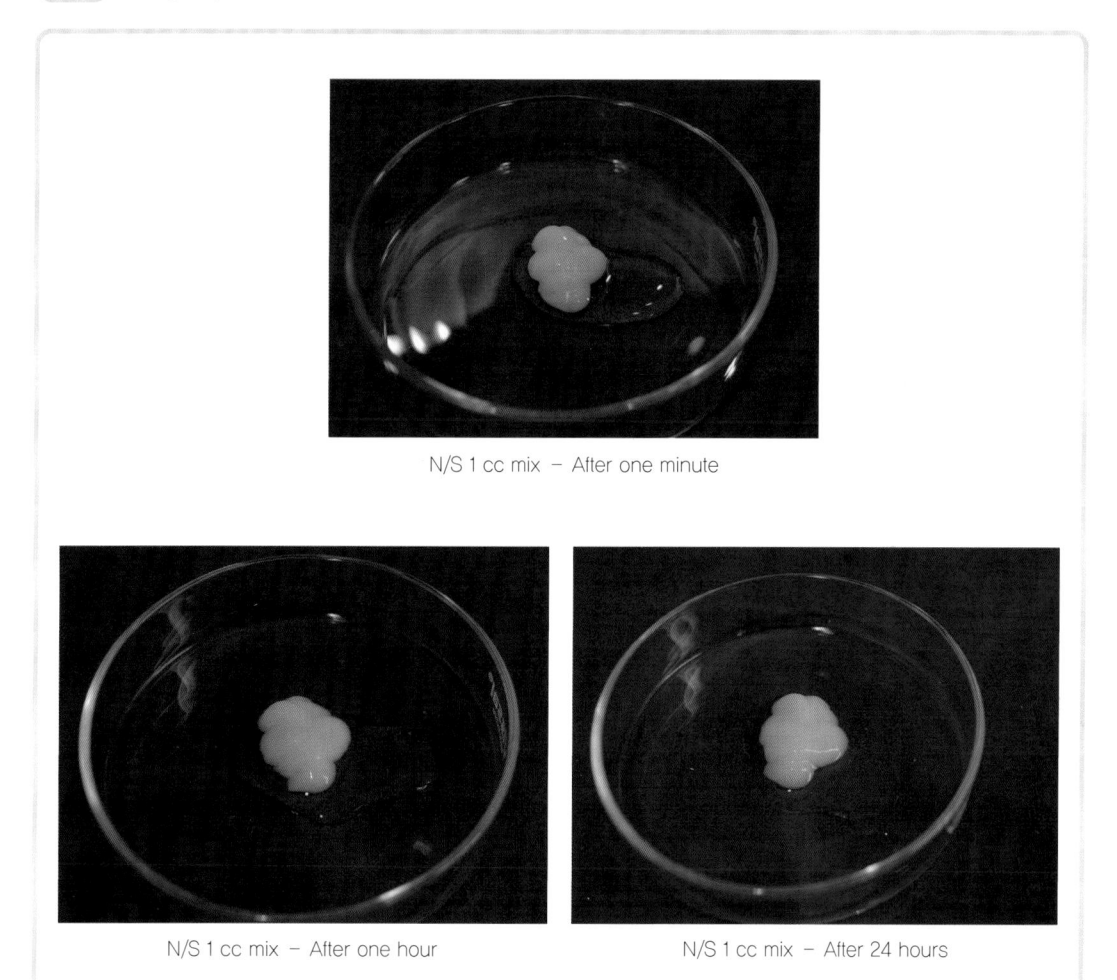

N/S 1 cc mix – After one minute

N/S 1 cc mix – After one hour

N/S 1 cc mix – After 24 hours

Polycaprolactone fillers also do not become readily dissolved in hyaluronidase since there is no visible decrease in viscoelasticity. Thus, when problems occur, they are more likely be treated with the elimination method rather than dissolving method.

Due to high longevity and ability to maintain shapes stably, polycaprolactone fillers have grown to be popular recently. Understanding the characteristics of these fillers is necessary to reduce the risk of clinical accidents and respond appropriately when confronting complications.

Reference

1. Ahmet Tezel & Glenn H. Fredrickson. The science of hyaluronic acid dermal fillers. J Cosmet Laser Ther. 2008;10(1):35-42.

2. K.Y. Park, H.K. Kim, B.J. Kim. Comparative study of hyaluronic acid fillers by in vitro and in vivo testing. J Eur Acad Dermatol Venereol. 2014; 28(5):565-8.

3. Timothy Corcoran Flynn MD et al. Comparative Histology of Intradermal Implantation of Mono and Biphasic Hyaluronic Acid Fillers. Dermatol Surg. 2011;37(5):637-43.

4. Narins et al. Clinical conference:management of rare events following dermal fillers-focal necrosis and angry red bumps. Dermatol Surg. 2006;32(3):426-34.

5. Hanke CW et al. Abscess formation and local necrosis after treatment with Zyderm or Zyplast collagen implants. J Am Acad Dermatol. 1991; 25(2 pt 1):319-26.

6. Hirsch et al. Successful management of an unusual presentation of impending necrosis following a hyaluronic acid injection embolus and proposed algorithm for management with hyaluronidase. Dermatol Surg. 2007;33(3):357-60.

7. Glaish AS. Injection necrosis of the glabella: protocol for prevention and treatment after use of dermal fillers. Dermatol Surg. 2006;32:276-81.

8. Kim et al. Vascular complications of hyaluronic acid fillers and the role of hyaluronidase in management. J Plast Reconstr Aesthet Surg. 2011;64(12):1590-5.

9. Joel L. et al. Treatment of hyaluronic acid filler-induced impending necrosis with hyaluronidase: consensus recommendation. Aesthet Surg J. 2015;35(7):844-9.

10. Signorini M. et al. Global Aesthetics Consensus: Avoidance and Management of Complications from Hyaluronic Acid Fillers-Evidence- and Opinion-Based. Review and Consensus Recommendations. Plast Reconstr Surg. 2016;137(6):961e-71e.

Safe Filler Injection Technique Demonstration
– using live imaging tools

Part
3

Basic Anatomy

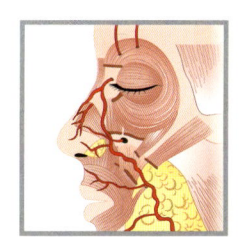

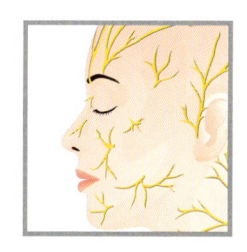

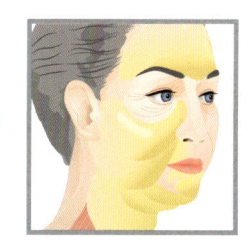

Safe Filler Injection Technique Demonstration
- using live imaging tools

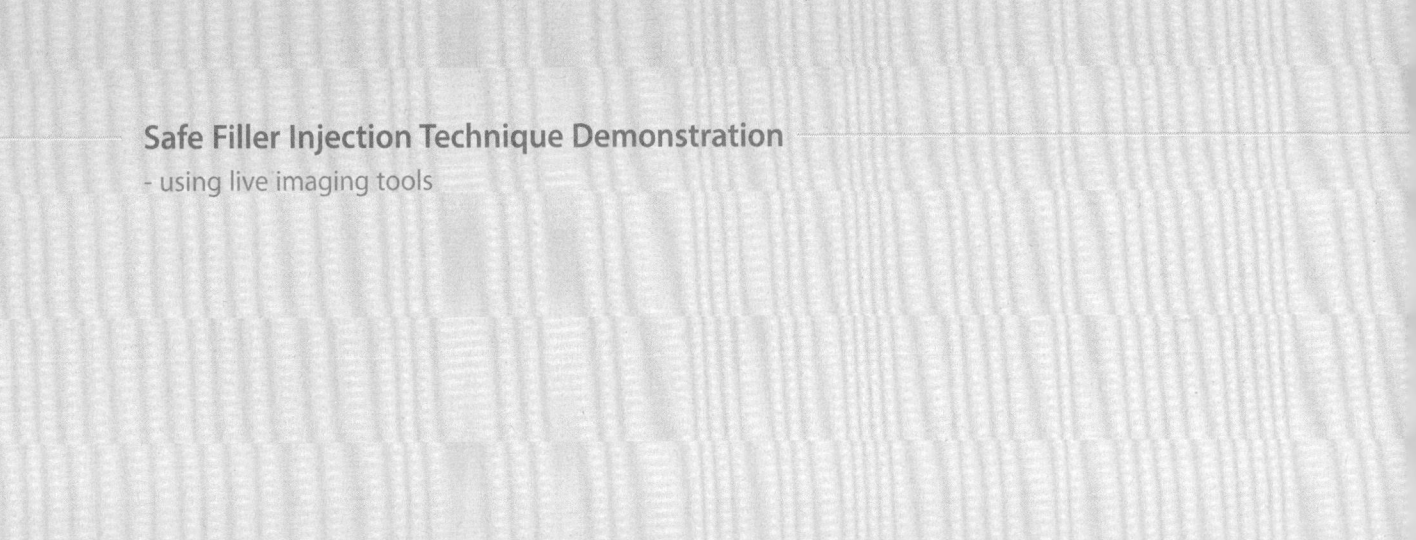

Part 3: Basic Anatomy

1. The Vasculature

1. The Facial Artery & Vein
2. Variations in the Facial Artery
3. The Supratrochlear Artery (STA) & Supraorbital Artery (SOA)
4. Superficial Temporal Artery (SfTA)
5. The External Carotid Artery & Internal Carotid Artery
6. Palpation of the Artery
7. Visual Inspection of Veins

2. Nerves

1. CN V (Trigeminal Nerve) – Sensory
2. CN VII (Facial Nerve) – Motor

3. Fat Compartments

1. Superficial Fat
2. Deep Fat

4. Muscles

1. Muscles around the Eyes
2. Muscles around the Mouth
3. Muscles of the Nose

5. The SMAS & Retaining Ligaments

1. The SMAS (Superficial Musculo-Aponeurotic System)
2. The Retaining Ligaments
   1) True Retaining Ligaments
   2) False Retaining Ligaments

Part 3

Basic Anatomy

••• The fundamentals of any procedure or surgery are anatomy. Performing procedures or surgeries without the fundamentals in anatomy is like looking for treasure without a map. Compared to other parts of the body, the face has more intricate functions, and accordingly, the structure of blood vessels, muscles and nerves is complex. Up until a few years ago, filler training focused on procedures. Now, after the occurrence of procedural side effects, more focus is being placed on anatomy. Many would select anatomy as one of the most tedious subjects in medical school. Medical school anatomy courses focused on understanding and memorizing the entire body from a single textbook filled with interminable text and complex terminology. Those who read this book, however, will have access to easy-to-understand illustrations from online journals and reference books. Therefore, the study of anatomy for safe and satisfactory filler procedures becomes simple and interesting. The same subject can be more easily understood by accessing diverse materials like actual anatomical diagrams, illustrations, videos, and medical figures.

The most important subject in filler procedures would be the facial vasculature which is also associated with the most severe complications. Moreover, for nerve blocks, the distribution of nerves must be understood. In addition, it is important to review the fat compartments, muscles, and connective tissues which make up the three dimensional structure of the face.

A thorough knowledge of facial anatomy is absolutely necessary, not only for filler procedures, but also for botulinum toxin and lifting procedures.

1. The Vasculature

••• There is no significant meaning in understanding just the two dimensional route of the facial vasculature. Knowledge of location of the important routes from a two dimensional view without an understanding of vessel depth is insufficient in avoiding vessels. Therefore, a comprehensive, three dimensional understanding of facial vasculature is mandatory. For example, it is important to know at which region the facial artery becomes superficial or at which regions the arteries that supply the forehead penetrate the muscles to course superficially.

1 The Facial Artery & Vein (Fig. 3-1)

- The facial artery branches from the external carotid artery and follows along the anterior border of the masseter muscle and courses to the oral commissure. In this region, the facial artery runs anteriorly to the facial vein.
- As the facial artery travels up from the angle of the mouth, it gives rise to the inferior labial artery.
- Thereafter when passing modiolus (chiasma of muscles around the mouth), the facial artery shows a superficial and tortuous route. It is at the place where the FA(facial artery), zygomaticus and risorius muscles diverges at the modiolus, the in between area of the ant. margin of the buccal fat pad. The facial artery becomes superficial and kinked in the empty space between fat and muscles. Pulsation of the artery can be visualized at times
- Next, as the facial artery courses superiorly, it gives rise to the superior labial artery (approximately 1.5 cm lateral to the mouth)
- As it passes the nasolabial fold, it branches into the lateral nasal artery which in turn gives rise to the angular artery.
- The angular artery, a terminal branch of facial artery, anastomoses with the dorsal nasal artery which is a branch of the internal carotid artery.
- The facial artery always runs anterior to the facial vein.
- The facial artery courses deeper than the upper lip elevator and zygomaticus major muscles. The superior labial artery is deep to the orbicularis oris muscle.

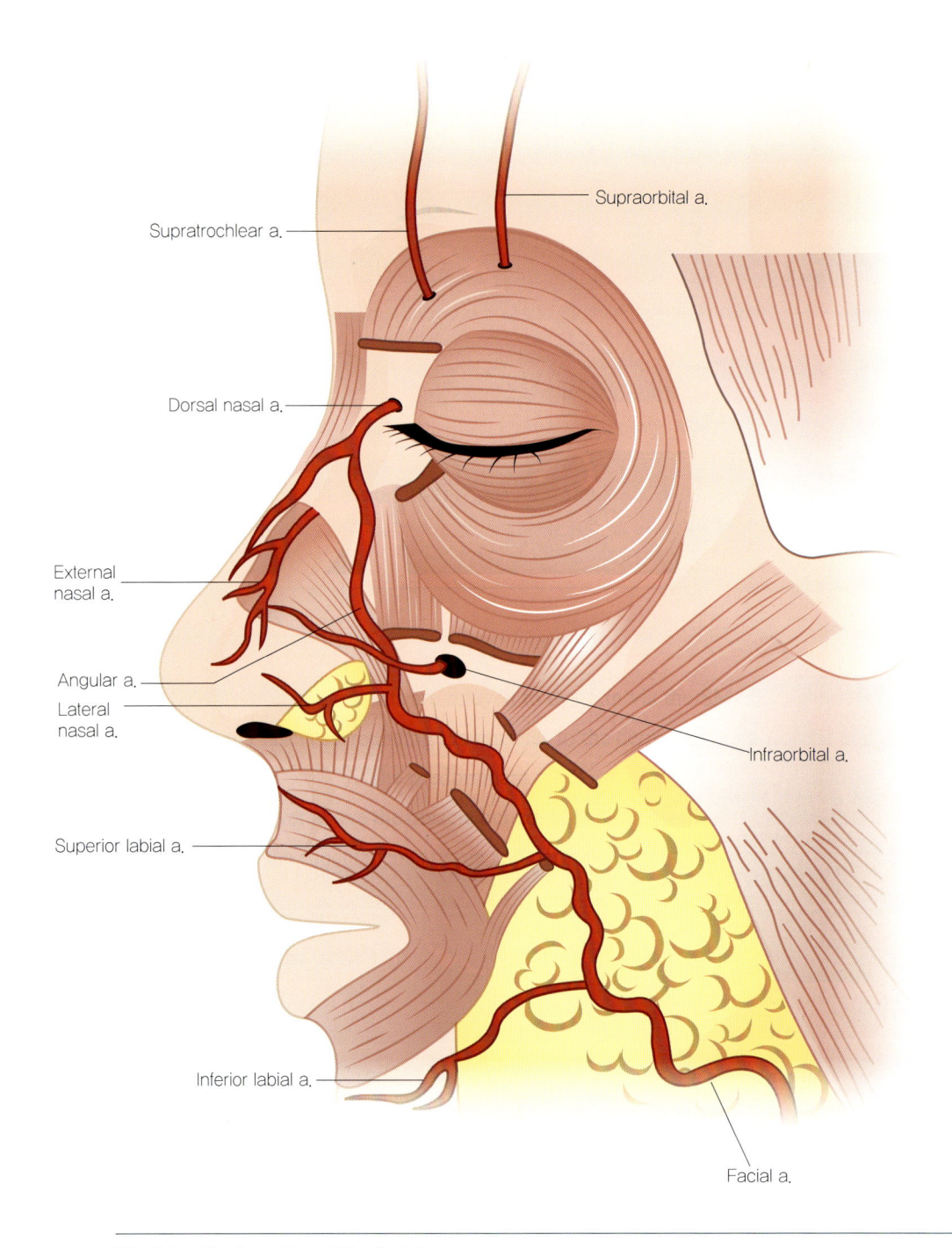

Safe Filler Injection Technique Demonstration – using live imaging tools

Fig. 3-1   The branches of the facial artery

2 Variations in the Facial Artery

Typically the facial artery gives rise to the angular artery which then continues as the dorsal nasal artery. However, in real life, there are many more instances of variations in the facial artery course than instances of the typical case as outlined above. The facial artery may terminate at the angular artery or it may branch into the lateral nasal artery and terminate there. The terminal artery of facial artery exists in many different forms. At times there are two facial arteries. In other cases, the artery courses up to the orbital region along the nasojugal groove (in this deviated pattern, the facial artery generally courses deep to the zygomaticus muscles, is located slightly deeper than the orbicularis oculi muscle. It is not superficial and courses along the nasojugal groove).

3 The Supratrochlear Artery (STA) & Supraorbital Artery (SOA)

The supratrochlear artery traverses a deep layer after exiting the supratrochlear foramen or notch, and then, after penetrating the corrugator muscle, it courses superficially.

The supraorbital artery traverses a deep layer after exiting the supraorbital foramen. After the supraorbital artery penetrates the corrugator muscle, it penetrates the frontalis muscle and then courses superficially. Compared to the supraorbital artery, the supratrochlear artery becomes superficial at an earlier point. (Fig. 3-2 and Fig. 4-8, 9)

4 Superficial Temporal Artery (SfTA)

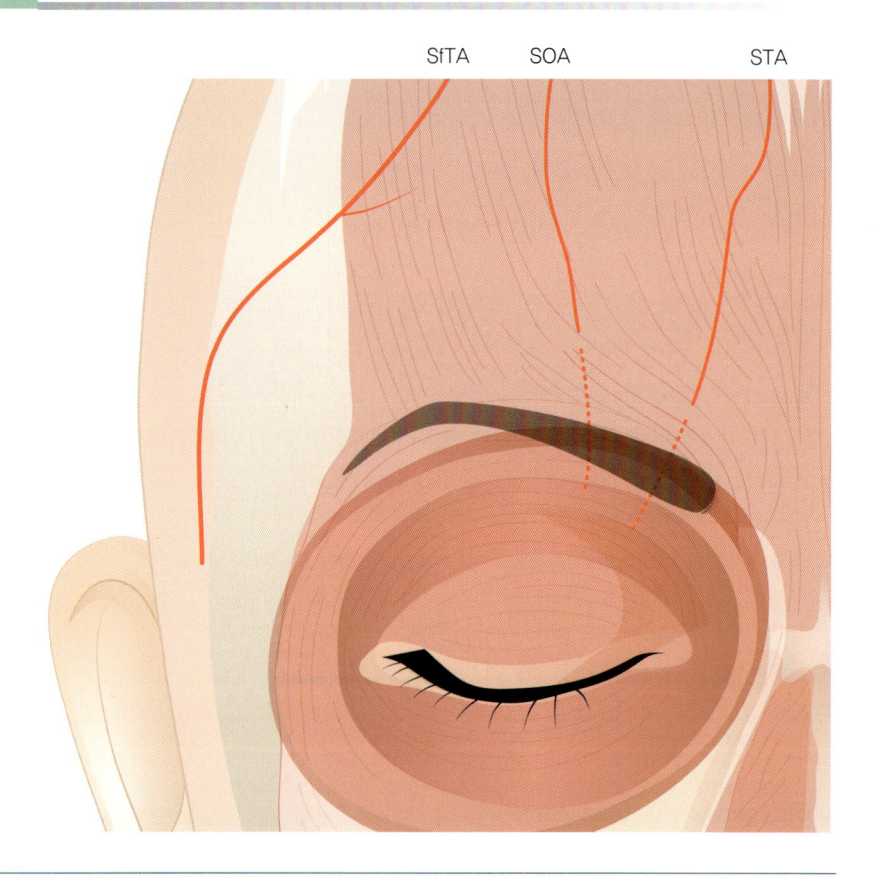

Fig. 3-2 Arteries of the forehead. STA: supratrochlear artery, SOA: supraorbital artery, SfTA: superficial temporal artery

Table 3-1   Branches of the facial artery

Branch	Origin	Course	Comments	Supplies
Inferior labial	Inferior to oral commissure	Deep to the DAO	In between the orbicularis oris muscle and mucosa	Glands of the lower lips, muscle, skin, mucosa
Superior labial	Superior to inferior labial artery	Along the upper lip margin	Gives rise to septal branch and alar branch	Glands of the upper lips, muscle, skin, mucosa, nasal septum, and alar
Lateral nasal	Proximal to superior alar groove	Medially across nose	Gives rise to alar branch	Skin of nasal alar, soft triangle, dorsum, tip
Angular	After lateral nasal artery branch	Along the side of the nose, up to the medial canthus	Anastomoses with dorsal nasal artery	Skin of cheeks, upper lip elevators, orbicularis oris muscle, nasal side wall

5 The External Carotid Artery & Internal Carotid Artery

If the filler is inadvertently injected into an artery during a filler procedure, this may cause dermal necrosis due to occlusion and worse, may lead to blindness. This complication arises because the angular artery, a branch of the facial artery, is connected to the internal carotid artery through the dorsal nasal artery. Through these anastomoses, the filler material can flow to the central retinal artery, a branch of the internal carotid artery. A potentially fatal case occurs when the material occludes a cerebral artery and causes a cerebral infarct.

The supratrochlear artery and supraorbital artery which supplies the forehead are terminal branches of the internal carotid artery. If the injection pressure is stronger than the normal blood flow, the filler material that has been accidentally injected into any one of these arteries may flow in a retrograde manner to cause blindness.

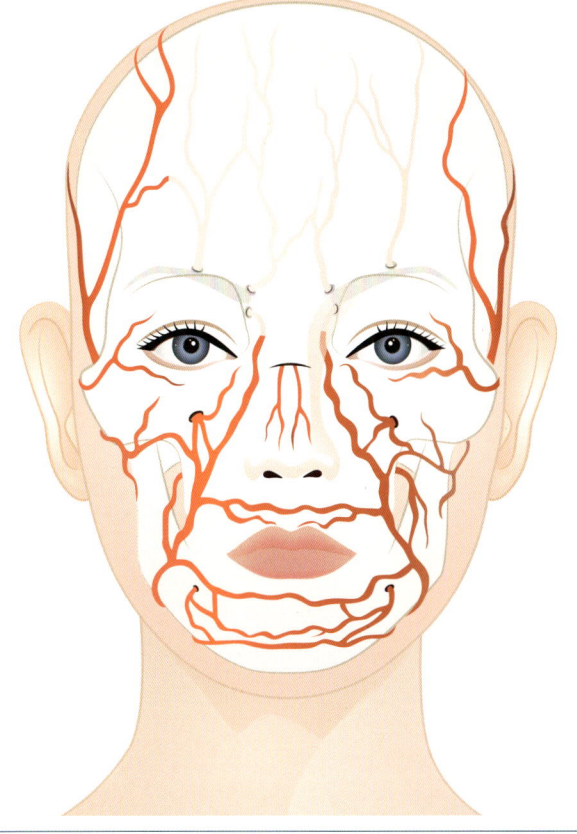

Fig. 3-3 **Anastomoses of the external carotid artery (red color) & internal carotid artery (apricot color)**

Safe Filler Injection Technique Demonstration – using live imaging tools

6 Palpation of the Artery

To avoid arterial injury when performing procedures in the orbital region, the artery should be inspected and palpated. In addition, the route of the facial artery can be determined to a certain extent by palpation. This serves as a useful guide in deciding the puncture point and entry route while treating the nasolabial folds. Occasionally, the pulsation of the facial artery can be seen.

Table 3-2 Danger zone and arterial pulses of the face

Artery	Palpation of pulse
Facial artery	When clenching the jaw firmly, pulse can be palpated at the anteroinferior border of masseter muscle
Facial artery	Palpated at one fingerbreadth lateral to the corner of the mouth
Angular artery	Palpated where the artery ascends from the side of the nose to the medial canthus
Superficial temporal artey	Palpated in front of the tragus at the superior border of the zygomatic process

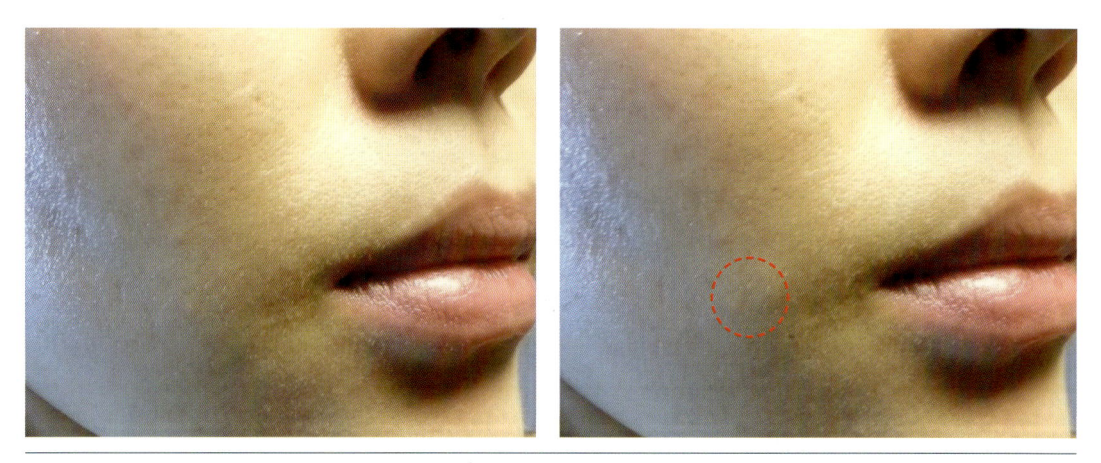

Fig. 3-4 In this case the facial artery pulse is seen without palpation. Lt: diastolic, Rt: systolic

7 Visual Inspection of Veins

Veins and arteries may get damaged during facial procedures due to the retrograde/anterograde movement of the needle or cannula within the injection layer. However, blood vessel injuries are made more commonly at the beginning of the procedure while making an entry point. As the skin is punctured, a vessel is also punctured, resulting in bleeding.

The regions of the face where the veins are most visible are the temples and forehead. Blood vessels in these areas are visible like the veins in most arms. They are more easily visualized in thinner people, while lying down, or under a light. Devices such as AccuVein (See No Bleeding Technique in Part 2) allow injectors to visualize the veins and their pathways in real time.

Confirming the routes of veins prior to procedures on the forehead and temples helps prevent bleeding during the procedure.

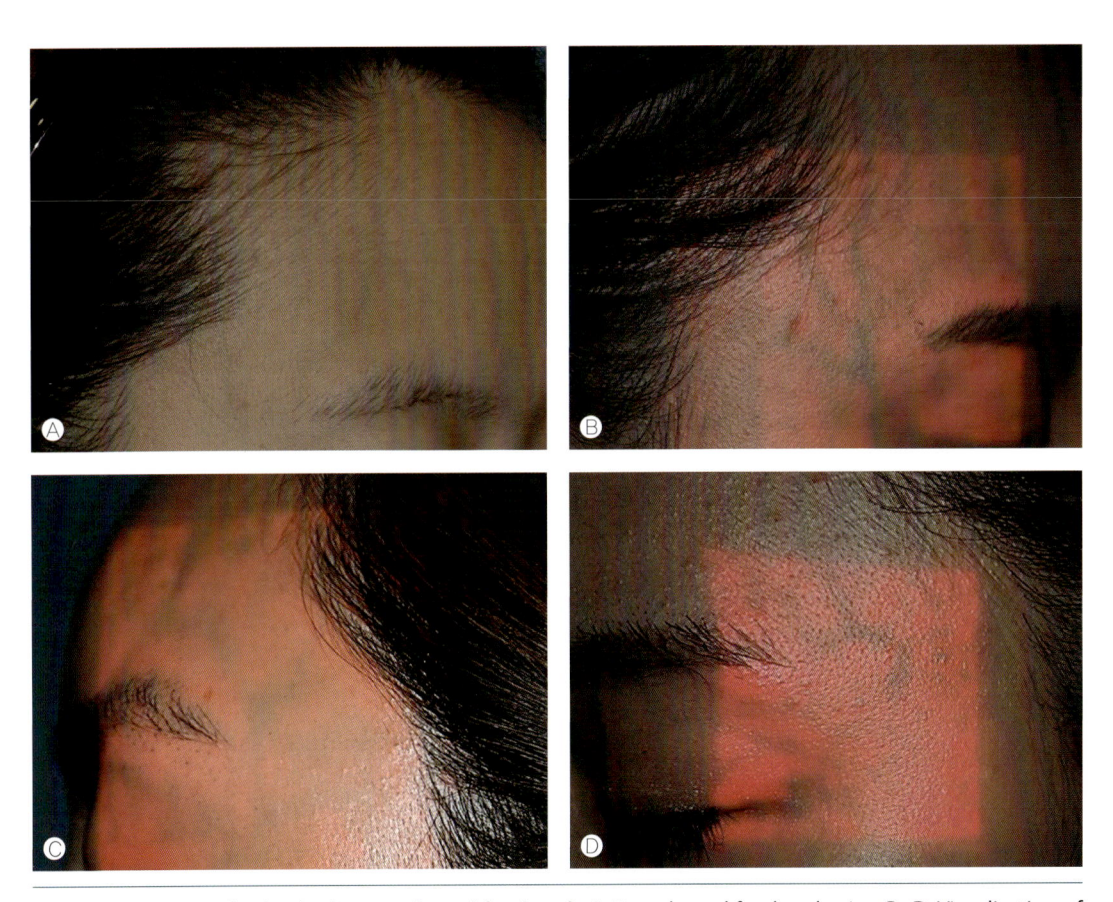

Fig. 3-5 **Pictures of veins in the temple and forehead.** A. Temple and forehead veins. **B~D.** Visualization of temporal and forehead veins using AccuVein

2. Nerves

••• From the 12 cranial nerves, the nerves that are important for filler procedures are cranial nerves V and VII.

1 CN V (Trigeminal Nerve) - Sensory

This is the nerve that is responsible for sensation in the face. CN V is divided into three branches, the ophthalmic division, (V_1), maxillary division (V_2), and mandibular division (V_3). The area that each division is responsible for (Fig. 3-6) and the distribution of the branches (Fig. 3-7) can be seen in the pictures below:

Ophthalmic division (V_1)

Maxillary division (V_2)

Mandibular division (V_3)

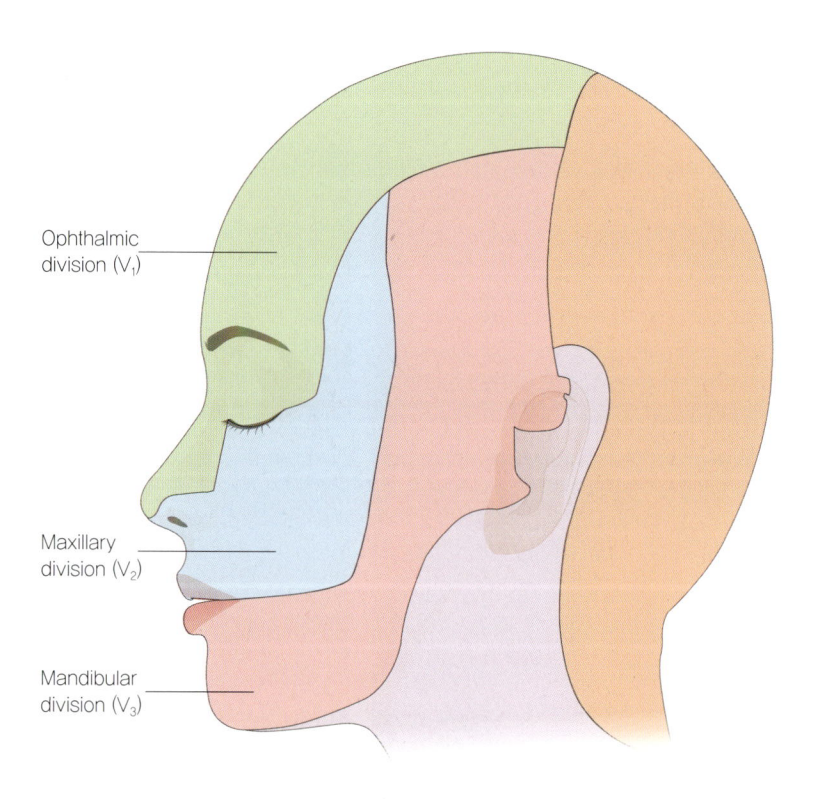

Fig. 3-6   Dermatome distribution of the trigeminal nerve

Supraorbital n.
Supratrochlear n.
Infratrochlear n.
ext. nasal branch of Ant. ethmoidal n.
Zygomaticotemporal n.
Zygomaticofacial n.
Infraorbital n.
Auriculotemporal n.
Buccal n.
Mental n.

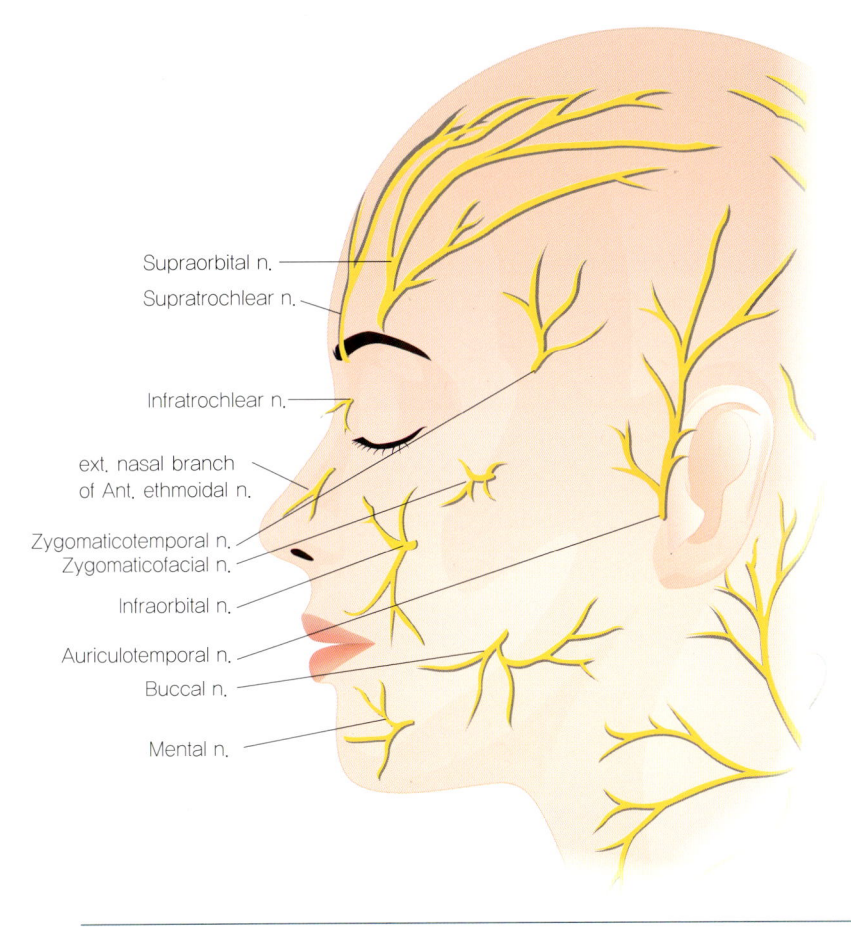

Fig. 3-7 **Branches of the trigeminal nerve**

There are times in which, in addition to applying topical anesthetic ointment, nerve blocks like lidocaine become necessary. A mild injury to the sensory nerve during needle procedures may lead to neuropraxia, which results in paresthesia and pain that lasts for a month or longer. These injuries are difficult to treat and although they may resolve spontaneously, NSAIDs are known to help.

The nerves that could be blocked with the filler procedures	• Forehead: Supratrochlear/supraorbital nerve • Temples: Zygomaticotemporal nerve • Nose: Ant. ethmoidal nerve, ext. nasal branch • Nasolabial folds: Infra orbital nerve • Retrognathism: Mental nerve

Safe Filler Injection Technique Demonstration – using live imaging tools

2 CN VII (Facial Nerve) - Motor

As open surgeries such as rhytidectomies are associated with a risk of injuring the facial motor nerves, extreme caution is required. However this risk is a lot smaller in filler procedures. In the process of administering a nerve block, a motor nerve may be affected resulting in a temporary impairment in motor function. However, in most cases motor function returns within 1~2 hours.

5 branches of the facial nerve
- Temporal branch (Frontal branch)
- Zygomatic branch
- Buccal branch
- Marginal mandibular branch
- Cervical branch

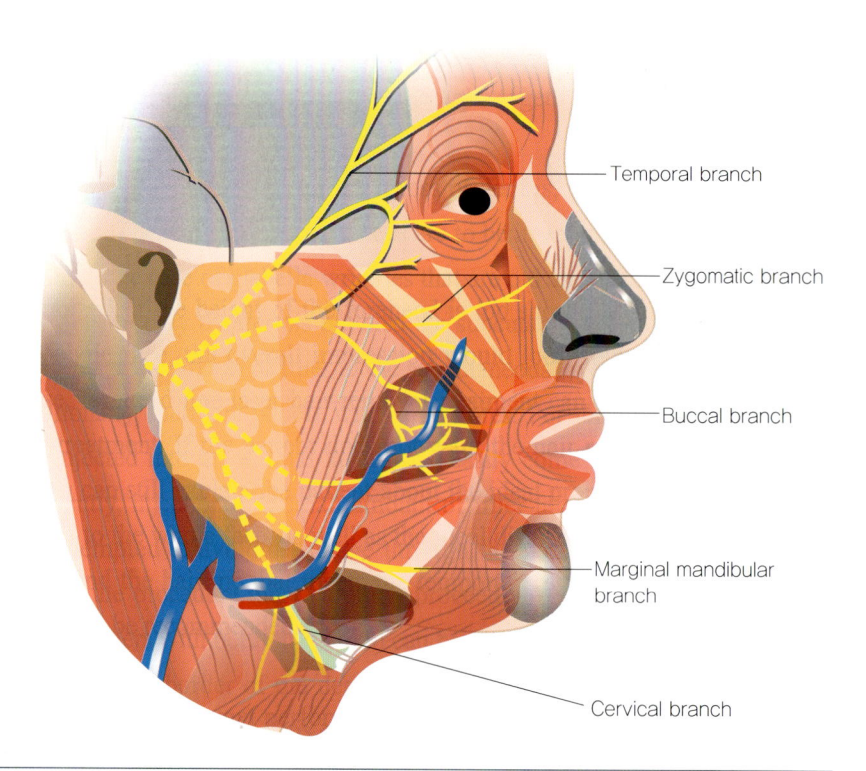

Fig. 3-8 5 branches of the facial nerve

Table 3-3 Motor innervation of head & neck

Branch of Facial Nerve	Muscle
Temporal branch	Frontalis
	Corrugator supercilii
	Temporoparietalis
	Orbicularis oculi (upper)
Zygomatic branch	Orbicularis oculi (lower)
	Procerus
	Nasalis (ala area)
	Buccinator
Buccal branch	Buccinator
	Depressor septi
	Nasalis (transverse)
	Zygomaticus major/minor
	Levator labii superioris
	Levator anguli oris
	Orbicularis oris (upper)
Marginal mandibular branch	Depressor anguli oris
	Depressor labii inferioris
	Risorius
	Mentalis
	Platysma (upper)
Cervical branch	Platysma (lower)

3. Fat Compartments

● ● ●   In the past, facial aging was attributed to decreased skin elasticity. Recently more focus is being placed on changes in fat volume and bone loss. The rates at which the fat compartments atrophy differ by region. The facial fat compartments are divided into superficial fat and deep fat. Fat compartments above the muscle or the SMAS layer are categorized as superficial fat and the fat compartments below, the deep fat.

1 Superficial Fat

The superficial fat compartments are related to the sagging caused by aging (Fig. 3-9). When injecting fillers into these compartments, it is recommended that only a small amount is injected. If a large amount is injected, the sagging may worsen. Superficial fat is divided into many fat compartments, as demonstrated by Pessa and Rohrich through cadaver dissections and dye staining technique(Fig. 3-10). The compartments are separated by either septae or retaining ligaments.

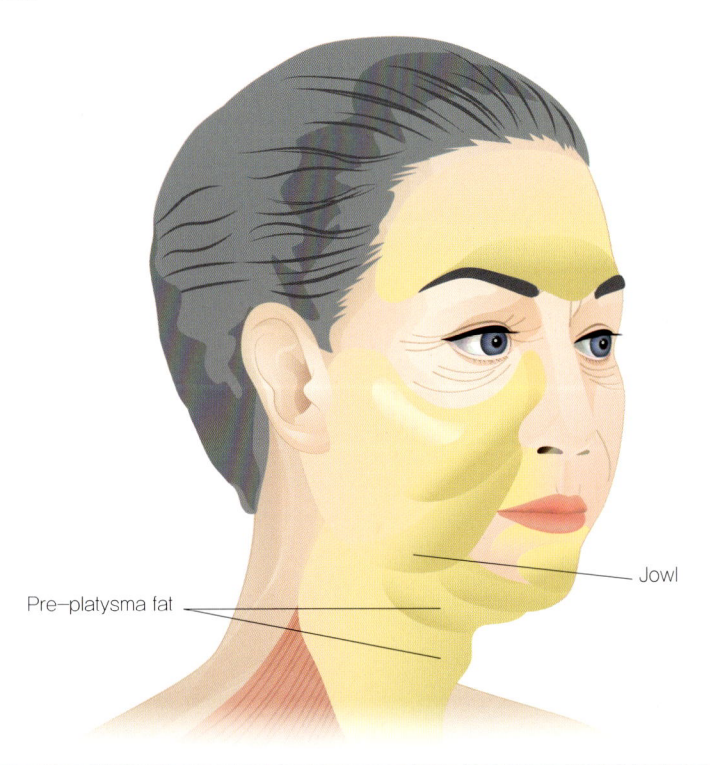

Fig. 3-9 Superficial fat

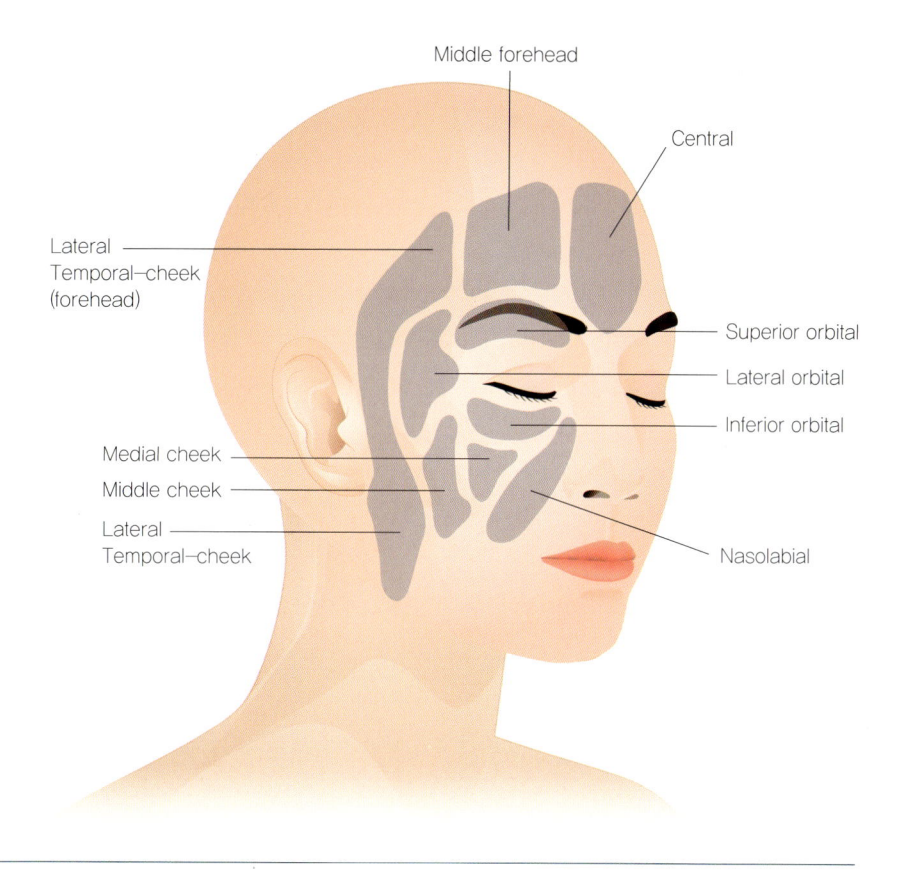

Fig. 3-10　**Superficial fat compartments**

2　Deep Fat

Fat atrophy occurs more markedly in the deep fat than in the superficial fat. Therefore, for volumizing purposes, it is more effective to inject into the deep fat. Also the deep fat is a safer layer to inject as there are fewer blood vessels here than in the superficial fat.

4. Muscles

●●● During filler procedures, injury to the facial muscles is extremely rare. Muscles divide superficial fat and deep fat and, in some areas, key blood vessels pass below the muscles. As such, it is important to know the location of muscles in relation to other structures such as blood vessels and fat. Moreover, appearance of scars can be reduced by making incisions parallel to the direction of the skin tension line (STL), which is the wrinkle created according to the movements of facial muscles. If you know the precise location of muscles, adverse effects associated with botulinum toxin procedures can also be avoided.

Facial muscles are thinner and flatter compared to muscles in other parts of the body. They have elevator and depressor functions with respect to the eyebrows and lips. They also have dilator and sphincteric functions with respect to the eyes and mouth (opening), which allow the formation of facial expressions. Combined use of fillers and botulinum toxin in the treatment of folds/skin creases with the knowledge of the muscle/s responsible for the formation of specific dynamic wrinkles will result in synergistic treatment effects.

1 Muscles around the Eyes

These include the frontalis, corrugator supercilii, depressor supercilii, procerus, and orbicularis oculi muscles.

2 Muscles around the Mouth

These include the zygomaticus major & minor, levator labii superioris (LLS), levator labii superioris alaeque nasi (LLSAN), risorius, orbicularis oris, depressor anguli oris (DAO), depressor labii inferioris (DLI), and mentalis muscles.

3 Muscles of the Nose

These include the compressor naris, dilator naris and depressor septi muscles.

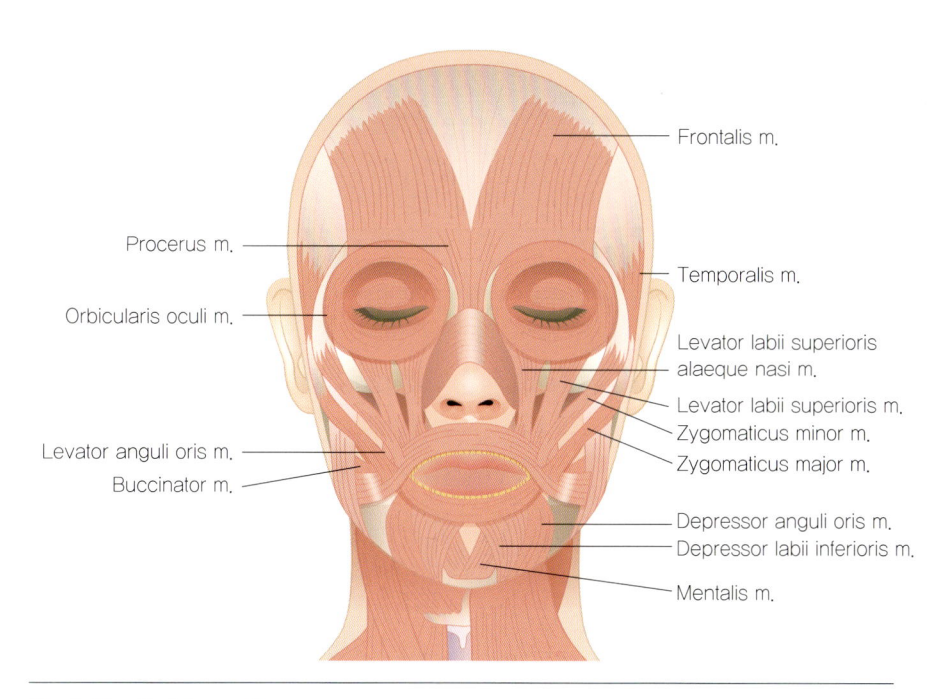

Fig. 3-11 Facial muscles

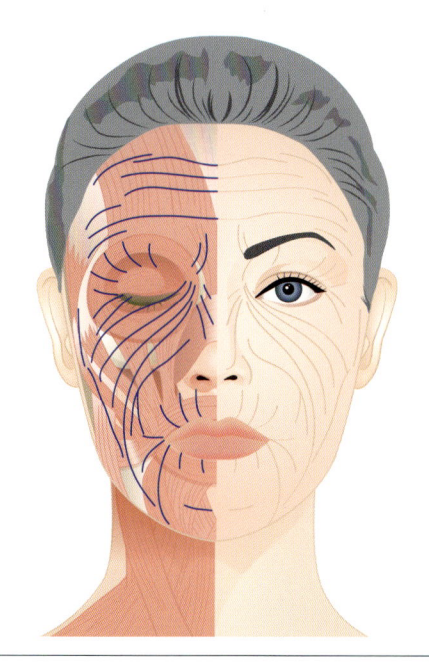

Fig. 3-12 Skin tension lines (STLs) & Muscles

5. The SMAS & Retaining Ligaments

● ● ●   The SMAS and retaining ligaments play a large role in facial sagging associated with aging. If the SMAS is a small pillar (small branch) that supports facial tissue, the retaining ligaments are analogous to large pillars.

It can be said that the most important structure in filler procedures is the facial vasculature. On the other hand, the SMAS and retaining ligaments are the most important structures for surgical and minimally invasive lifting procedures. However, these structures are important in filler procedures as well. Unlike in other regions, when trying to pass the needle or cannula through these structures, resistance will be felt. Hence a general understanding of the location and functions of the SMAS and retaining ligaments is necessary.

1 The SMAS (Superficial Musculo-Aponeurotic System)

The SMAS was first defined by Mitz and Pevronie in 1976. Since then, the scope of its meaning has expanded, but has not yet been completely established.

In a broad sense, the SMAS can be understood as the layers of tissue that envelop the facial muscles. It is well developed from the forehead to the occiput, temples, and lateral cheeks but not as well developed in the medial region of the midface (Table 3-4).

In a narrower sense, the SMAS, refers only to a system in the lower and mid face. In this definition the system is connected in a single plane spanning through the neck (platysma), face (SMAS), temporal area (temporo-parietal fascia), and forehead (galea aponeurotica).

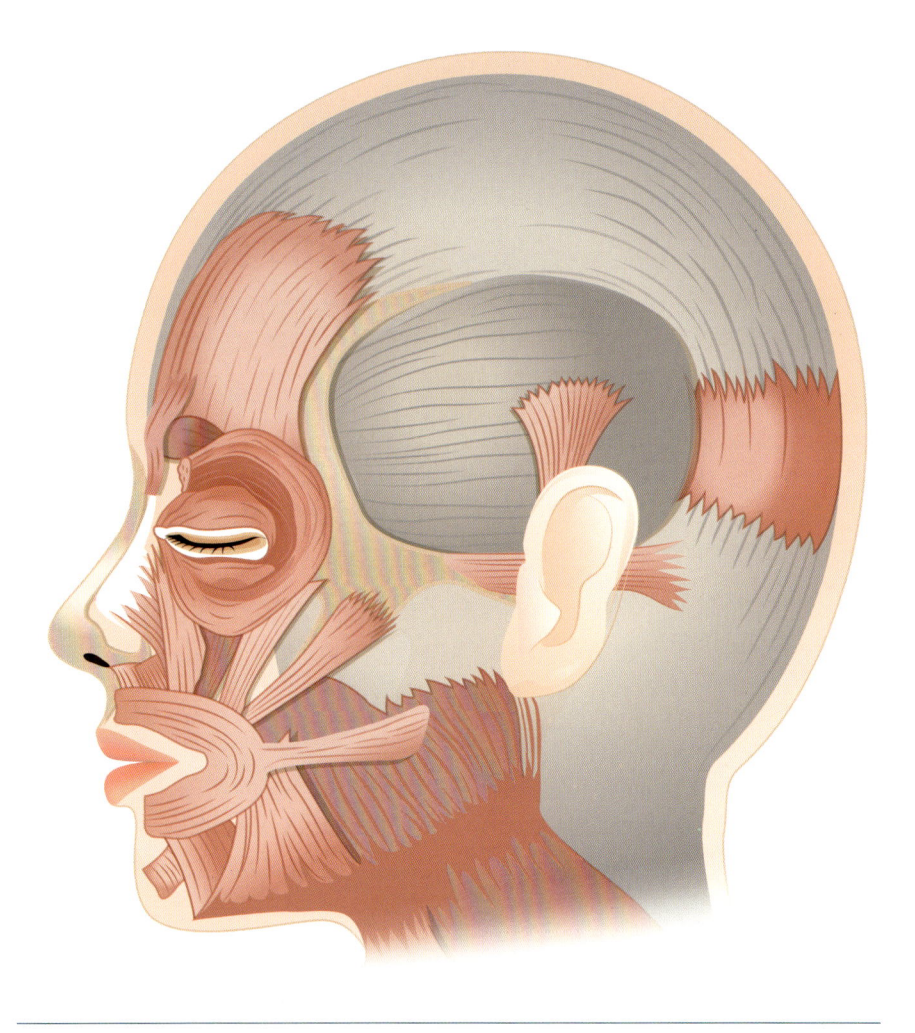

Fig. 3-13   Facial Muscles & Aponeurosis

Table 3-4   SMAS attachment by facial region

Region	SMAS attachment site
Posterior (occiput)	Inserts into the mastoid process and SCM. Envelops occipitalis m.
Superior (scalp)	Forms galea aponeurotica and connects to occipitofrontalis m. Almost no muscle fiber.
Forehead	Envelops frontalis m.
Temporal scalp	Continuous with superficial temporal fascia
Zygomatic arch	SMAS is not connected below or above this region. Muscles below and above serve different functions.
Cheek	Part of the deep SMAS meets the parotid/masseteric fascia
Anterior (neck)	Connects to the superficial cervical fascia. Envelopes the platysma m.
Midfacial region	Not developed

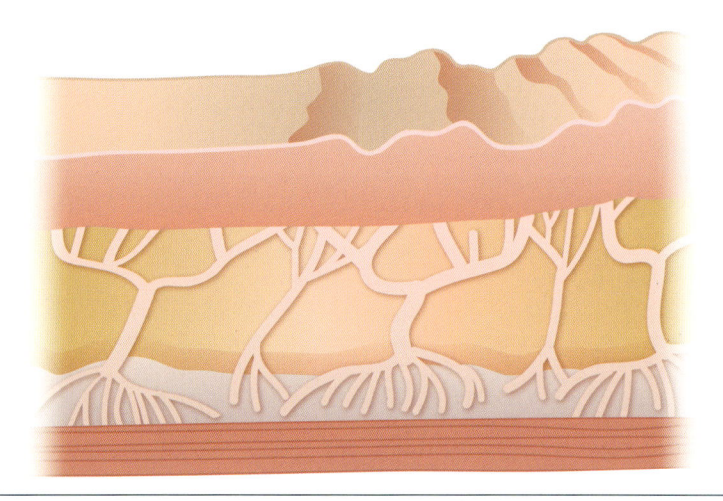

Fig. 3-14　Three dimensional structure of the SMAS

The muscle movements are relayed to the skin via the SMAS. It connects the superficial fascia surrounding the muscles to the dermis through fibrotic connective tissue (Fig. 3-14). The predominant view is that the SMAS does not consist as a single layer above the muscle but consists as a unit of many branches spread throughout the subcutaneous tissue and dermis.

2　The Retaining Ligaments

The retaining ligaments, which can be thought of as large pillars that support soft tissue, are divided into two types depending on the function.

1) True Retaining Ligaments

- These ligaments originate from the bone and insert into the dermal layer. They also have a strong bearing power.
- These structures are more easily confirmed.
- The retaining ligaments include; the orbital ligament, zygomatic ligament, maxillary ligament, and mandibular retaining ligament.
- Zygomatic ligament (McGregor's patch)
  : Originates from inferior border of the zygomatic arch, posterior to the origin of the zygomaticus minor muscle, and inserts into the dermis.
- Lateral orbital thickening
  : Orbital retaining ligament is thicker in the superolateral portion of the orbital rim.
- Mandibular ligament
  : Originates from the mandible bone connecting to the origin of the depressor anguli oris muscle before inserting into the dermis.

2) False Retaining Ligaments

- The false retaining ligaments insert into the superficial/deep fascia of muscles and do not have a strong bearing power.
- They are diffuse condensations of fibrous tissue.
- More susceptible to the effects of gravity. More prone to stretch and sagging.
- Platysma-auricular ligament and masseteric-cutaneous ligament coincide with the areas that sag the most in the face, as seen in Fig. 3-15.
- Masseteric-cutaneous ligament
  : Originates from the anterior border of the masseter muscle through SMAS and inserts into the skin of the cheek. Thins gradually with aging and sags, resulting jowl formation.
- Platysma-auricular ligament
  : Located at the border of the area below the earlobe and lateral temporal-cheek fat compartment

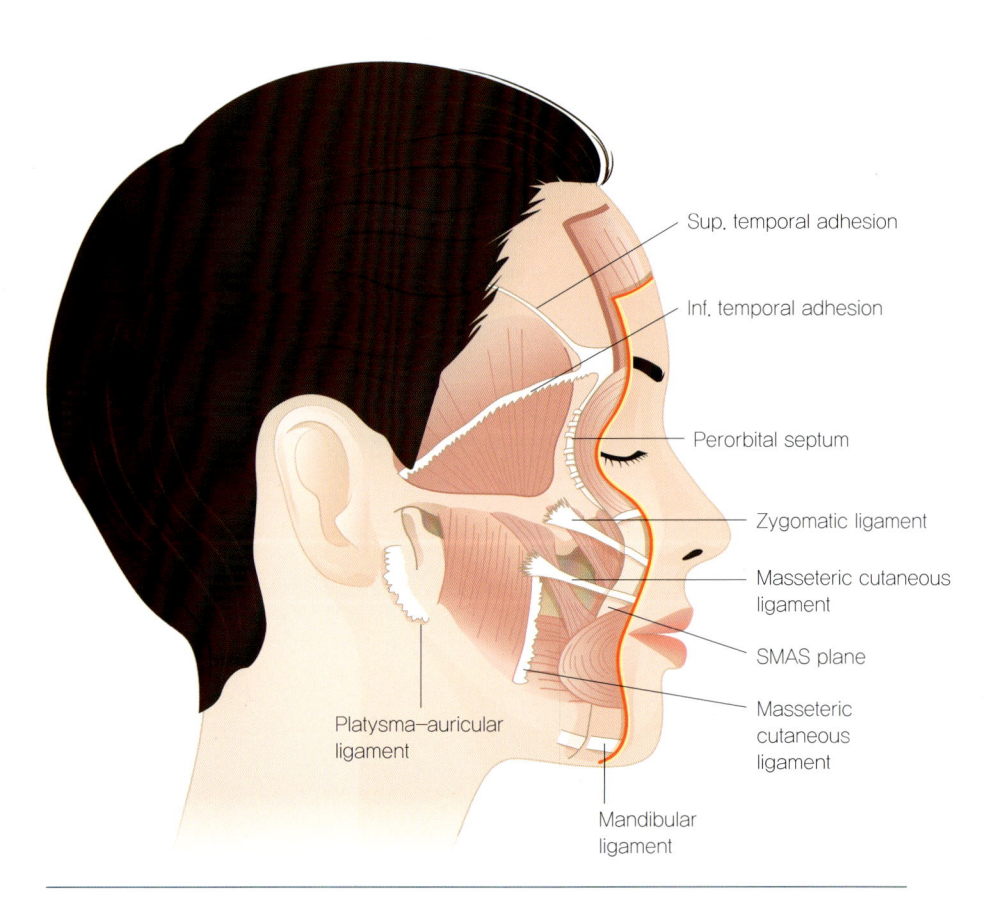

Fig. 3-15 **Retaining ligaments of the face**

Safe Filler Injection Technique Demonstration
– using live imaging tools

Part
4

Filler Treatment
for Each Facial Area

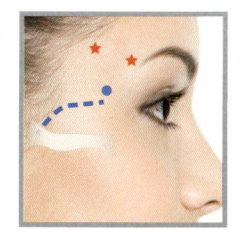

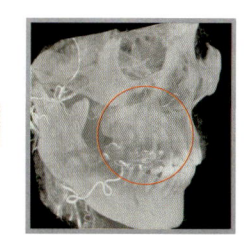

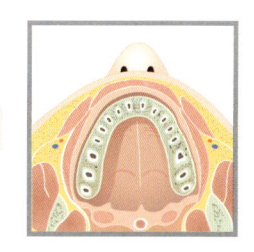

Safe Filler Injection Technique Demonstration
- using live imaging tools

Part 4: Filler Treatment for Each Facial Area

Upper Face

1. Forehead
2. Glabella
3. Temples

Mid Face

4. Nose
5. Nasolabial Folds
6. Cheek (Upper Cheek and Lower Cheek)
7. Dark Circles
8. Lower Eyelid Pretarsal Augmentation
9. Sunken Eyes

Lower Face

10. Chin
11. Marionette Line
12. Lips

Part 4

Filler Treatment for Each Facial Area

Upper Face

1. Forehead

1 Beauty

Determinants of beautiful forehead »
1. Height of the Forehead & Hairline
2. Convexity of the Forehead

The determinants of beautiful forehead is summarized as above.

Firstly, the ideal length of the forehead is 1/3 of the vertical length of the entire face (Fig. 4-1). Even if a forehead with a dent or hollow region is sufficient-

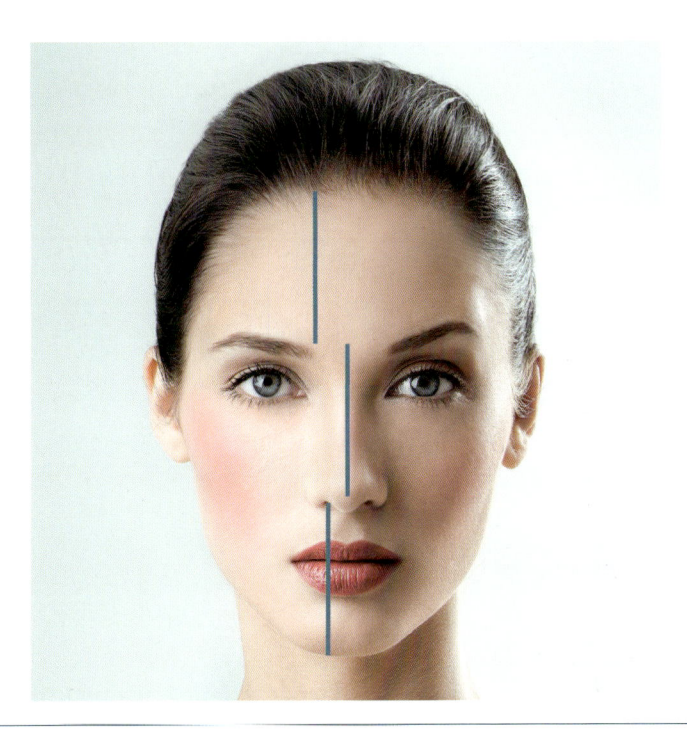

Fig. 4-1 **Ideal ratio of the face.** One third of the vertical length

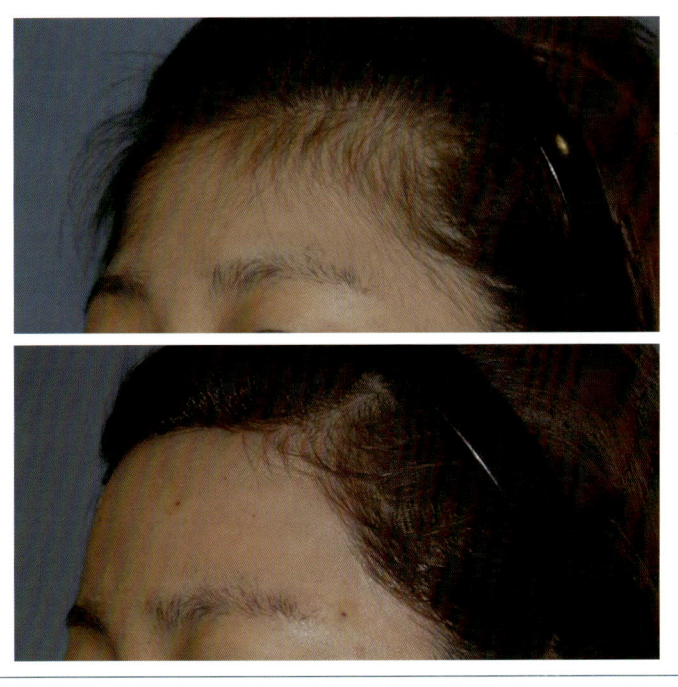

Fig. 4-2 **Change of hairline** (Top: before, bottom: after hair removal and filler procedures)

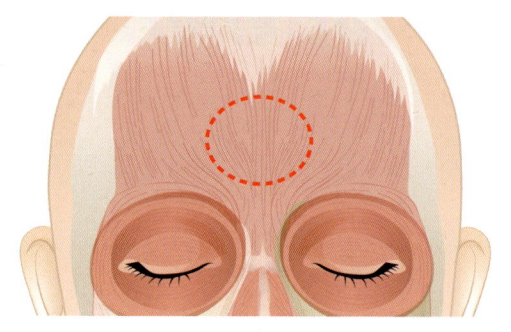

Type I Central concavity (depression at the center)

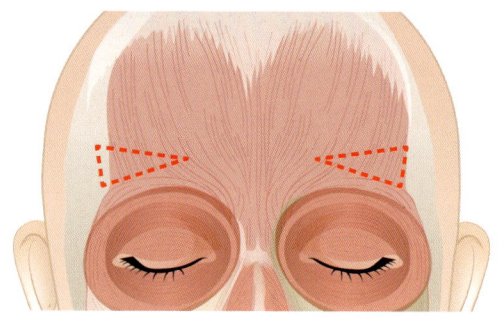

Type II Bilateral concavity (depression at the sides)

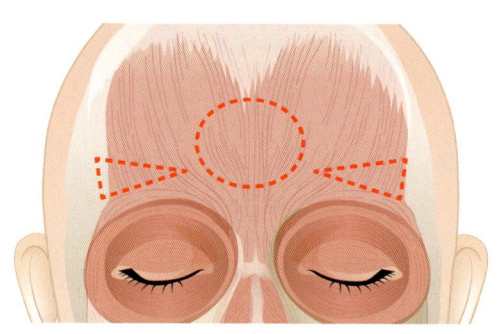

Type III Mixed type (Combination type)

Fig. 4-3   Forehead shape classification depending on the location of depression - illustrations

ly volumized, if the height of the forehead is too short compared to the length of the whole face, the overall impression would look somewhat cramped. In this case, forehead line laser hair-removal treatment can be recommended pre- or post-treatment. If the patient does not want the hair removal-treatment, the physician can still explain the patient about the ideal proportion of the forehead compared to the whole face, as well as the ideal distance between the end of the eyebrow and the hairline that meets the temporal crest. Trimming of the baby hair can also be recommended.

The authors of this text perform shaving using an electric razor prior to the hair removal procedure, and most of the time, they find patients satisfied with their treatment results with their new hairline after the procedure. (Fig. 4-2)

Type I Central concavity (depression at the center)

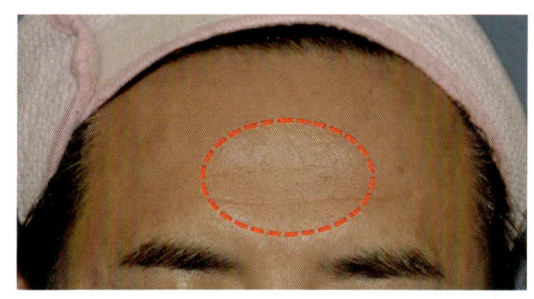

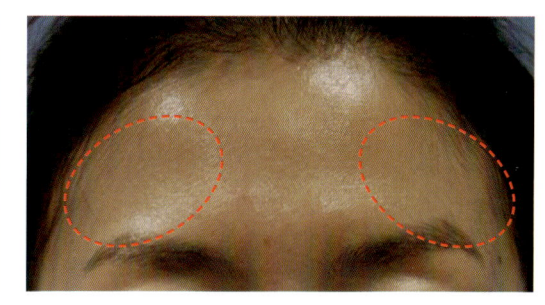

Type II Bilateral concavity (depression at the sides)

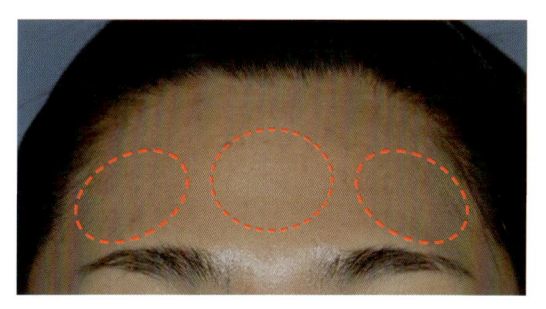

Type III Mixed type (Combination type)

Fig. 4-4 Forehead shape classification depending on the location of depression - Figures

Furthermore, with respect to convexity of the forehead, it is ideal to have the entire area nicely padded without any sunken regions, however, the patient's preferences on the desired volume and the desired location of improvement must be confirmed prior to the procedure. The sinking of the forehead is classified into three types depending on the location and degree as seen in Fig. 4-3 and 4-4. Entry points differ in each case when performing the procedures. Type I is the most common area for procedures that appears in both men and women. In order to have the forehead that shines when looked at directly from the front, there should not be any hollow regions present in the center. In the case of young adults, an ideal forehead can be made simply by replenishing the sunken areas. However, in the case of elderly people, where layers of thick wrinkles are present, it is almost impossible to create an ideal beautiful forehead only by volumization.

For this situation, treatment for fine wrinkles must be accompanied effectively. A combination of fillers, which are small in particle size and easily spreadable, and botulinum toxin that represses excessive movements of the frontalis muscle must be used together to bring out the best result. Here, it is important to remember that, for those who uses the forehead to open the eyes due to ptosis, caution must be taken not to cause sagging of the eyebrows after the botulinum toxin treatment.

In regards to convexity at large, an S-line view from the side as well as the overall convexity from a 45 degree angle are very important for creating a beautiful forehead. This is the reason why it is necessary to adjust the sunken areas near the temples as previously mentioned in the forehead shape classification type II.

If the shape of the forehead is dissatisfied, hairstyles such as those exposing the forehead or up-dos tend to be avoided trying to hide the forehead. Then, the hidden forehead makes the face look wider due to the increased width-to-length ratio of the visible face, only showing the area from the chin to the eyebrows. For patients who come to consult about their forehead, it is helpful to explain these concepts. Use figures to show that, the entire face will look slimmer and more radiant after the procedure. Even for patients who come for other procedures, a simple patient analysis regarding their forehead could encourage them to revisit for forehead filler procedures later.

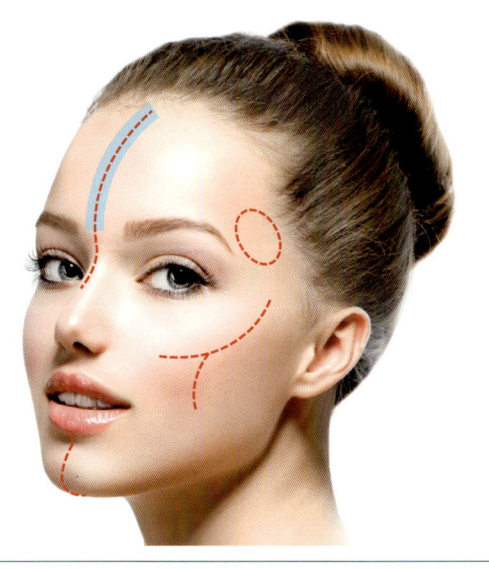

Fig. 4-5 The forehead is to be nicely filled without any hollowness and to have convex curve from the side view.

2 Anatomy

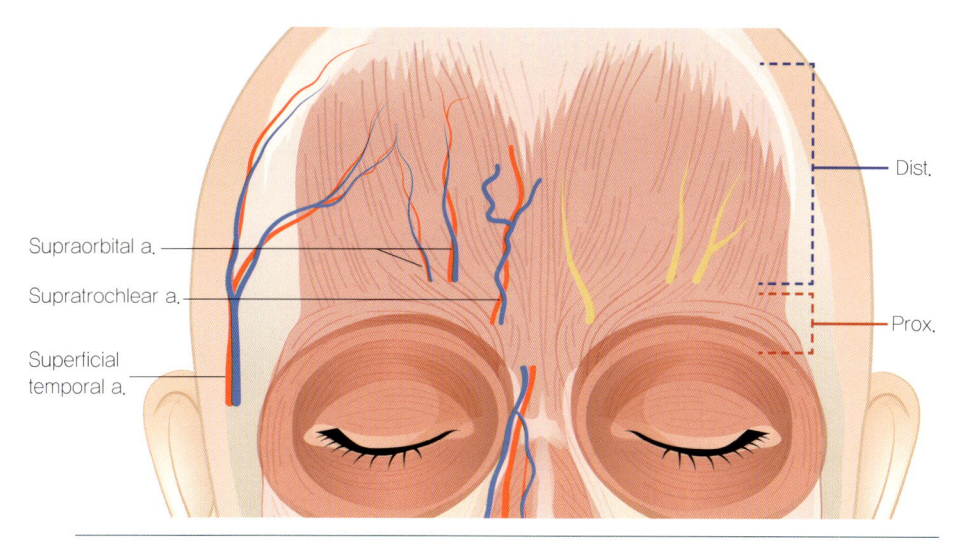

Fig. 4-6 Blood vessels in the forehead -Supratrochlear artery (STA) & supraorbital artery (SOA). Depth of the frontal vessel (based on the eyebrow), proximal: deep, distal: superficial

Supraorbital a.
Supratrochlear a.
Superficial temporal a.
Dist.
Prox.

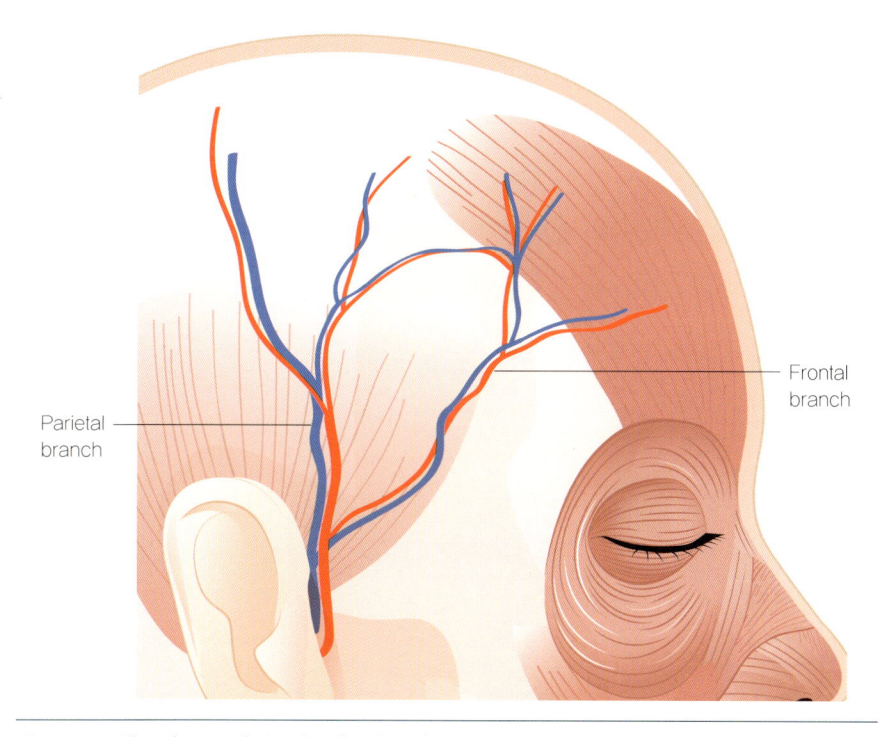

Fig. 4-7 Blood vessels in the forehead-Superficial temporal artery (SfTA). Begins approximately 3 cm from the end of the eyebrows. Frontal branch of the SfTA.

Parietal branch
Frontal branch

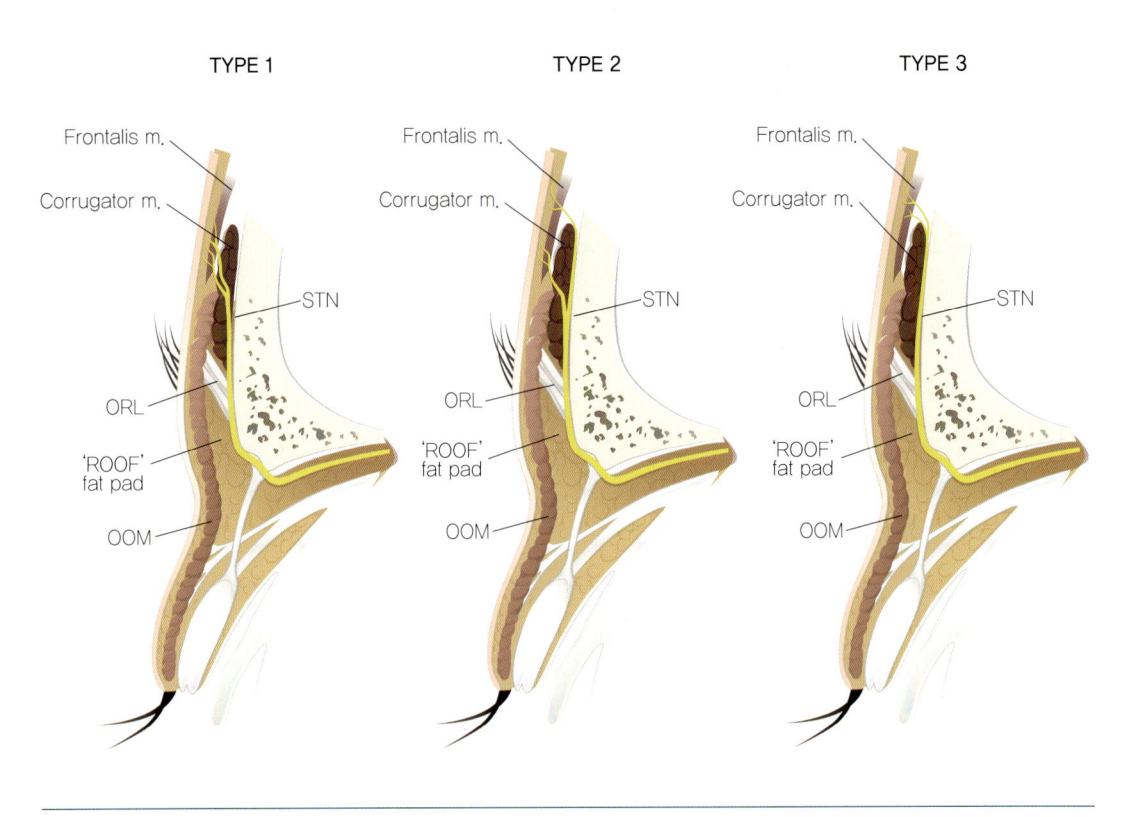

Safe Filler Injection Technique Demonstration – using live imaging tools

Fig. 4-8 Cross section of nerves in the forehead (Supratrochlear nerve).
STN: Supratrochlear Nerve, ORL: Orbital Retaining Ligament, OOM: Orbicularis Oculi Muscle
ROOF: Retro- Orbicularis Oculi Fat

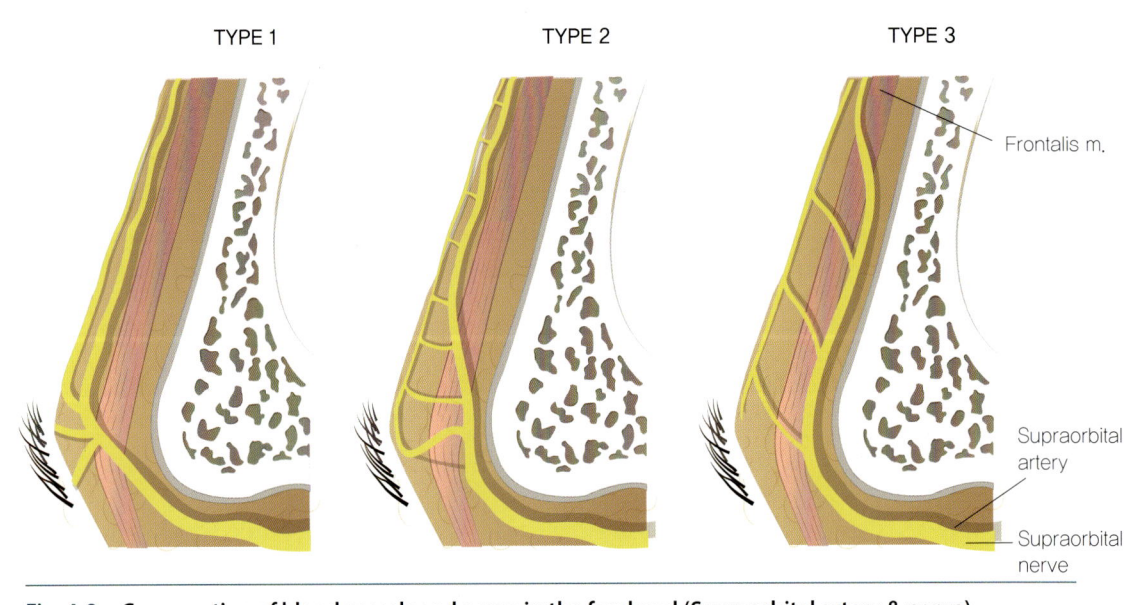

Fig. 4-9 Cross section of blood vessels and nerve in the forehead (Supraorbital artery & nerve)

The supratrochlear artery coming out of the supratrochlear foramen embeds itself into the deep layer, and then once it reaches and penetrates the corrugator m., it becomes superficial.

Likewise, the supraorbital artery coming out of the supraorbital foramen embeds itself into the deep layer. It penetrates and passes through the corrugator m., or penetrates the frontalis m. after passing the corrugator m., and then becomes superficial. The supraorbital artery produces more branches than the supratrochlear artery. (Fig. 4-6, 8 and 9)

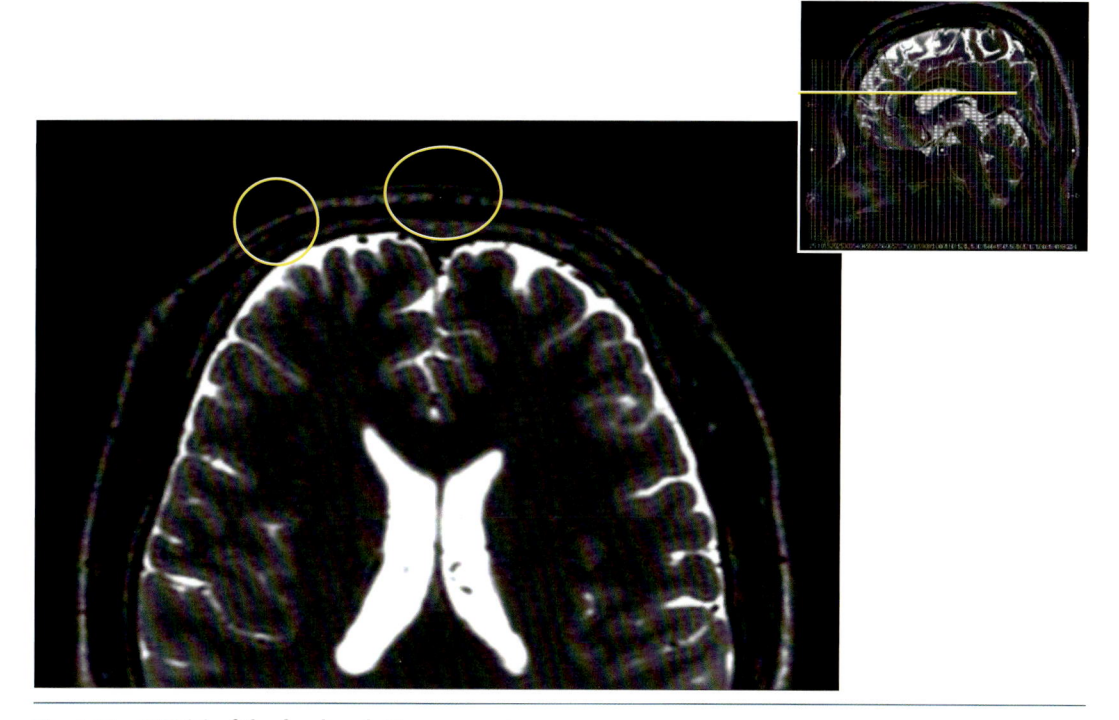

Fig. 4-10 **MRI (1) of the forehead** - Transverse view

- The MRI transverse view shows sunken areas (yellow circle) at the top of the forehead.
- When the inside of the left circle on the MRI T2W image is observed closely, we notice two fat layers showing relatively high signals. The outer (superficial) layer is subcutaneous fat and the inner (deep) layer is the fat above the periosteum. In between these is the frontalis m. By looking into the central area (the circle in the center), it can be seen that many blood vessels pass through the subcutaneous fat layer. These images show in the region superior to the corrugator m. it is safe to inject fillers deep to the frontalis m.

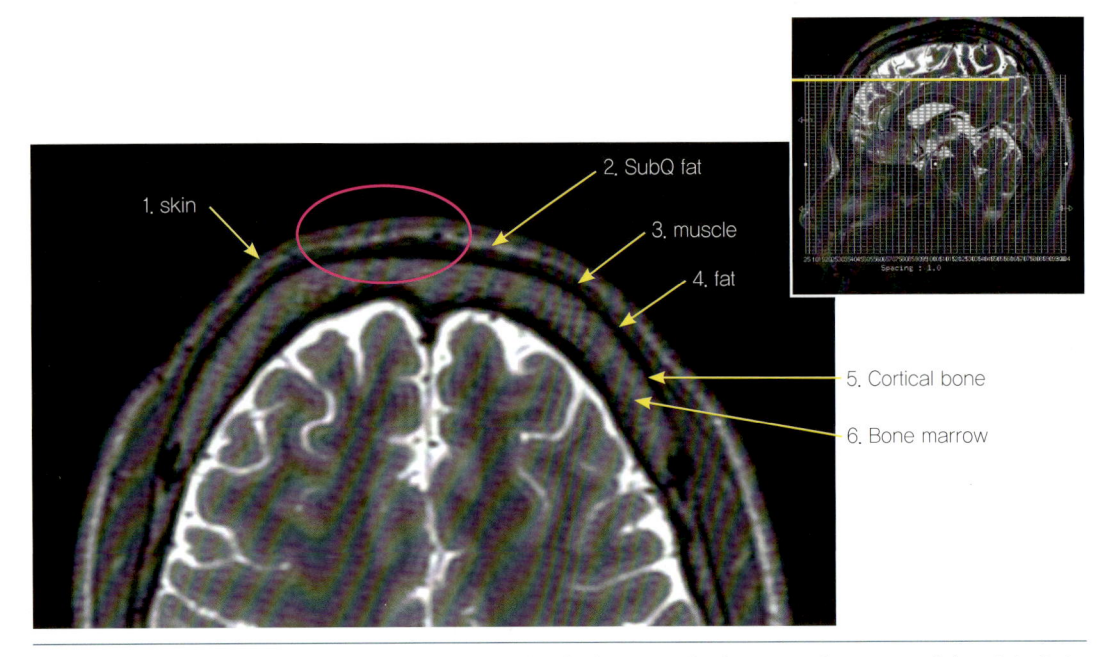

Safe Filler Injection Technique Demonstration – using live imaging tools

Fig. 4-11 MRI (2) of the forehead. **(1)** Skin. **(2)** SubQ fat layer - By looking into the center of the pink circle, it can be seen that thick veins mostly pass through the subcutaneous layer. Arteries are not very detectable with MRIs, but their depths mostly coincide with that of the veins. **(3)** Muscles - Underneath the fat, there are muscles (frontalis m.) shown as relatively darker compared to the fat. **(4)** Fat layer underneath the muscle – This is the layer targeted for filler injection in the forehead. It is not very distinguishable because it is thin. It is shown brighter on the lateral side. **(5)** Bone cortex – It appears as dark, which makes it difficult to distinguish the cortex from muscles. **(6)** Bone Marrow – This is the area with moderate signals reflected in light grey. It is considered the center of the skull.

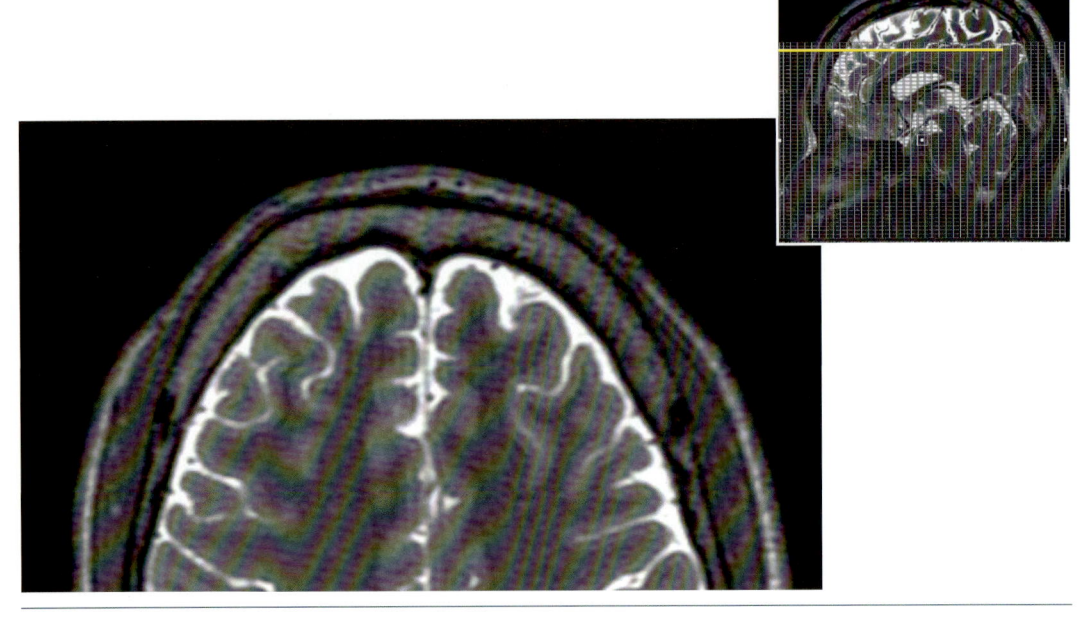

Fig. 4-12 **MRI (3) of the forehead**

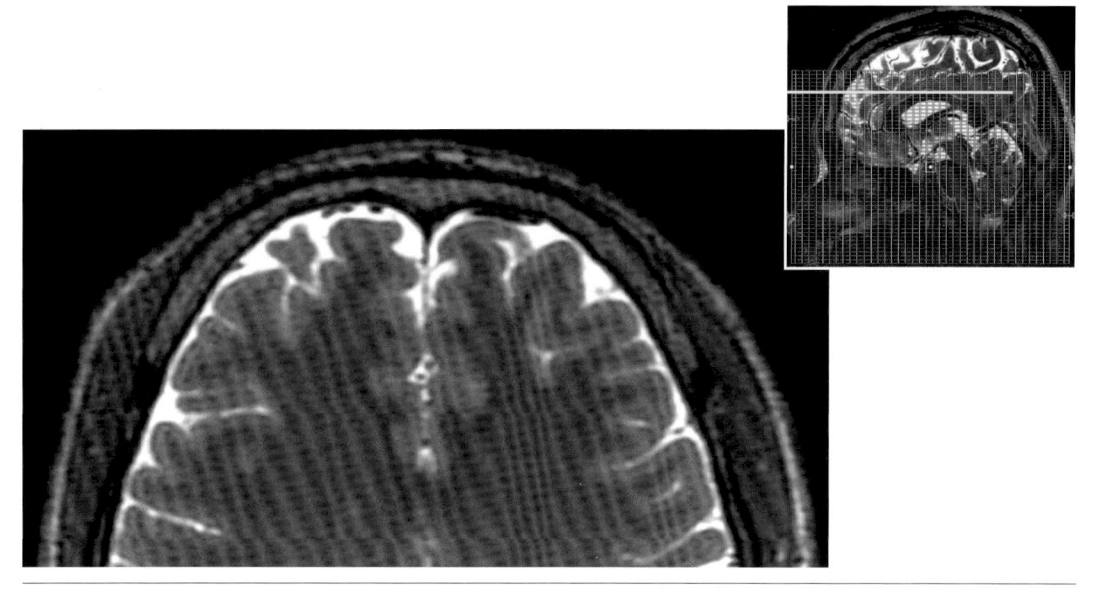

Fig. 4-13　MRI (4) of the forehead

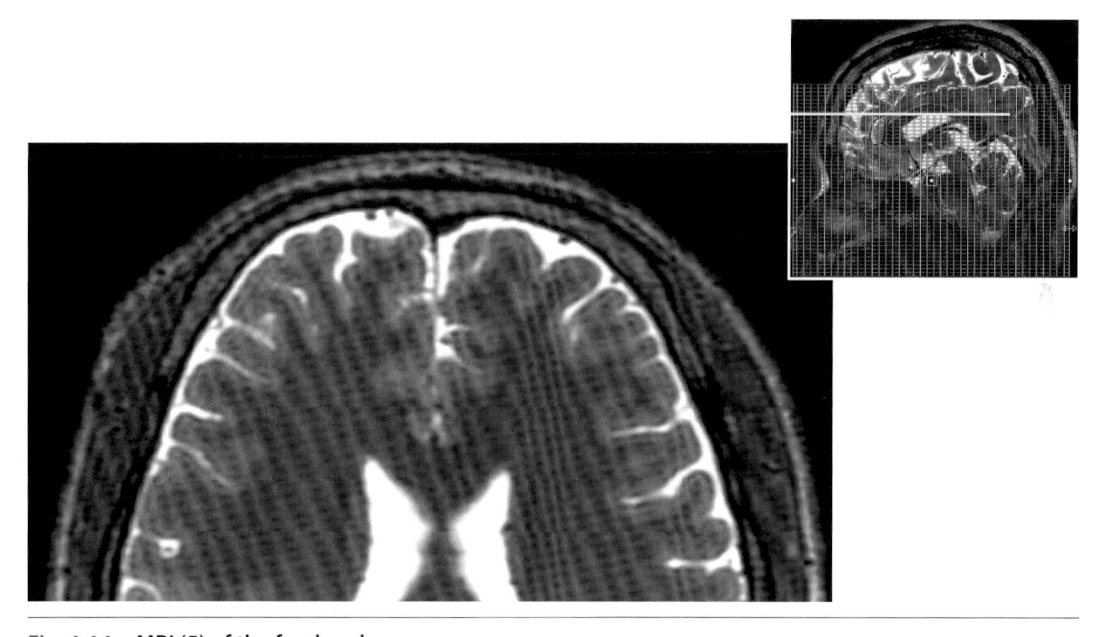

Fig. 4-14　MRI (5) of the forehead

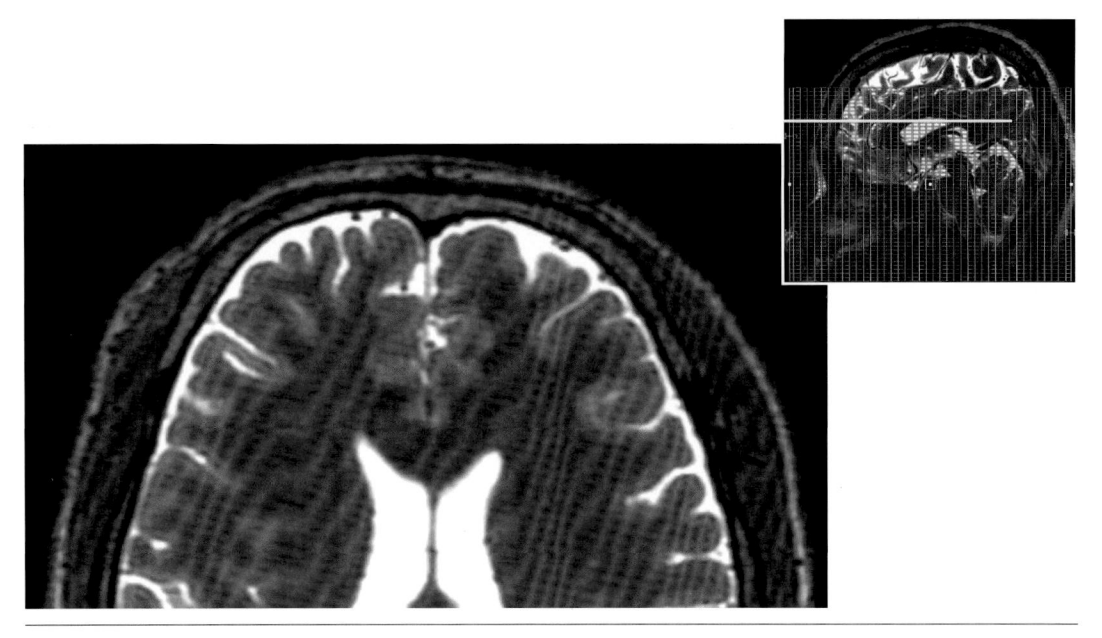

Safe Filler Injection Technique Demonstration – using live imaging tools

Fig. 4-15 **MRI (6) of the forehead**

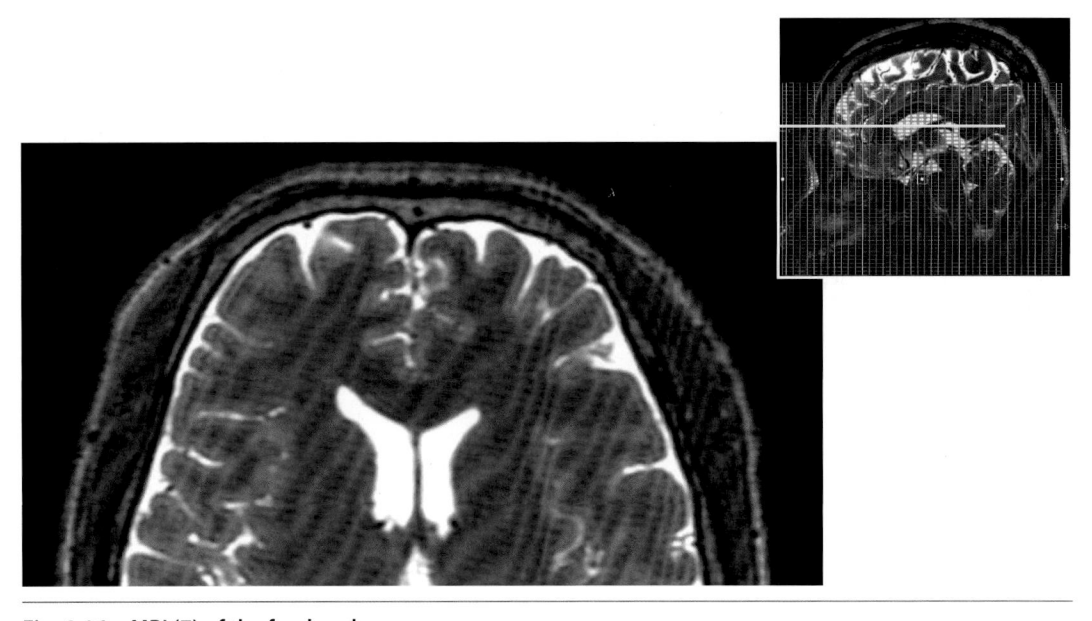

Fig. 4-16 **MRI (7) of the forehead**

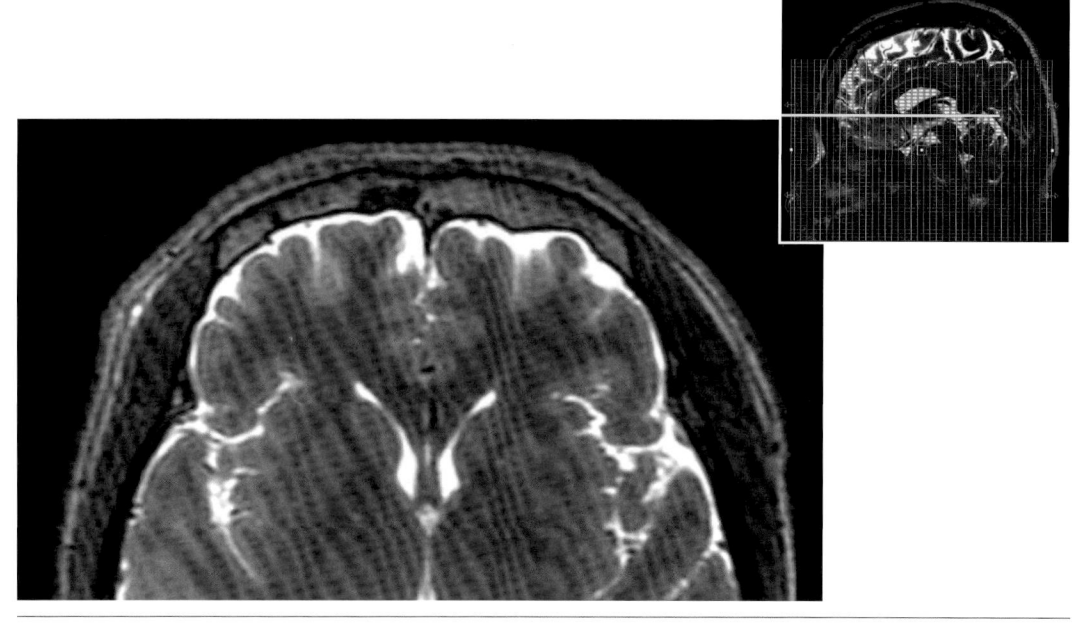

Fig. 4-17 MRI (8) of the forehead

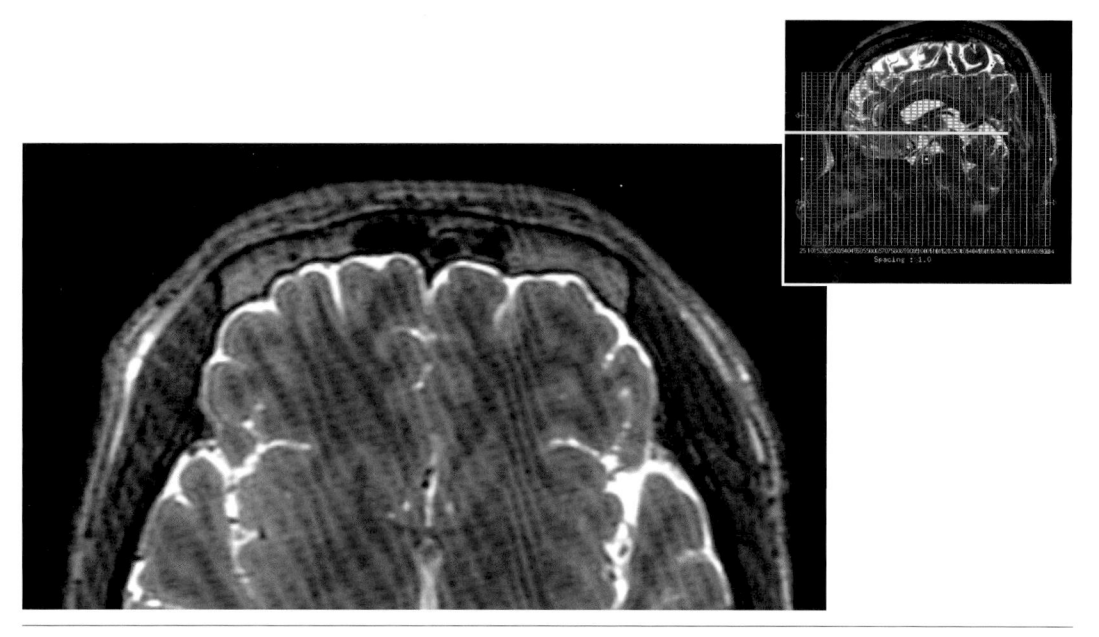

Fig. 4-18 MRI (9) of the forehead

> **Imaging explanation**
>
> - The major blood vessels in the forehead exist in the subQ fat layer. Due to the thickness of the veins, significant amount of bleeding can occur when they are damaged. Arteries that are small in width and hardly visible also exist in the subQ fat layer.
>
> - There is a submusclar fat layer below the muscle layer. In the MRI image, it is visible in the lateral section but not so much in the medial section. It is a good target layer for injecting fillers.
>
> - Since the muscle layer and the submuscular fat layer are very thin, it is tricky to inject fillers along the layer. It is likely for the needle to move unintentionally towards the subcutaneous fat layer. It is necessary to perform the procedures with confidence with respect to the deep layer.

3 Choice of Filler

1) Concavity of the Forehead

It is best to use fillers with high viscosity that demonstrate volumizing effects on top of the periosteum.

The biphasic fillers are useful for quickly creating an ideal augmented shape, but due to their relatively low moldability they should always be injected well at once with caution, especially for unexperienced users. In contrast, the monophasic fillers are easier to mold, but have the disadvantage of potentially becoming bumpy due to external forces even within a few days post procedure. When monophasic fillers somewhat harden, typically three to four weeks after the procedure, a second procedure can be done to reshape the forehead as desired. After accumulation of many real-life experiences and the sufficient understanding of the properties of fillers, the physician may effectively use monophasic fillers in the forehead with confidence.

2) Fine Wrinkles

It is advisable to use fillers with mid to low viscosity.

4 Demonstration of Technique

1) Entry Point

In forehead procedures, physicians inquire most about the location of the entry point. This is also the case for procedures on the glabella and the temples. Entry points are normally considered two dimensionally. In our face, blood vessels, nerves, muscles and fat exist between the skin and the bones and, accordingly, any entry point may be dangerous or safe depending on how deep the cannula or needle is inserted. Therefore, this book places emphasis on learning the location of entry points and the depth at which blood vessels and nerves are located underneath entry points.

In addition to entry points, methods for avoiding scars must be considered. Safety is based on having studied the depth and direction of blood vessels and nerves. Scars can be avoided through cautious use of a cannula and the selection of an appropriately sized cannula.

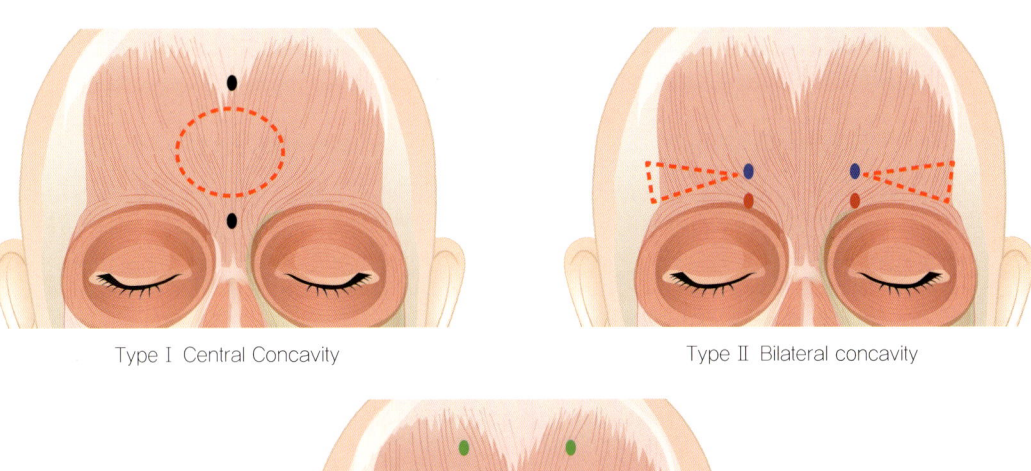

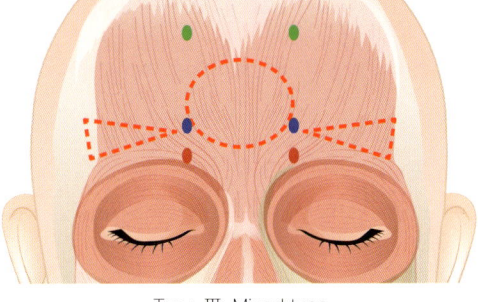

Type I Central Concavity

Type II Bilateral concavity

Type III Mixed type

Fig. 4-19 Entry points depending on the classification of forehead concavity

(1) Black Entry Points

These points can be targeted when the area of convexity in the forehead is small and centered. There is some degree of variation, but in general the blood vessels and the nerves are positioned in the deep layer below the corrugator m. and in the superficial layer above the corrugator m. Therefore, after making an entry route through the deep layer below the frontalis m. the targeted area can be filled. It is advisable not to inject fillers unnecessarily below the corrugator m.

(2) Blue Entry Points

These points are the spots that allow a cannula to access most places in the forehead via a linear path. It has the advantages of causing minimal bruising and being convenient in terms of making space for fillers but also has an increased risk of leaving a mark in the center of the forehead. In order to prevent such mark, the smallest cannula can be used and decrease the size of the entry point as much as possible.

(3) Green Entry Points

These points are helpful for accessing a wide area. After entering into the deep layer and freeing up space, an injection with cannula can be done. However, accidents can occur if fillers are injected into blood vessels in the opposite direction of the blood flow. This can be prevented by carefully freeing up space within the tissue and then steadily injecting fillers little by little with controlled pressure.

(4) Red Entry Points

These points have the advantage of hiding scars as the entry points fall within the eyebrows. It is relatively safe to perform procedures at these spots because the direction of injection is upward, which coincides with the flow of blood vessels. For entry, a point that lies between the supratrochlear artery and supraorbital artery should be selected.

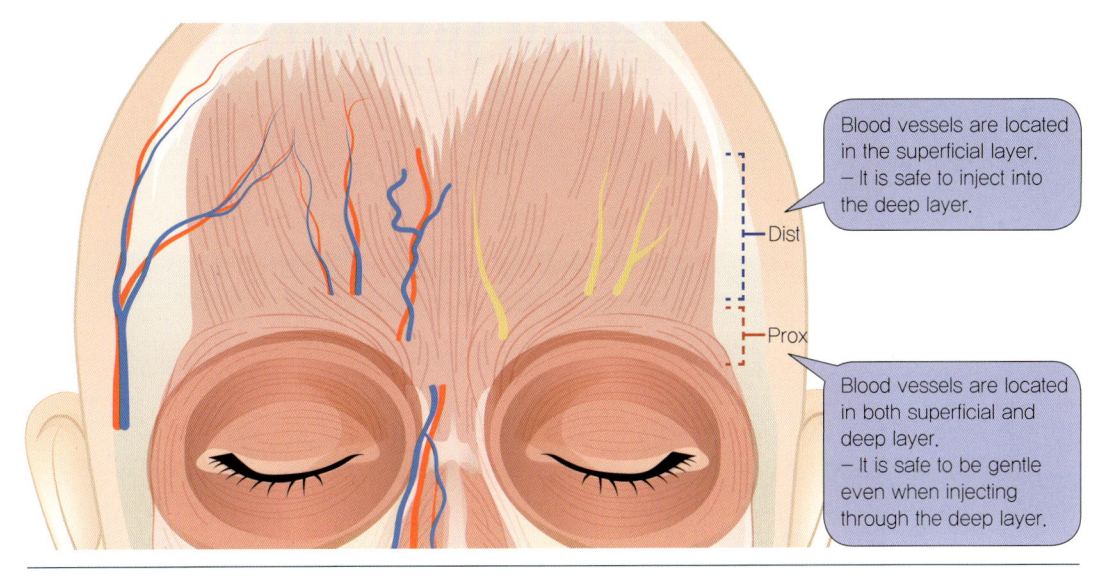

Fig. 4-20 Dispersion of blood vessels and nerves

Blood vessels are located in the superficial layer.
– It is safe to inject into the deep layer.

Blood vessels are located in both superficial and deep layer.
– It is safe to be gentle even when injecting through the deep layer.

2) Injection Method-DPS

- Above the superior line of demarcation of the corrugator m., where arteries and veins lie in the superficial layer, injection into the deep layer below the frontalis m. is considered safe.
- In the area around the corrugator m., arteries and veins lie in both the deep and superficial layers. In order to prevent accidents, such as blindness, injection into the deep layer via a transverse approach or vertical approach in the direction of the proximal to the distal regions can be performed.
- Below the border line of frontalis m., procuring space through separating the area without bleeding is essential for filler injection and molding.

3) Perpendicular Pulling Method

- Consider the location and depth of nerves and blood vessels.
- Mark visible veins with a pen or marker.
- Check the degree of pressure in the syringe by shooting a small amount of filler in the air.
- After perpendicularly puncturing the area above the corrugator m. in 1.5~2 cm intervals, touch the bone with the needle.
- Inject at the touch position or at the position slightly pulled back (0.1 mm), depending on negative pressure.
- After injection, spread out the filler by pressuring.

5 Complication

1) Dermal Necrosis

Skin necrosis can occur in the targeted area from direct injection into the supratrochlear artery, supraorbital artery, superficial temporal artery or extravascular compression (see Blood Vessel Complications 1-8 of Part 5).

2) Blindness

Blindness can occur in the event that fillers are accidently injected into the supratrochlear artery or the retrograde supraorbital artery blood flow, moving to the ophthalmic artery and then entering into the retinal artery. It is difficult to recover this symptom even with rapid treatment. (see Blindness, 3-1, Part 5).

Both of these complications are likely to happen especially to those who do not have much knowledge on blood vessel anatomy. Hence, thorough knowledge on the location and depth of the relevant arteries can easily prevent such events.

SUMMARY of Forehead

A
- Location and depth of the supratrochlear artery and veins/nerves
- Location and depth of the supraorbital artery and veins/nerves
- Position of the superficial temporal artery

B
- Hollowness above both sides of the supraorbital rim and hollowness above the glabella should be corrected to create an ideal forehead.
- Augmention of the forehead should be completed in the manner that the center shines from the front. (The degree of convexity at the center should be selected according to patient preference).
- Augmention of the forehead should be completed in the manner that it appears as a smooth curve from the lateral view.
- In general, there should be no sunkenness in the forehead. It should have a round shape.

C
- Because a large amount of filler needs to be injected, a filler with high viscosity should be used.
- Make sure that the filler doesn't diluted by bleeding.
- To fill-in wrinkles on the forehead, a filler with medium to low viscosity should be used.

D
- Perpendicular pulling injection method: After touching the bone with the needle, perform the injection by shooting upwards and then flatten by pressing.
- DPS Method: Make space in the area below the frontalis m., separate, and inject fillers.

X
- In the danger zone of blood vessels perform procedures slowly, making sure to bypass blood vessels.

2. Glabella

••• One of the facial areas that results in patient dissatisfaction, especially for patients in their 40s to 50s, is the glabella. There are cases where they want to adjust the concavity of the glabella in a similar way to adjust the concavity at the center of the forehead, and there are cases where they want to adjust fine wrinkles, which result from the contraction of dermis. Sufficient communication with the patient prior to a procedure is necessary in order to promote satisfaction and ensure that the procedure is being done in the desired area. For instance, it is advisable to discuss patient expectations and concerns while looking in a mirror prior to procedures. Besides, in case of deep wrinkles, the dents made in the dermis do not flatten to perfectly match normal skin regardless of the type of filler used. Therefore, prior to a procedure it is important to explain what can be expected by spreading the wrinkled area with two fingers for image simulation. Since many patients visit their clinic to resolve concavity and wrinkles in the glabella only with botulinum toxin, it is necessary to briefly explain the difference between filler and botulinum toxin procedures.

Moreover, in many cases, concavity and wrinkles are both present in the forehead, in which case, performing procedures together leads to a much better result.

Concavity in glabella is caused by a loss of dermis, which is the primary target of fillers. Therefore, filler substances are to be injected into the dermal layer. However, in the case of glabella wrinkles that are old and severely deep, it is not unusual for not only the dermis but also the subcutaneous tissue to be concave. For such feature, addition of filler to the subcutaneous layer may be necessary.

Additionally, there are people with large pores. For these people, when fillers are injected into the dermal layer, they easily come out through the pores. Consequently, injection of a small amount of filler into the subcutaneous layer can be attempted to avoid a leakage through the pores. As soon as a leakage is noticed, the procedure must carefully proceed into deeper area. In this case, combining fillers with botulinum toxin can be used for resolution.

Dissecting the border of the dermal and subcutaneous layers for separation can help improve wrinkles. This can be done with a cannula.

1 Beauty

1) Concavity of Glabella vs Frown Lines

The concavity of glabella occurs due to the innate concavity of the bone structure of the glabella itself or due to a reduction of fat volume. If this area is concave, the line connecting to the forehead is not smooth.

2) Good to Understand as Part of Forehead Wrinkles for Performing Procedures

Frown lines are normally vertical, and is often known as a (JII) shaped wrinkle. They are symmetrical left and right in some cases and in other cases one of many vertical wrinkles is more distinct.

Frown lines become more severe with aging, between young people and old people, the degree of wrinkles differs and, depending on the age, the amount of filler required differs. The MERZ AESTHETICS Scales is a handy tool during consultations. For example, when consulting with a scale 4 patient who requests an injection of the amount required for a scale 1 patient, it can be used to explain the patient's current status and the differences in the amount required for adjustment (Fig. 4-21).

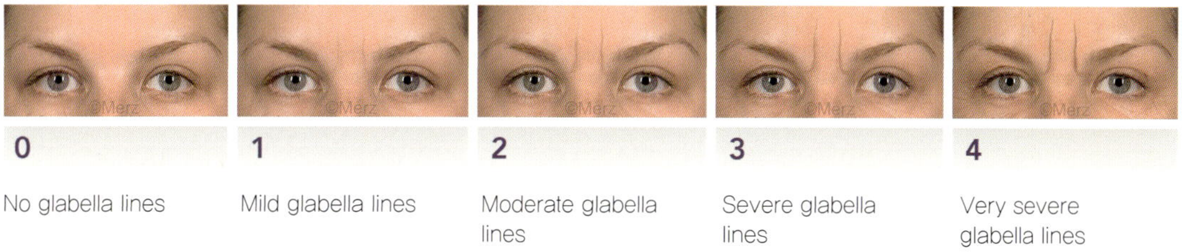

0	1	2	3	4
No glabella lines	Mild glabella lines	Moderate glabella lines	Severe glabella lines	Very severe glabella lines

Fig. 4-21 MERZ AESTHETICS Scales (Glabella-at rest).
Copyright© (2009) Merz Pharmaceuticals
Flynn, et al. Validated assessment scales for the upper face. Dermatol Surg. 2012;38(2 Spec No.):309-19.

2) The Curve along the Forehead-Glabella-Radix and Degree of Convexity

Fig. 4-22 shows the ideal degree of convexity.

Current beauty trends include creating a profile with a smooth and gradual S line curve starting from the forehead and continuing to the glabella.

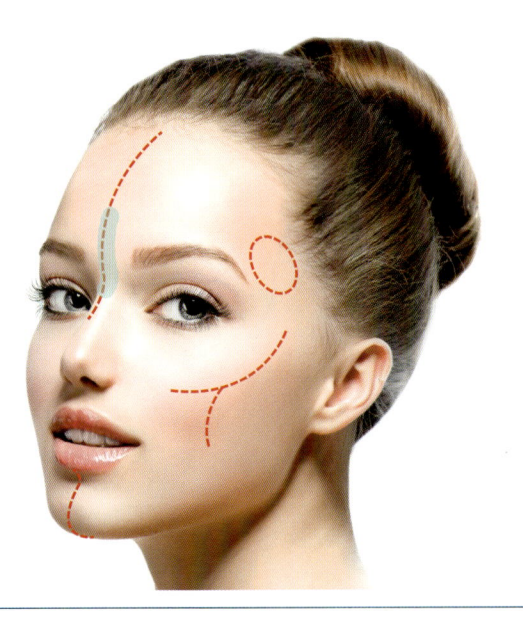

Fig. 4-22   S-line curve from the forehead to the glabella

2 Anatomy

Frown lines form due to excessive muscle contraction of the corrugator m. and procerus m. of the eyebrows.

There are many blood vessels and nerves dispersed in this region. As the supratrochlear artery, vein, and nerve exit the notch they course through the deep layers. After passing the corrugator muscle, they then course superficially. When treating just the frown lines, it is best to inject fillers with small particles into the dermis layer. However, if filler seeps out through the pores, filler can be injected after careful dissection of the top most layer of the subcutaneous layer and ensuring there was no bleeding.

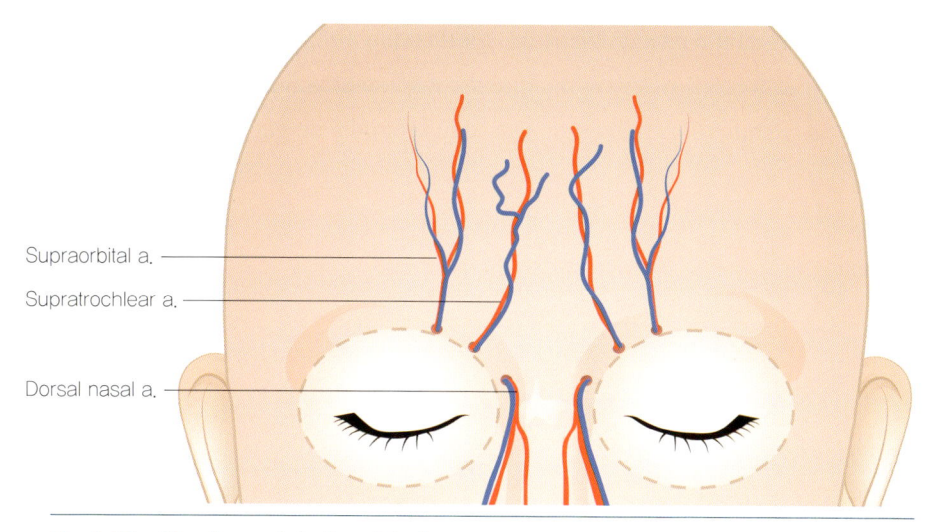

Fig. 4-23　Blood vessels in the glabella

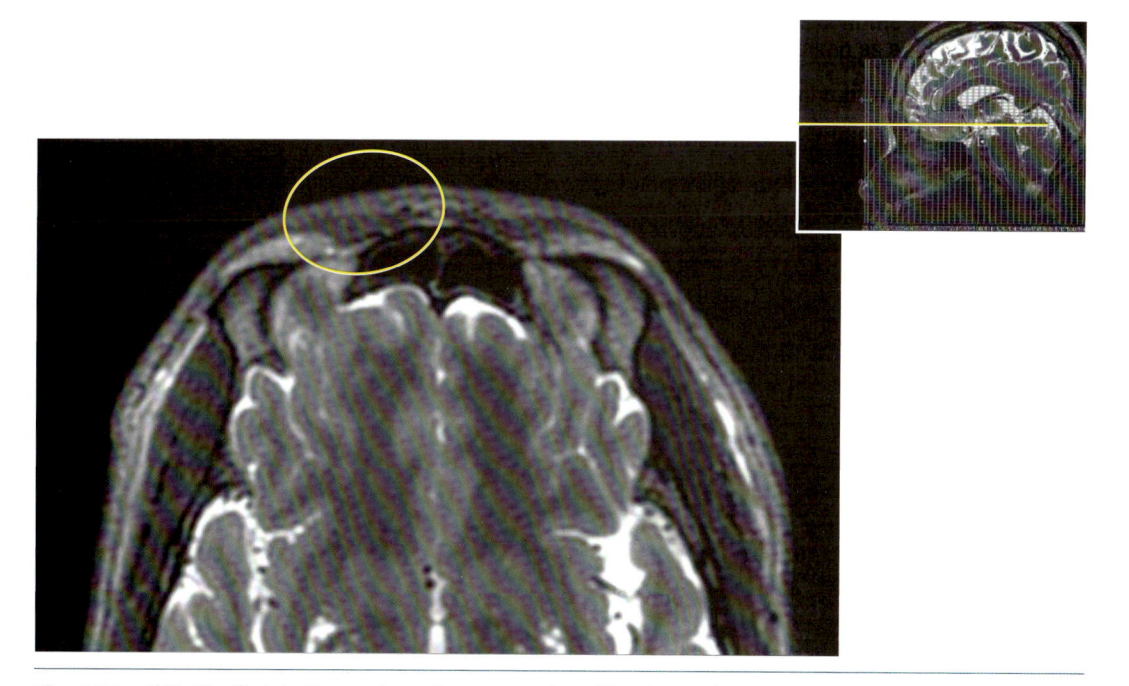

- Supraorbital a.
- Supratrochlear a.
- Dorsal nasal a.

Fig. 4-24　**MRI (1) of glabellar region.**　Transverse view. Blood vessels coursing the subcutaneous fat layer and corrugator m. can be seen.

Filler Treatment for Each Facial Area

Be cautious of the intercanthal vein (see anatomy of the nose. 4-2, Part 4).

As seen in the yellow circle in Fig. 4-24, the supratrochlear vessels penetrate the central portion of the corrugator muscle. From the point the vessels exit the corrugator muscle, they begin to course superficially. Some of the veins course through the junction between the subcutaneous fat layer and muscle. By administering with botulinum toxin, we can decrease the volume of filler.

As there is anatomical variation in this region, procedure must be performed gently. To ensure patient safety, filler should be injected in the superior direction towards the head (distal to the supratrochlear artery). In the event of intravascular injection directed superiorly will result in skin necrosis. On the other hand, injection in inferior direction towards the foot may result in intravascular administration of the filler into the proximal arterial flow which may cause occlusion of retinal artery (see Blindness. 3-1, Part 5). With cannulas, it is recommended that space is procured in advance and to confirm for absence of bleeding prior to filler placement. With needles, injection into the dermis layer seems to be comparatively safe, but as stated above, the filler seeps out through the pores in many cases.

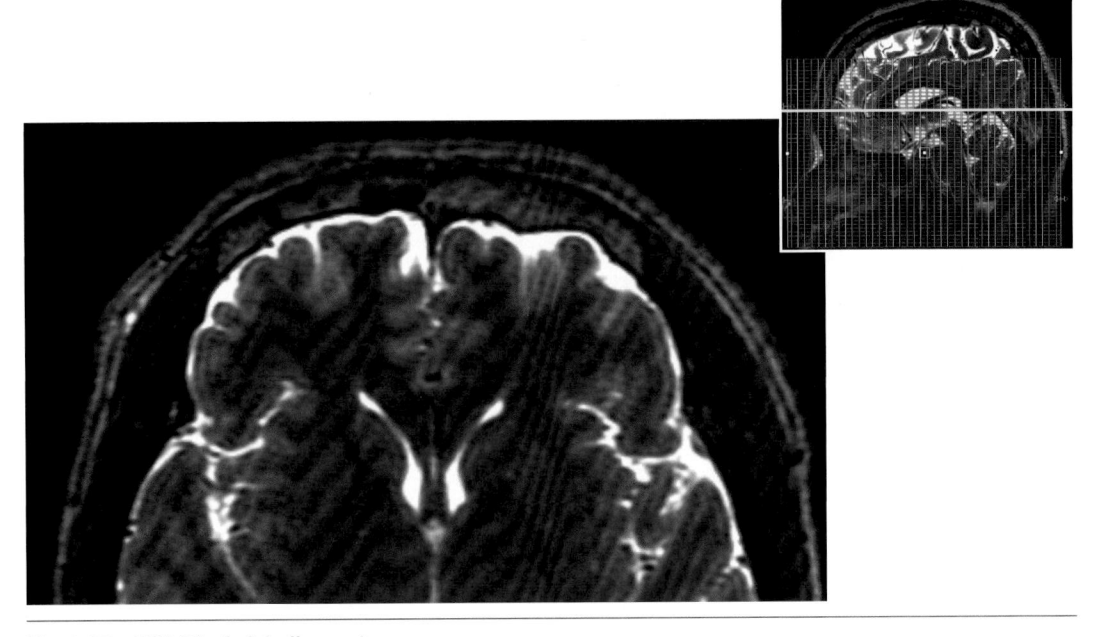

Fig. 4-25 MRI (2) of glabellar region

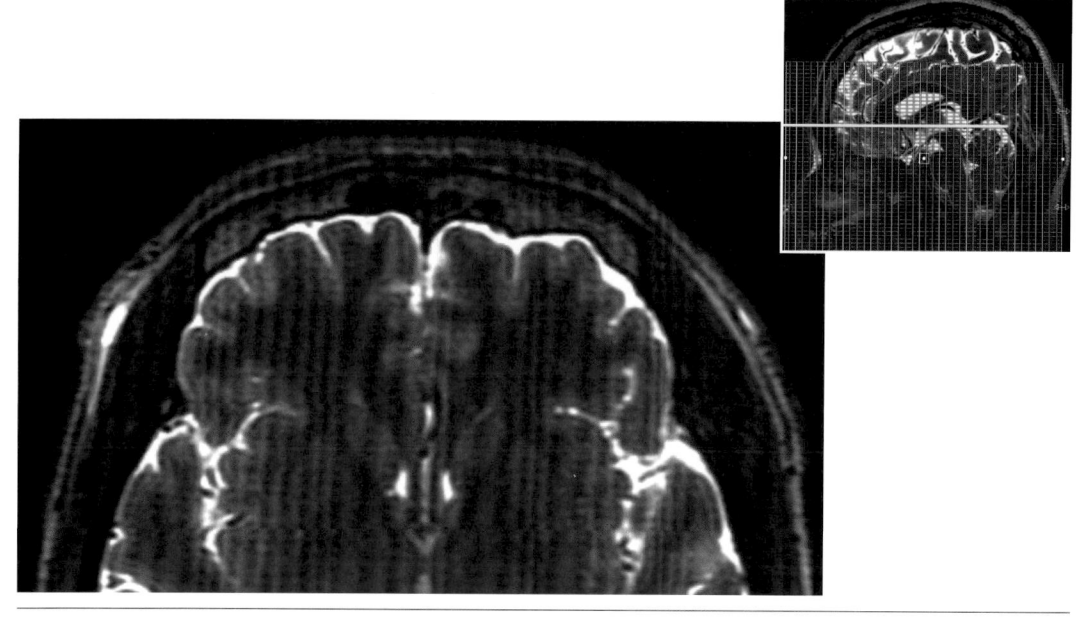

Fig. 4-26　MRI (3) of glabellar region

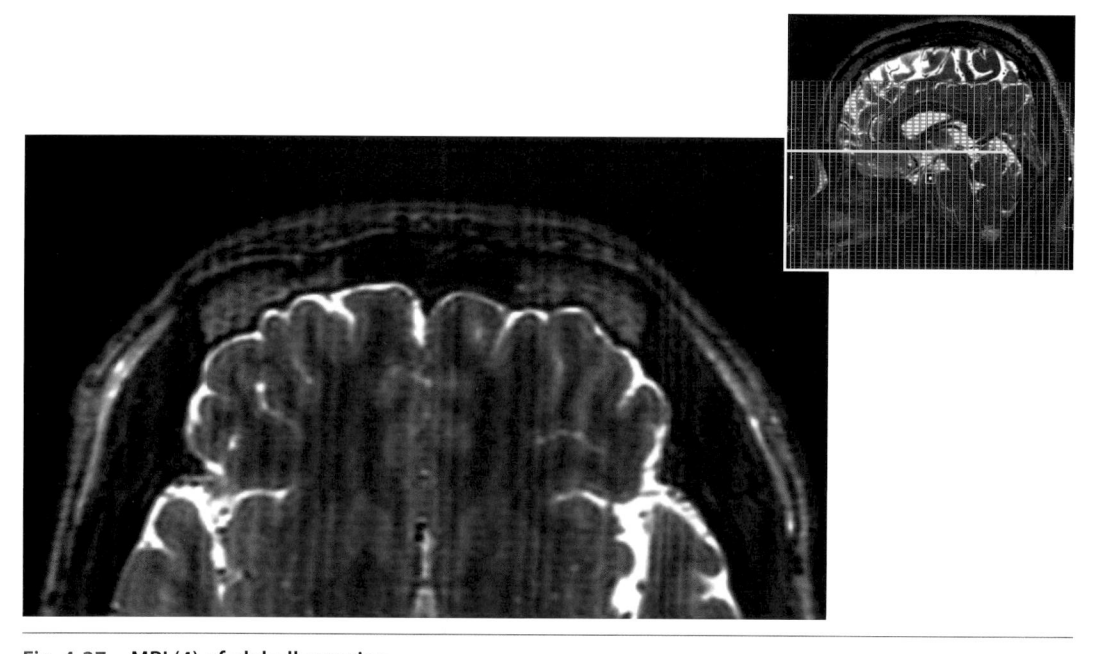

Fig. 4-27　MRI (4) of glabellar region

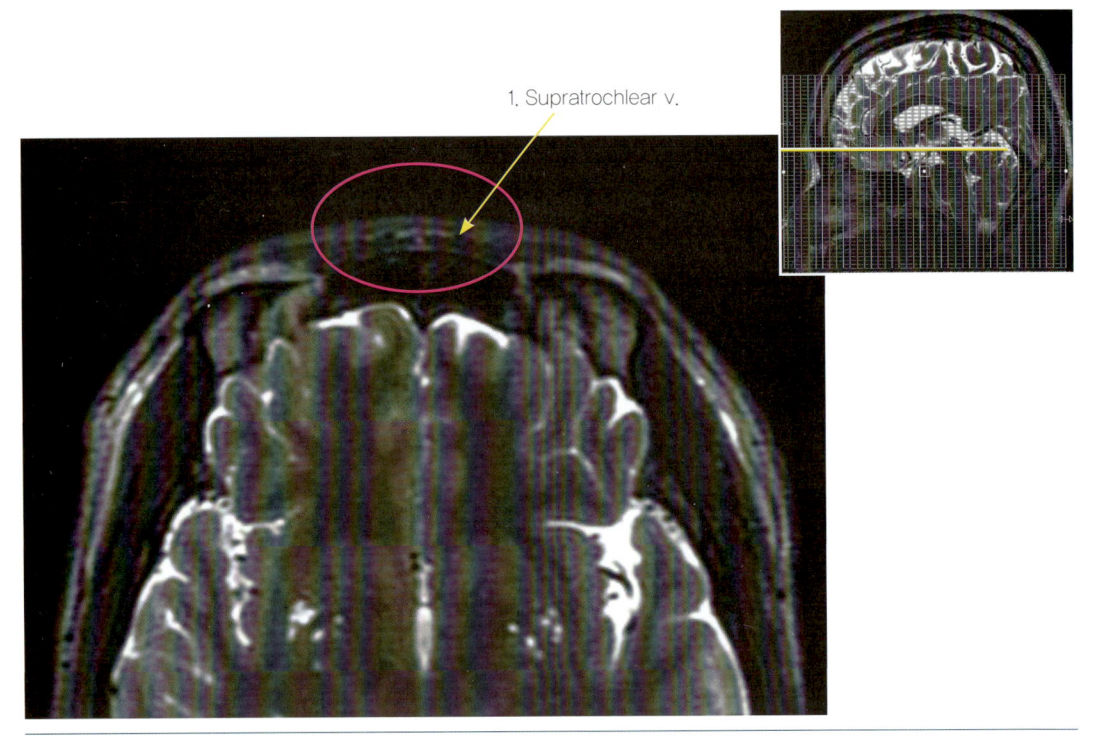

Safe Filler Injection Technique Demonstration – using live imaging tools

Fig. 4-28 **MRI (5) of glabellar region**

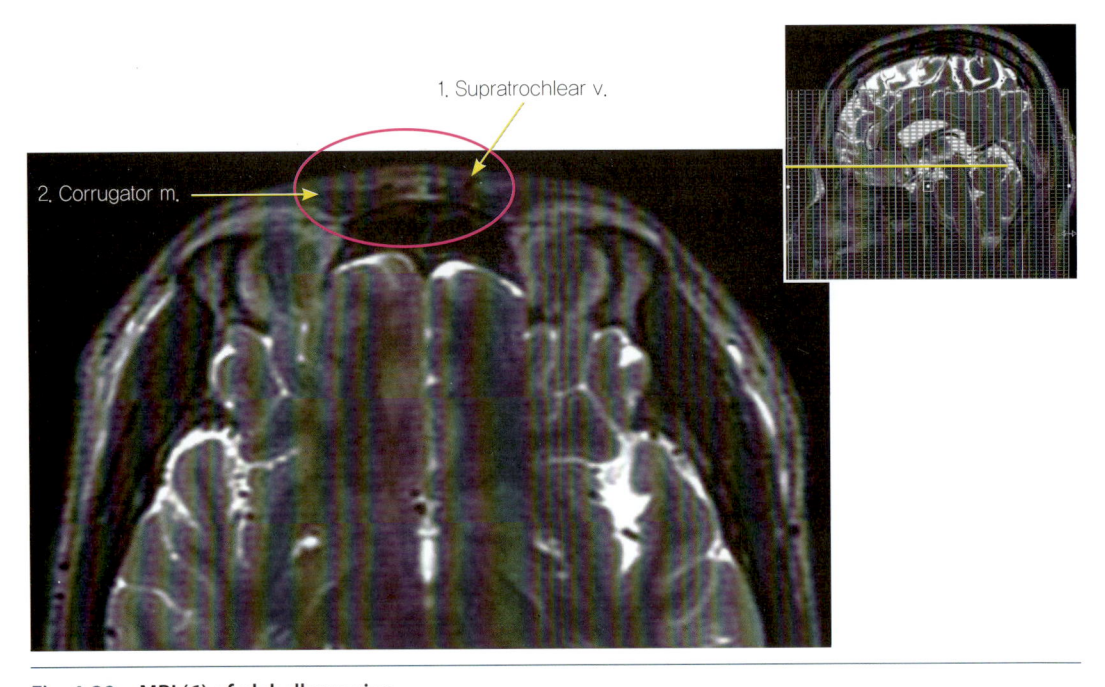

Fig. 4-29 **MRI (6) of glabellar region**

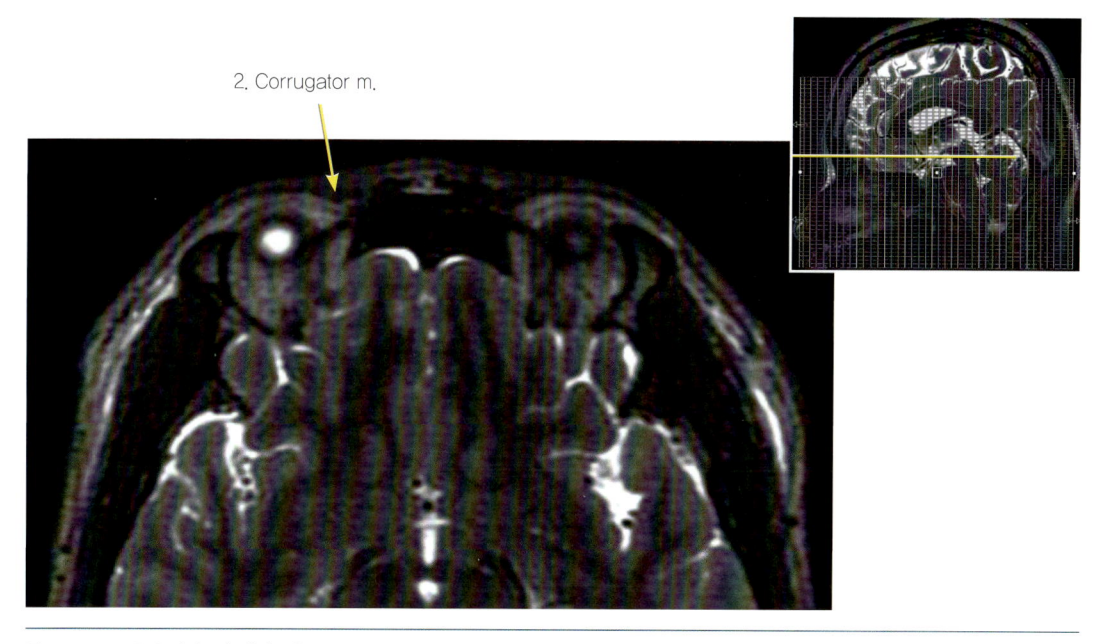

Fig. 4-30   MRI (7) of glabellar region

> **Imaging explanation**
> - The main blood vessels penetrate the corrugator m. and then course superiorly.
> - As they pass the forehead region, the blood vessels move to the superficial fat layer areas. Caution must be taken with respect to supratrochlear artery and vein.
> - The injection of fillers into the dermis or the dermal subcutaneous junction is generally safe.
> - Injection into deep layers or middle layers is riskier due to variation. Caution is required when injecting in these layers.

3 Choice of Filler

1) Bone Concavity or Fat Atrophy

Fillers with high viscosity that can provide volumizing effect when injected immediately above the periosteum are recommended.

Due to their characteristics, biphasic fillers are more suitable for creating the desired shape. However, caution must be taken for those who lack experience. Due to the softer characteristic of monophasic fillers, when pressure is applied in the treated region after the procedure, depressions or indentations may form. However, these fillers are easier to mold.

2) Frown Lines

- It is good to use fillers with mid to low viscosity.

4 Demonstration of Technique

1) Frown Lines

- It is good to use fillers with mid to low viscosity.
- Use the retrograde linear thread technique.
- After injection, massage the treated area.
- Regardless of filler type, the deeper furrows in the dermis may not completely smoothen out to match the adjacent, normal skin
- In patients with large pores, inject into deeper layer.

2) Bone Concavity or Fat Atrophy

Despite the rich vascular and nerve network, injections administered centrally into the deep layers are relatively safe.

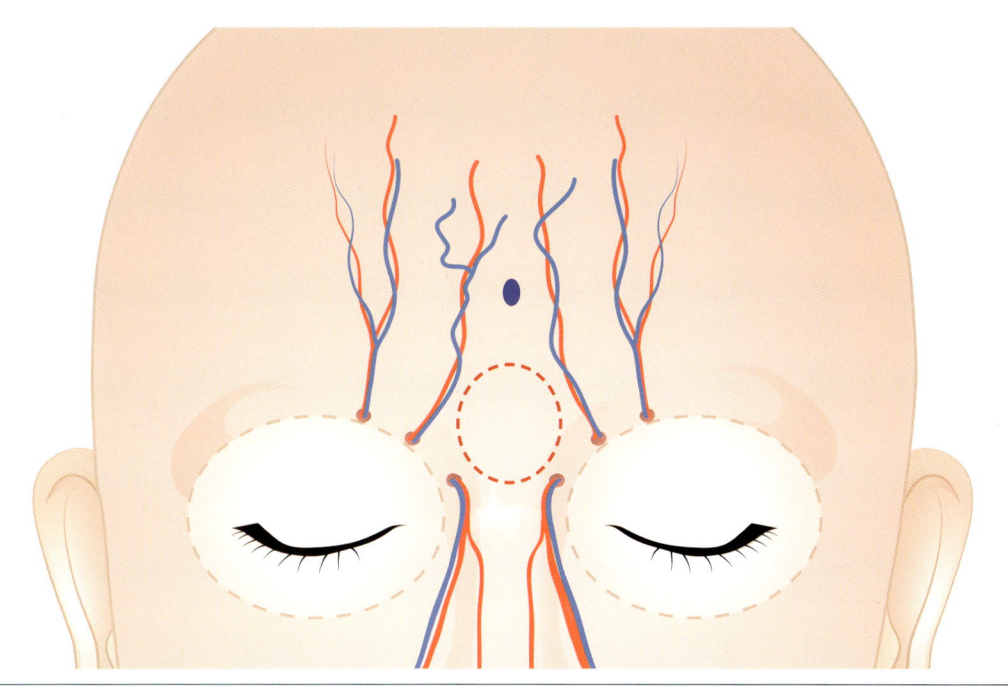

Fig. 4-31 Cannula procedure: Entry point (blue dot) and treatment area (region within the red dashed circle)
There are cases in which veins are clustered around the recommended entry point. In such cases, the entry point can be made further up or down.

5 Complications

Similar to complications that occur with forehead procedures. Intravascular accidents involving the supratrochlear artery may occur.

1) Dermal Necrosis

Skin necrosis can occur due to direct injection into the supratrochlear artery or extravascular compression (see Vascular Complications in 1-8, Part 5).

2) Blindness

Blindness can occur if fillers are accidentally injected into the supratrochlear artery or supraorbital artery and flow to the ophthalmic artery by retrograde flow and then into the retinal artery. Once symptoms occur, recovery is difficult even with active intervention (see Blindness in 3-1, Part5).

SUMMARY of Glabella

A
- Supratrochlear artery and vein
- Intercanthal vein

B
- Create a smooth curve connecting the forehead and the glabella without depressed region (S line)
- In patients presenting with both depressed region and wrinkles, treat simultaneously

C
- Depressed region – Filler with high viscoelasticity
- Wrinkles – Filler with low viscoelasticity

D
- Superficial layer (treatment of depressions in dermal layer): Filler may seep out through large pores (Needle linear pulling backward method)
- It is possible to inject into the superficial subcutaneous layer but caution must be taken (DPS method)
- Botulinum toxin treatment of the procerus, corrugator muscles must be performed in advance

X
- Blood vessel danger zone – Must proceed slowly avoiding the blood vessels
- Deep (below the frontalis m. – Using the perpendicular pulling method, proceed after bone touch)
- Within the dermis (needle – liner pulling backward method), superficial subcutaneous layer (DPS method)
- Deep subcutaneous layer, deep to the corrugator m. is a danger zone

3. Temples

1 Beauty

Compared to other facial regions, the temples are less frequently subject to procedures. This is partially due to the fact that patients do not request this procedure as they are able to hide their temples with their hair. It is also partially due to the fact that surgeons do not recognize the necessity of this procedure. However, in the case of temporal hollowness, the facial shape is not ideal. Furthermore, if temporal hollowness is compounded with a pronounced zygomatic arch, the cheek bones can appear more prominent. Correction of the temples is therefore necessary for facial balance and harmony.

2 Anatomy

Compared to other regions, the temples consist of many layers and each layer has different blood vessels. An accurate understanding is necessary, especially if the filler needs to be injected around the large blood vessels such as the sentinel vein or middle temporal vein. If an accident occurs, it can lead to pulmonary embolism through venous drainage. Therefore, special caution must be taken.

1) Three Layers of Temporal Fascia

The fascia surrounding the temples consists of three layers: the temporo-parietal fascia, superficial layer of the deep temporal fascia, and deep layer of the deep temporal fascia (superficial to deep). The terminology varies in literature but the terminology above is used most frequently. The temporo-parietal fascia (TPF) is also called the superficial temporal fascia. The TPF is immediately below the subcutaneous layer and the two layers of the DTF are above the temporalis muscle. During lifting surgery, targeted space is generally procured by separating the TPF and the superficial layer of the DTF. The two layers separate relatively easily.

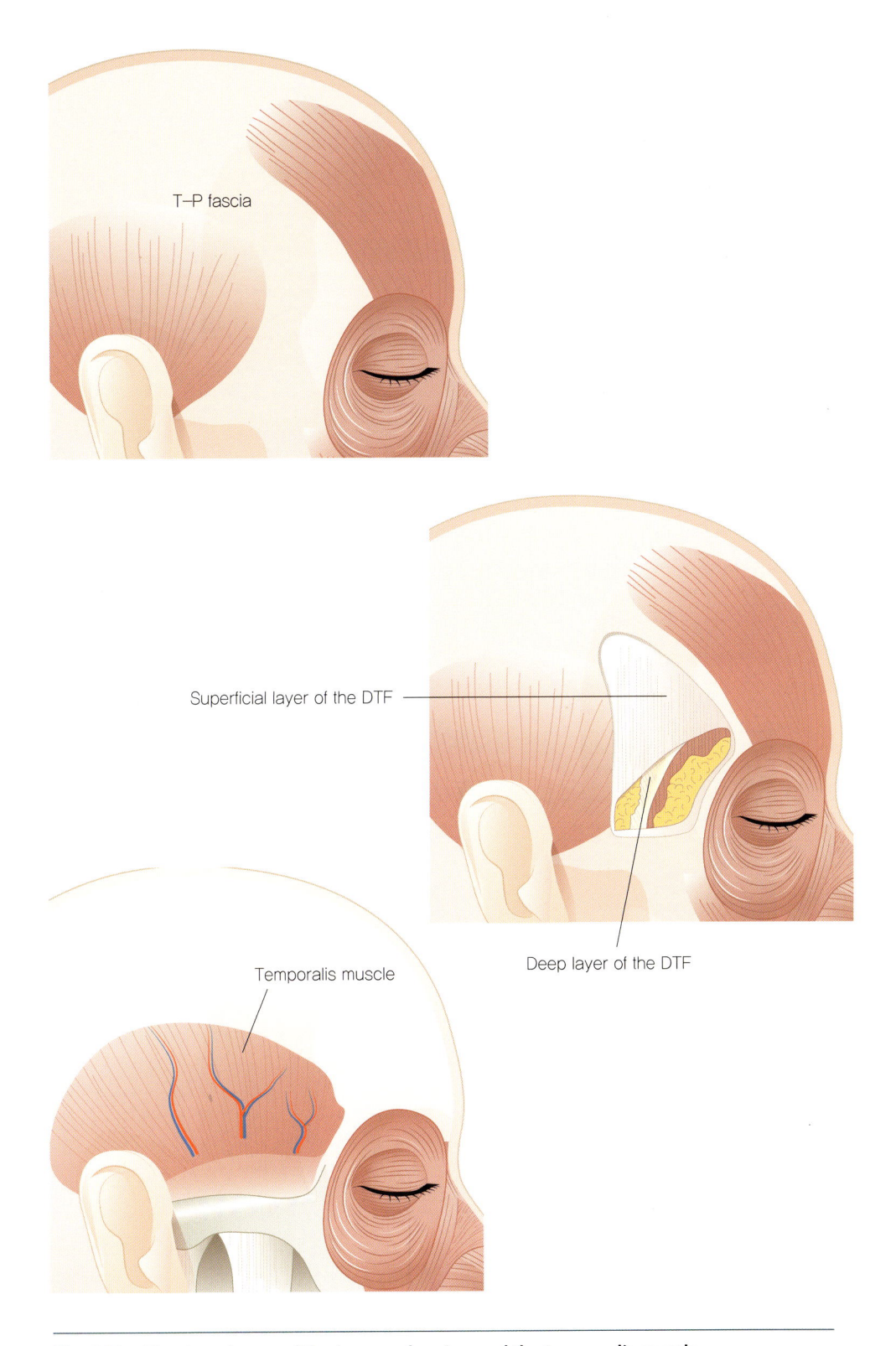

Fig. 4-32 The three layers of the temporal region and the temporalis muscle.
T-P fascia: temporo-parietal fascia, DTF: deep temporal fascia

2) The Superficial Temporal Artery and Vein and Deep Temporal Artery and Vein

The arterio-venous system of the temple includes the superficial temporal artery and vein in the superficial layer and the deep temporal artery and vein that come up from below the muscles. Both arteries branch out from the external carotid artery (ECA). The superficial temporary artery (STA) branches out directly from the ECA and the deep temporal artery (DTA) branches out from the maxillary artery, which is a branch of the ECA.

The STA is located in a layer above the temporo-parietal fascia (the TPF surrounds the STA). It divides into two branches, the frontal and parietal. These branches supply the forehead and crown, respectively. The DTA supplies the temporalis muscle, but there are variations in the blood vessels and the areas they supply.

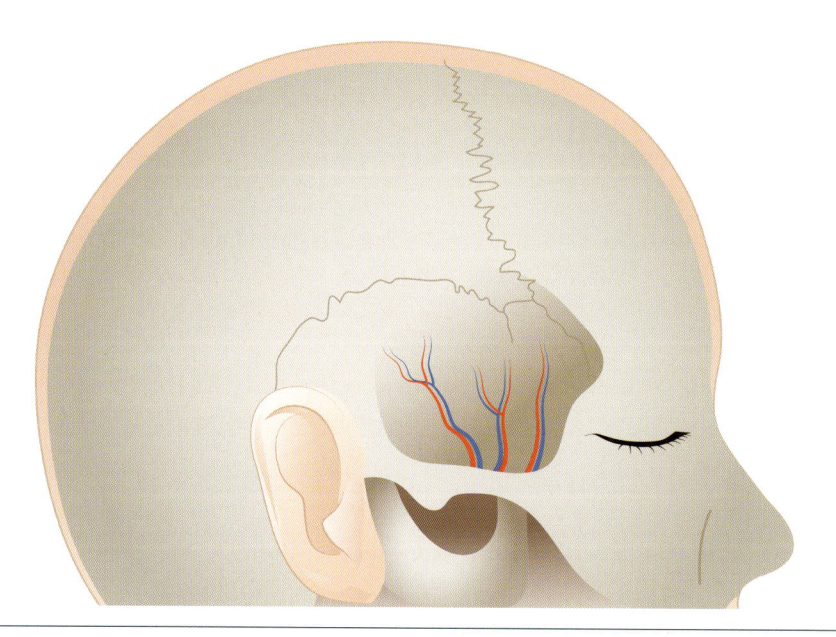

Fig. 4-33　Deep & superficial artery/veins of the temple

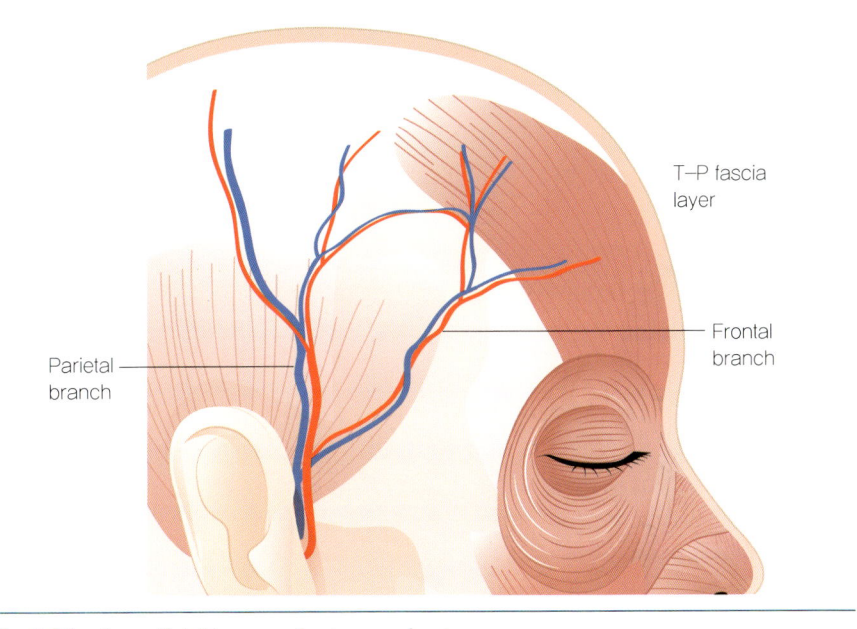

Fig. 4-34 Superficial temporal artery and vein

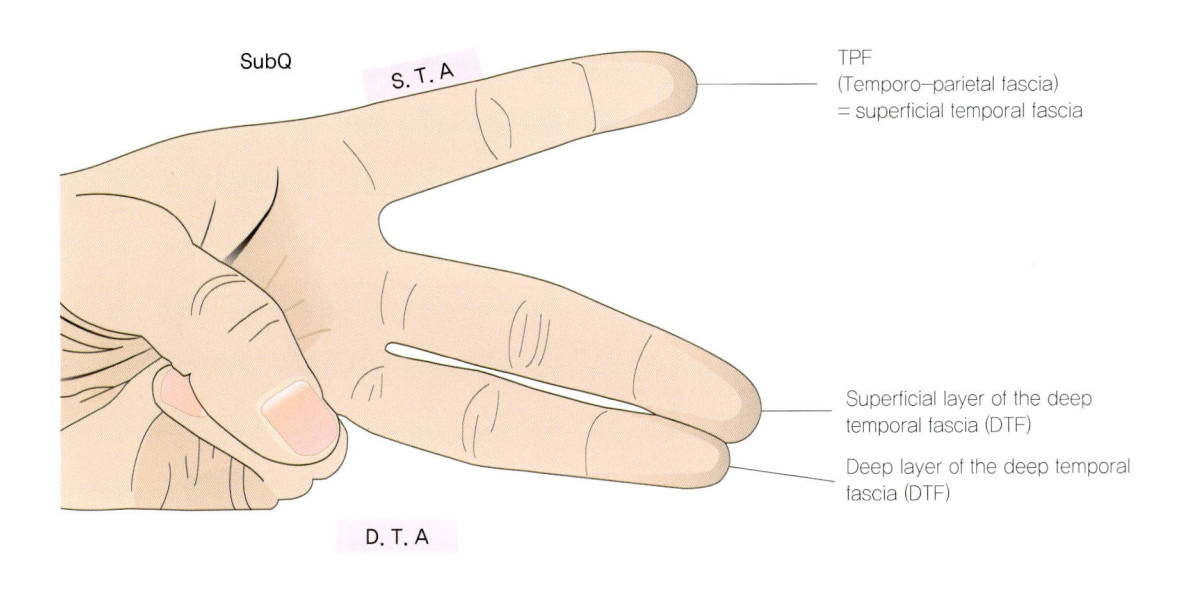

Fig. 4-35 Cross section of the temple and layers of the temple
SubQ: Subcutaneous tissue, STA: Superficial temporal artery, DTA: Deep temporal artery

3) Temporal Fat

In order to understand the structure of the temples properly, the cross sections in the illustrations above must be understood.

4) Sentinel Vein

The sentinel vein is a distinct structure from the superficial/deep temporal veins and is an important landmark in lifting surgeries. In lifting academia, the purple column (Fig. 4-37 and 4-38) seen in space between the TPF and DTF (layer of tissue separated in endoscopic surgery) is referred to as the sentinel vein. However, according to the anatomy field, the sentinel vein penetrates the point where is 2.5 cm lateral to orbital rim (Fig. 4-39) and then goes up to the lateral eyebrow and temporal crest (Fig. 4-36). It is also called the medial zygomatico-temporal vein and has a thickness of approximately 1.9 mm. The sentinel vein is visible in people with less subcutaneous tissue, in the supine position, or in cases when the venous pressure is increased by valsalva maneuver. Patients tend to examine the treated area more often after procedures, so it is good to have patients see their reflections and check their sentinel veins prior to proceeding with the procedure.

This is to minimize patient complaints that blood vessels in the temples seem to bulge out after the correction of the temples.

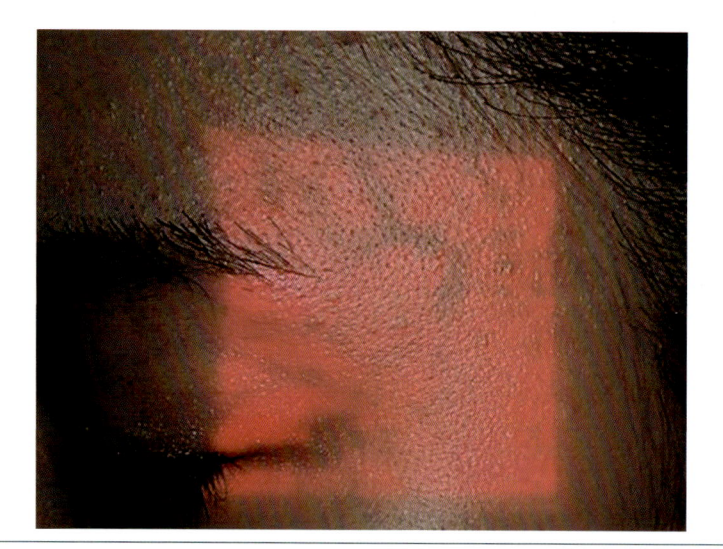

Fig. 4-36 Course of the sentinel vein as seen on the surface

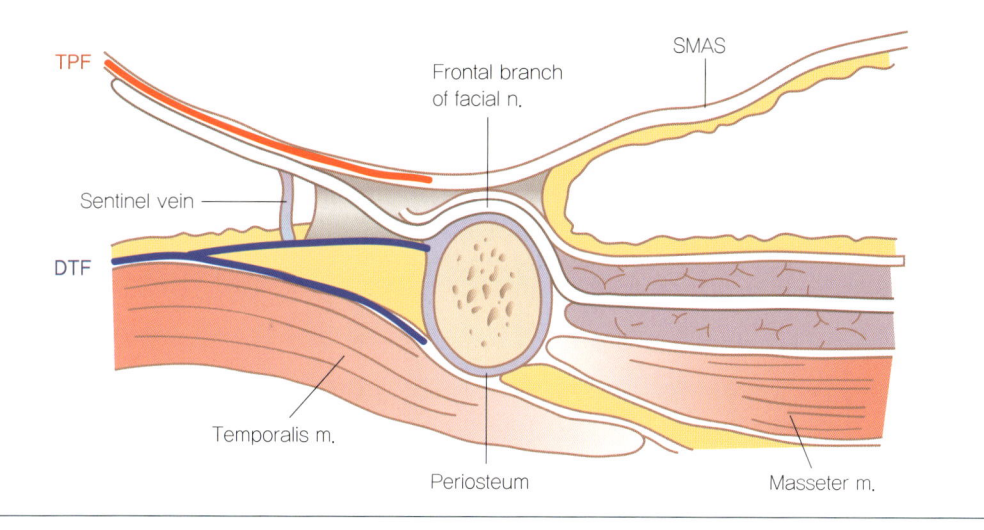

Fig. 4-37   Cross section of where the sentinel vein passes

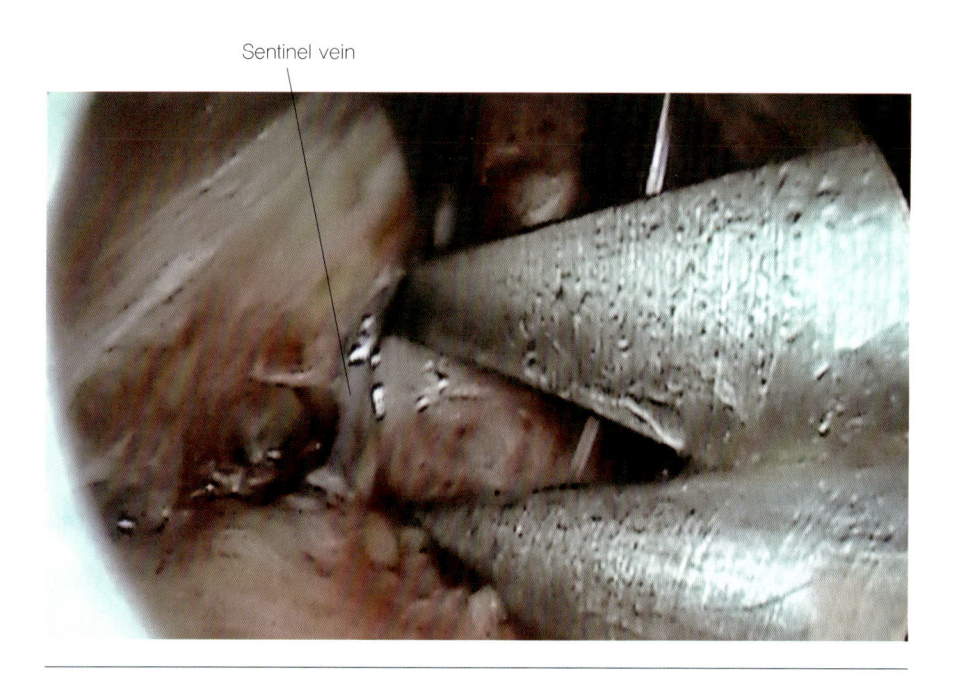

Fig. 4-38   Cross section where the sentinel vein passes

(Source: Dr. Il Koo Kim of Meducation K)

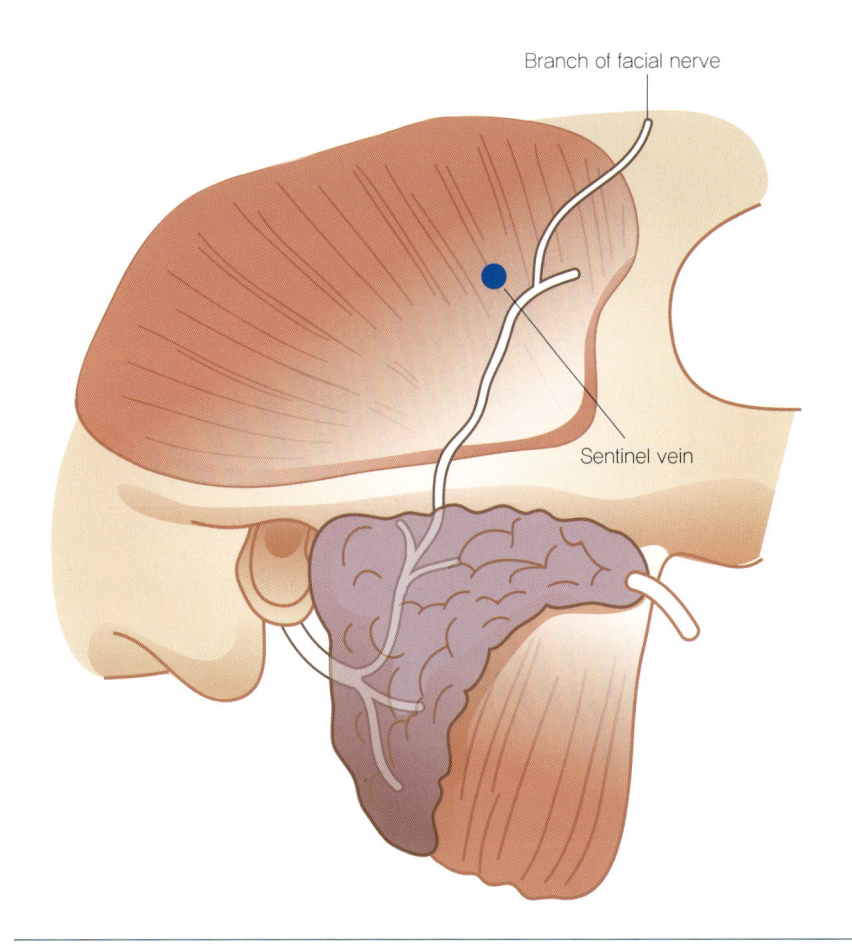

Safe Filler Injection Technique Demonstration – using live imaging tools

Fig. 4-39 Point where the sentinel vein exits (blue dot)

5) The Middle Temporal Vein

The sentinel vein penetrates the superficial layer of the DTF and connects with the middle temporal vein (MTV). The MTV is located within the temporal fat pad between the superficial layer and deep layer of the DTF (Fig. 4-41). Its internal diameter is approximately 3~5 mm and it drains through the superficial temporal vein (Fig. 4-40).

The sentinel vein and the MTV, large caliber veins, are the largest veins in the face. If any one of these veins is punctured and accidental intravascular injection of filler material occurs while treating the temple region, pulmonary embolism can result. The filler embolus flows through the jugular vein into the heart and eventually to the pulmonary artery. Based on recent reports, there have been three cases of pulmonary embolism after fat injection into the temple region. In one of these, the patient was under general anesthesia and died as a result.

In contrast to other areas of the face, the temples contain complicated layers and an arterial and venous system. Accordingly, a thorough understanding of anatomy must be obtained prior to proceeding with any procedures.

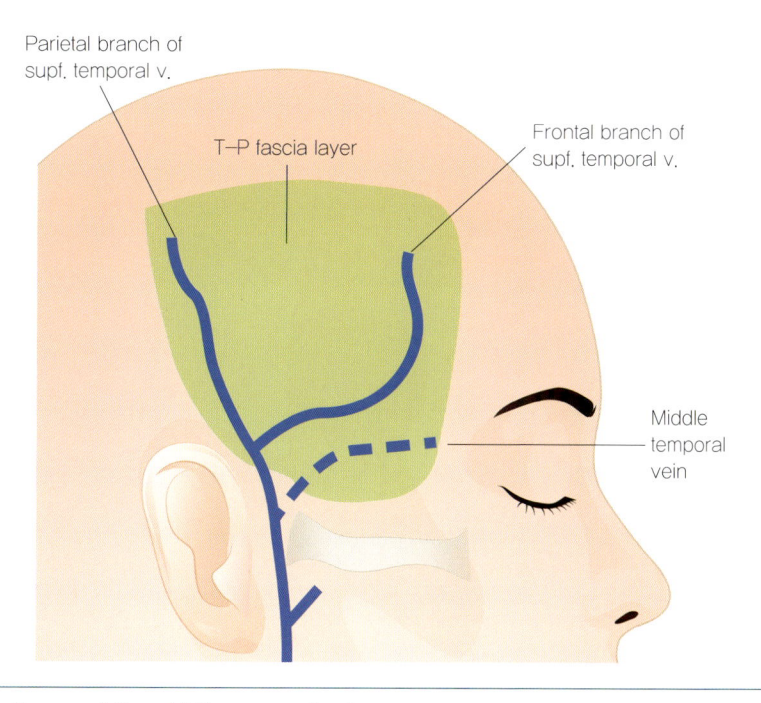

Fig. 4-40   Course of the middle temporal vein

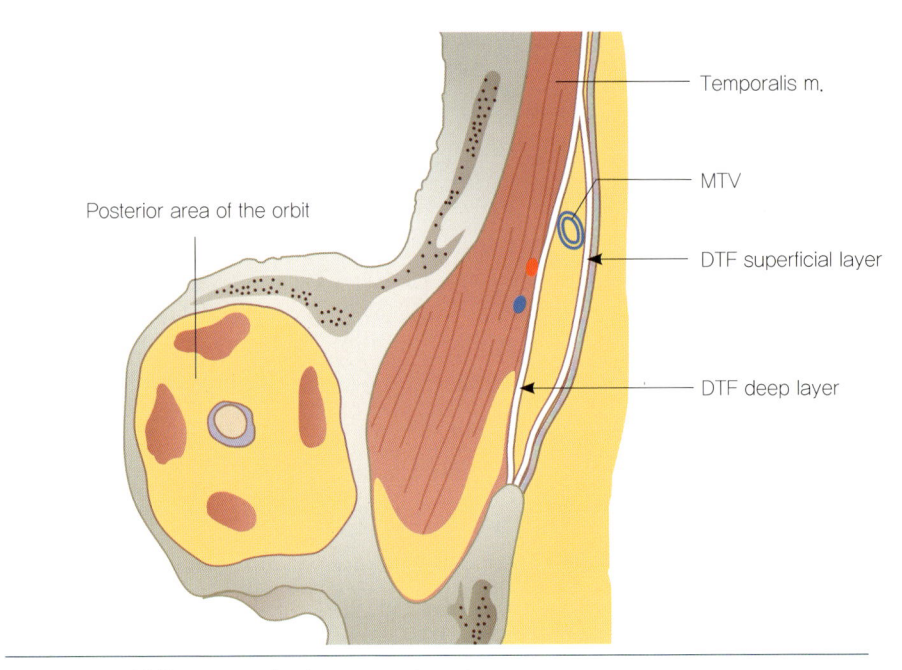

Safe Filler Injection Technique Demonstration – using live imaging tools

Fig. 4-41 Middle temporal vein - coronal section

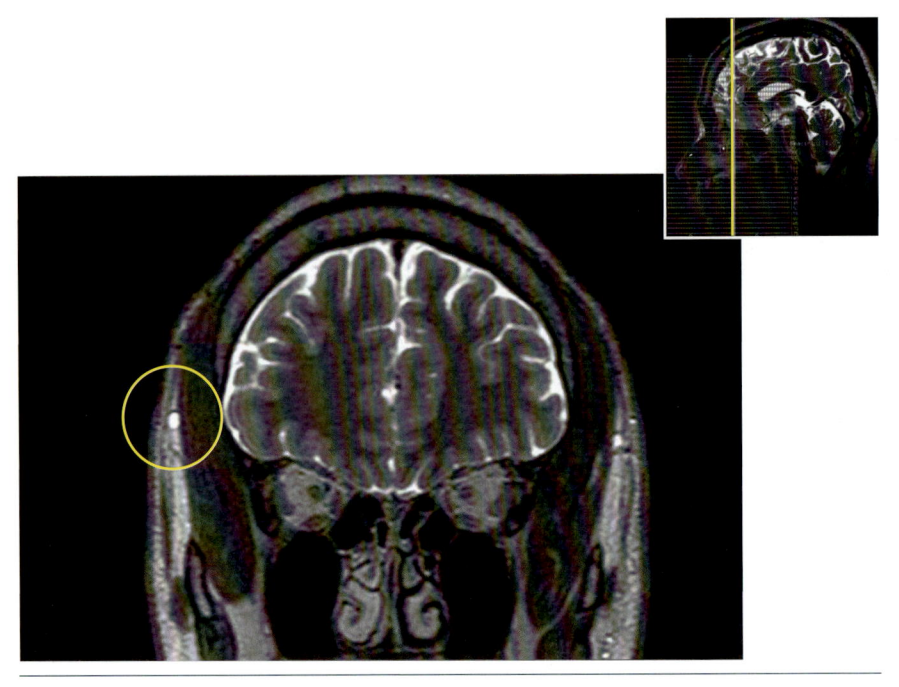

Fig. 4-42 MRI of the temples (1) - coronal view

Compared to a needle, a cannula does not guarantee safety. Regardless of the equipment used for injection, it is important to select an entry point that minimizes vessel puncture and to administer an appropriate volume in the injection layer.

The high signal seen in the circle is the middle temporal vein. The image shows its location between the superficial layer and the deep layer of the deep temporal fascia. As this is a very thick blood vessel, it is easily damaged. Only after a thorough review of the important landmarks for avoiding complications should the injection layer be selected.

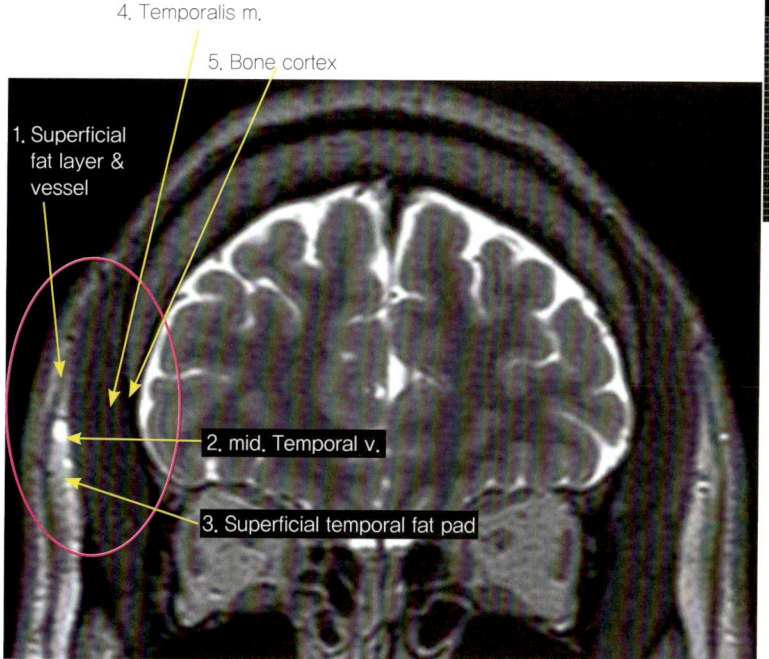

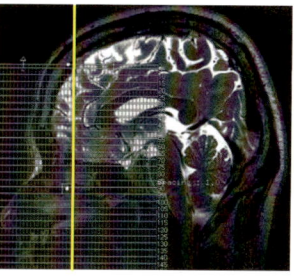

Fig. 4-43 MRI of the temples (2). 1. This shows the superficial fat area around the temples and the vessels that pass through the layer. 2. The middle temporal vein is shown in another fat layer that is distinct from the superficial fat layer. In the deep temporal fascia, the temporal fat pad is located between the superficial and deep sections. 3. The temporal fat pad mentioned above. 4. The temporalis can be seen easily. 5. The temporal bone cortex can be observed in black.

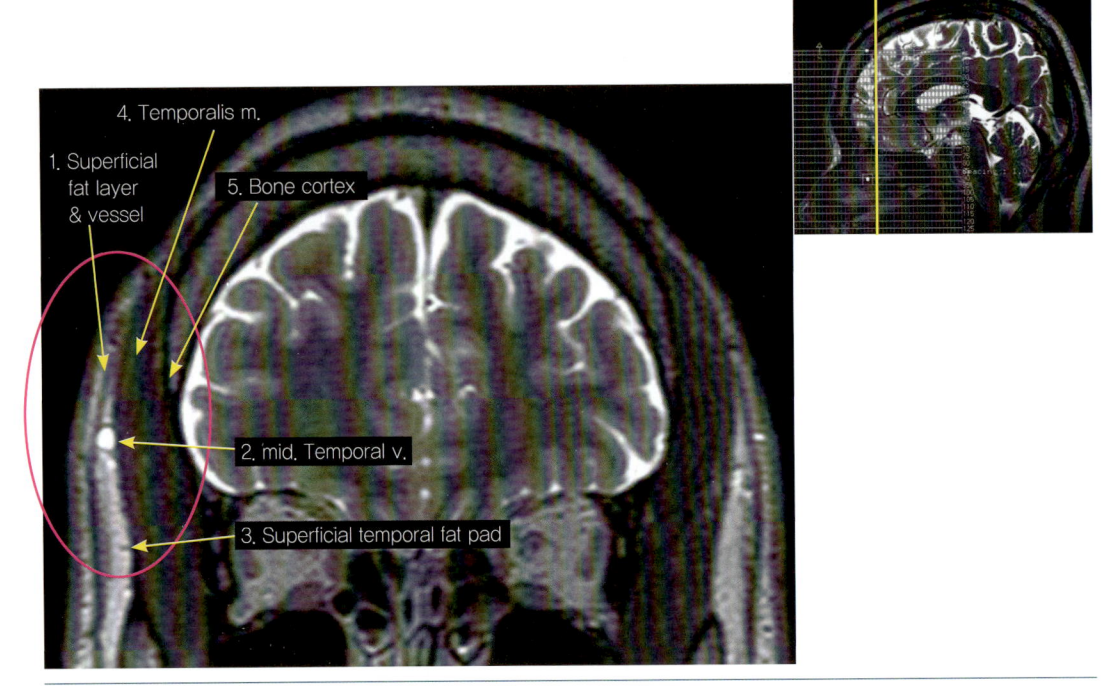

Safe Filler Injection Technique Demonstration – using live imaging tools

Fig. 4-44   MRI (3) of the temples

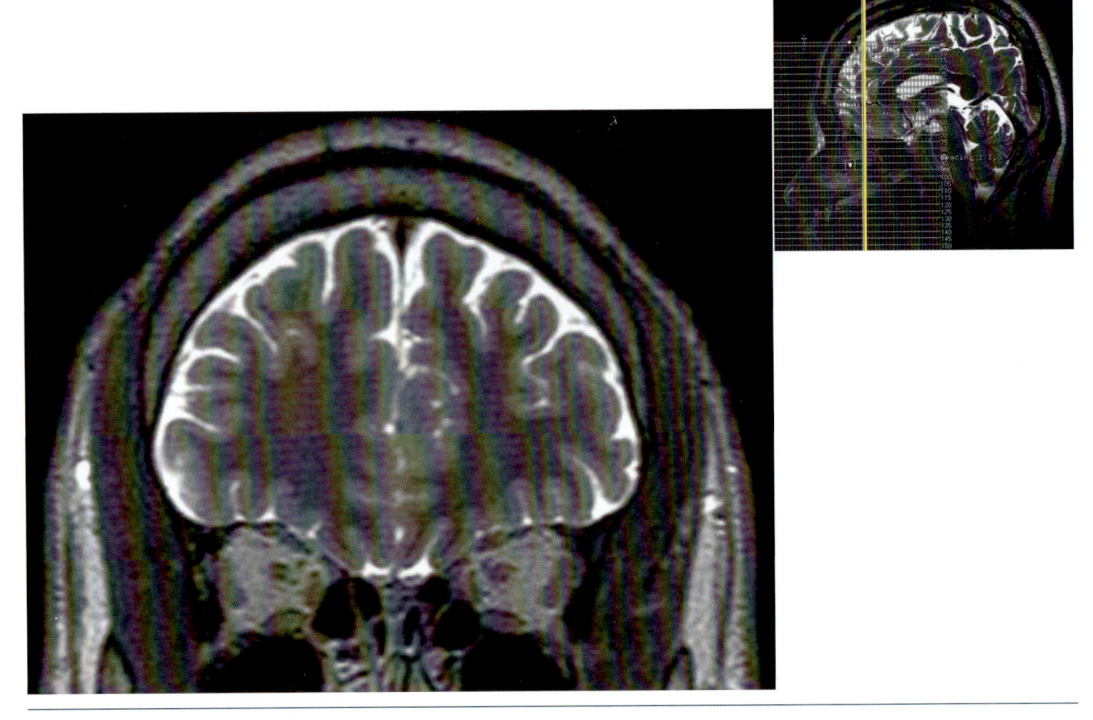

Fig. 4-45   MRI (4) of the temples

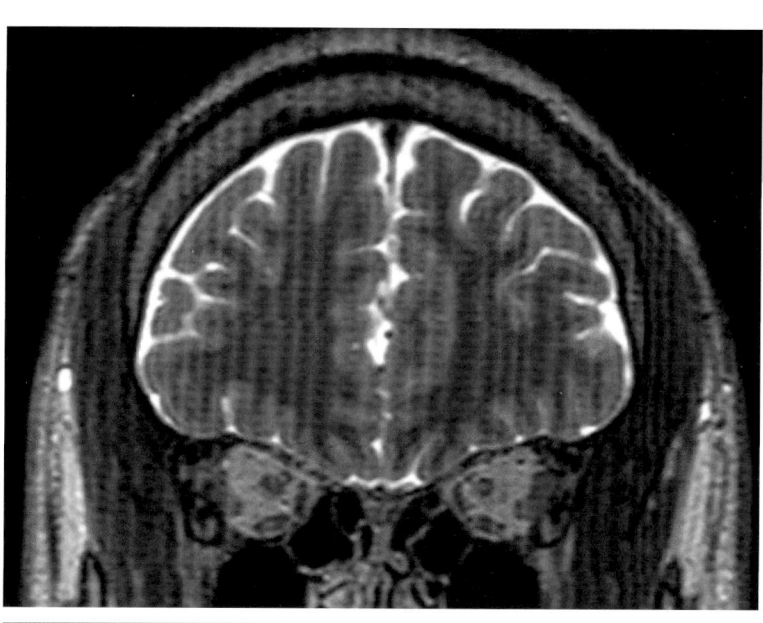

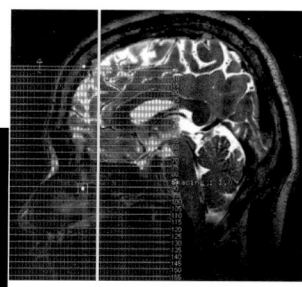

Fig. 4-46　MRI (5) of the temples

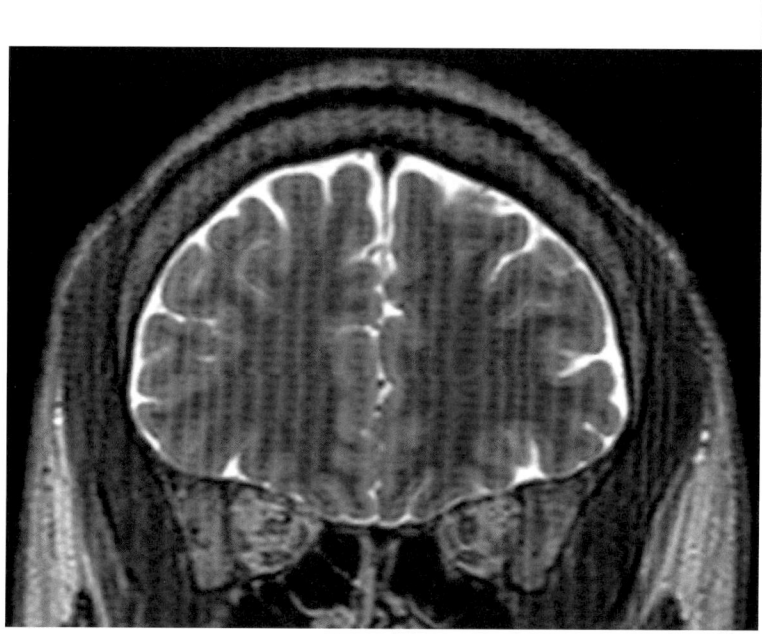

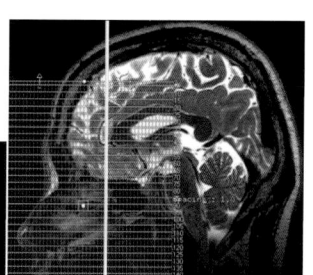

Fig. 4-47　MRI (6) of the temples

> **Imaging explanation**
> - Standards on injection depth must be established as many vessels, including the mid temporal vein, pass through this region.
> - In general, it is best to inject fillers very deeply below the temporalis muscle.
> - Alternatively, it is also safe to inject into the layer located between the superficial temporal fascia and deep temporal fascia.

3 Choice of Filler

1) Deep Injection

High viscosity fillers, which can implement volumizing effects just above the periosteum, should be used.

2) Superficial Injection

Mid to high viscosity fillers must be used.

4 Demonstration of Technique

The boundaries of temple are defined as zygoma at the bottom and temporal crest anterosuperiorly. Due to this structure, there is no need to concern for the filler substances migrating below or above its targeted area at the time of injection.

Depending on the layer in which fillers are injected, either of superficial injection and deep injection, is recommended in general.

Firstly, superficial injection is a method that uses a cannula to inject into the layer lying between the TPF and DTF. With accurate targeting skills followed by gentle injection into the layer, the risk of puncturing the vessel can be minimized and satisfactory augmentation can be achieved with a small amount of

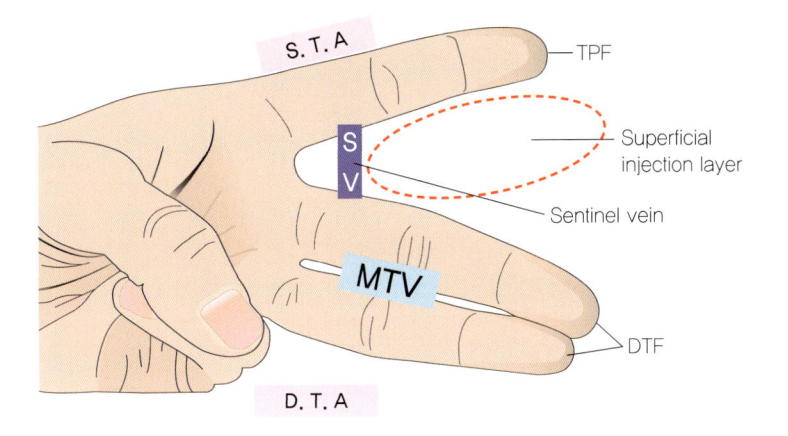

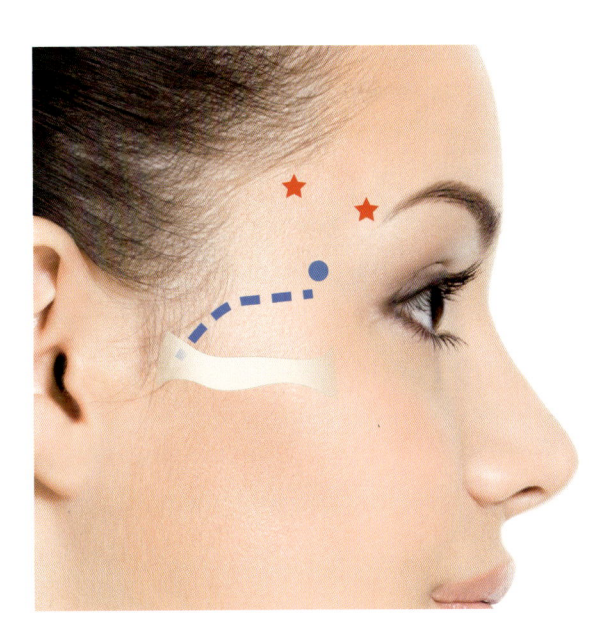

Fig. 4-48 Superficial injection layer & entry point of the temples
Blue dot: sentinel vein, Blue dotted line: Middle temporal vein, Red star: entry point,
SV: Sentinel Vein, MTV: Middle Temporal Vein

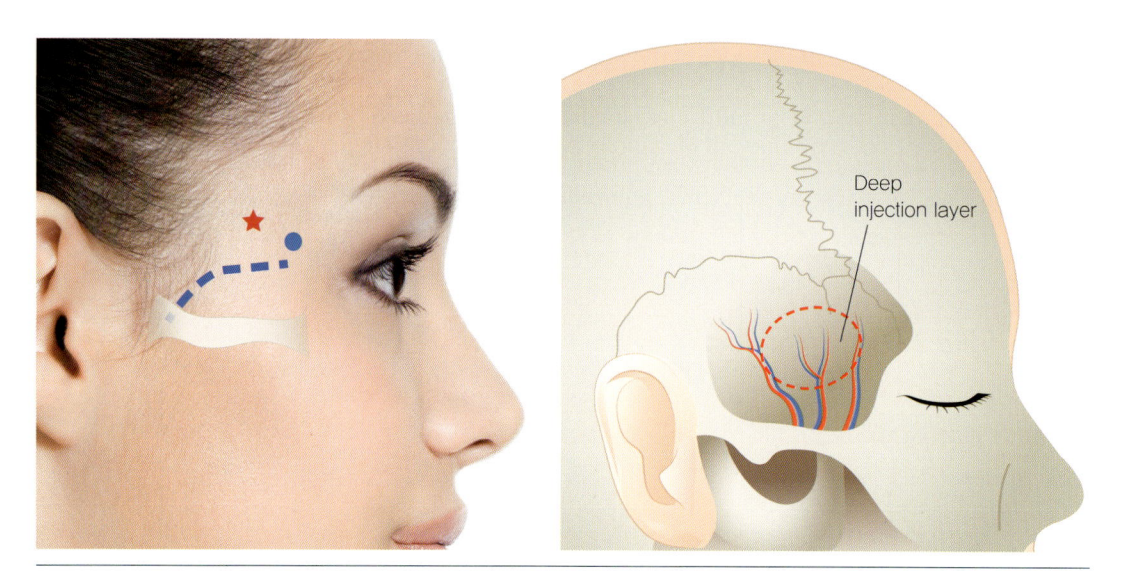

Fig. 4-49 Deep injection layer & entry point of the temples.
Blue dot: sentinel vein, Blue dotted line: Middle temporal vein, Red star: entry point

filler. However, it is often difficult to target the layer accurately. If an injection is made between the two layers of the DTF or into the layer right below the DTF, filler migration into the prezygomatic space or buccal fat is possible. We should note that it is more difficult to target injections into the fat layer between the two layers of the DTF because MTV is passing through this region in the horizontal direction. If a fan technique is used for injection, it is possible for the cannula to face and hit the MTV.

Secondly, after inserting a needle either perpendicularly or at a slight angle, inject filler deeply on the supraperiosteum level after performing the bone touch. The needle must not be withdrawn after the bone touch because this may allow injection into the blood vessel. Recently, there was a case report on blindness right after the treatment on the temporal area using this method; accordingly, an injection must be made after aspiration was confirmed upon bone touch. Moreover, there is a possibility that a vessel is damaged after the needle passes through the multiple skin layers, so it is recommended to check whether there is hematoma immediately after the procedure. If the injection is to be made deeply, a greater amount of filler is needed for augmentation.

Any physician can effortlessly bring similarly effective results for this type of injection than for superficial injection.

5 Complications

1) Bruises and Hematoma

- Since there are many developed arteries and veins in the temporal area bruises and hematoma can occur easily.
- At the puncture point, bleeding can easily occur from the sentinel vein at the lateral margin of the eyebrow. It is helpful to check the location of blood vessels visually prior to the procedure.
- For superficial injections, watch out for bleeding of the superficial temporal artery and vein. Since the artery can be palpated at the hairline, check the location of the artery prior to the procedure.
- For deep injections, watch out for bleeding of the deep temporal artery and vein.

2) Blindness

- Blindness has been reported after procedures around the temporal.
- Regardless it is a needle or cannula, gently make an insertion with it and be cautious not to inject any filler substances into the blood vessels (see Complication – Blindness, Part 5).

3) Embolism

- Although it is uncommon, some studies have reported cases of embolism after autologous fat transplantation.
- In the event that blood vessels are injected into via the sentinel vein or the middle temporal vein, the largest veins in the face, pulmonary embolism can occur through the external jugular vein affected by venous drainage (see Complication – Pulmonary Embolism, Part 5).

SUMMARY of Temples

A

- Three layers of Fascia
  - → TPF (Temporo-Parietal Fascia)
  - → Deep temporal fascia (DTF) superficial layer
  - → Deep temporal fascia (DTF) deep layer
- Location of the superficial temporal artery & vein and deep temporal artery & vein
- Location of the sentinel vein and middle temporal vein

B

- The face is not ideal with the presence of temporal hollowness.
- In case of severe hollowness, the shape of the face appears as the number 8, making the person look ill and old.
- Make the facial line starting from the temples to the zygomas and cheeks into one smooth curve.

C

- HA filler

  deep injection: Filler with high viscosity

  superficial injection: Filler with mid- to high viscosity

- Fillers with very low viscosity are subject to migration. Even though temporal area exhibits relatively low muscle movement, it is connected to areas with buccal fat, or the prezygomatic space that may allow relocation of fillers.

D

- Superficial injection
  - Insert a cannula between the TPF and DTF.
  - Safely augment the face with a small amount of filler.
  - Be aware that this layer is difficult to target with high accuracy.
- Deep injection
  - Inject filler with a needle just above the supraperiosteum of the deep layer.
  - Be cautious of bruises and hematomas; a large amount filler is required.
  - Anyone can get a good result.

X
- Temporal area has plenty of blood vessels and nerves present.
- Be cautious of big bruises. They usually occur when the superficial temporal artery & vein and deep temporal artery & vein are damaged.
- Be cautious of pulmonary embolism. They occur after injection into large blood vessels, such as the sentinel vein and middle temporal vein.

Mid Face

4. Nose

• • •   Rhinoplalsty using fillers dramatically transforms the face with a simple procedure. This is an area that is most in demand, usually learned at the beginner stage together with the nasolabial folds. However, dermal necrosis from excessive augmentation of the nose tip and ophthalmology complications such as blindness from intravenous filler injection near the radix area can result from the nose treatment. Therefore, a thorough understanding of anatomical structure is required prior to performance. If a dramatic transformation post plastic surgery is desired, it is not always advisable to recommend filler procedures to the patient. Therefore, it is necessary to carefully consult with patients before the procedure.

Proceed with nose filler treatment when
- Surgery is not desired
- A natural improved look with a slight change is desired
- No down time is desired

Do not proceed with nose filler treatment when
- An extreme change in the nose height is desired
- Expected surgical results are greater than the results possible in real life.

1 Beauty

Criteria for an Ideal Nose	1. The length of the entire nose is 1/3 of the length of the entire face (same as the height of the forehead) 2. The horizontal width of the nose is 1/5 of the horizontal width of the entire face 3. Naso-frontal angle is 115 to 130 degrees 4. Naso-labial angle is 90 to 95 degrees for men and 95 to 105 degrees for women

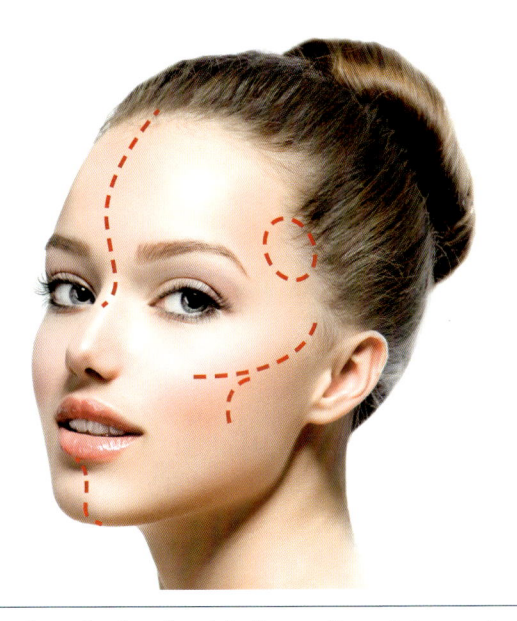

Fig. 4-50 S-line starts from forehead – glabella – radix and then ends at the nose by coming out straight.

2 Anatomy

There are five types of nose filler procedures, depending on the area of augmentation.

- radix
- dorsum
- nasal tip
- columella
- nasolabial angle

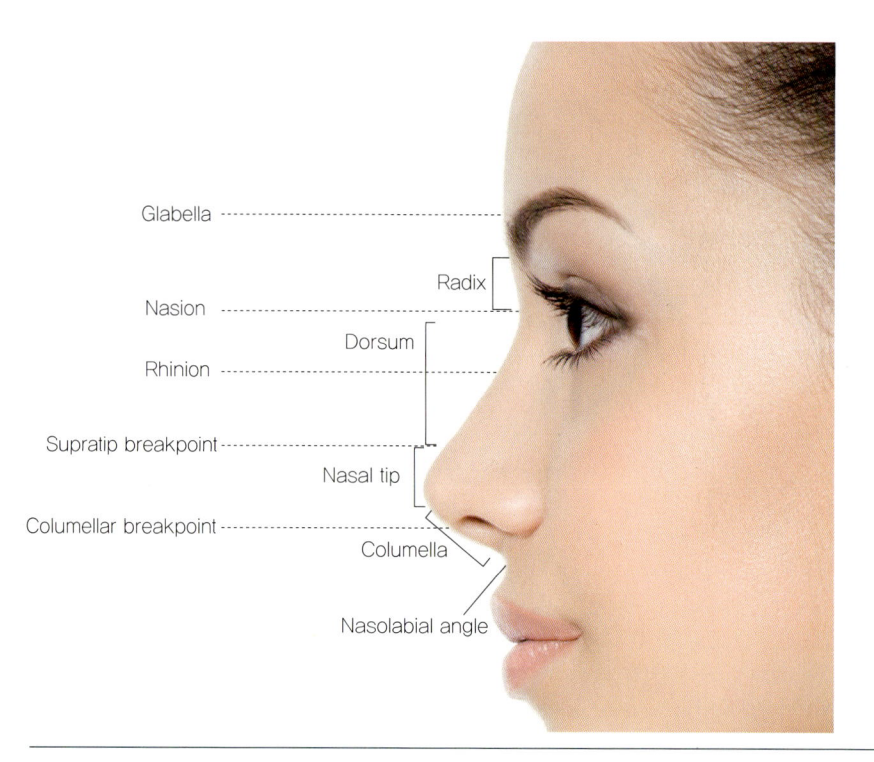

Safe Filler Injection Technique Demonstration – using live imaging tools

Fig. 4-51 **Five divisions of the nose**

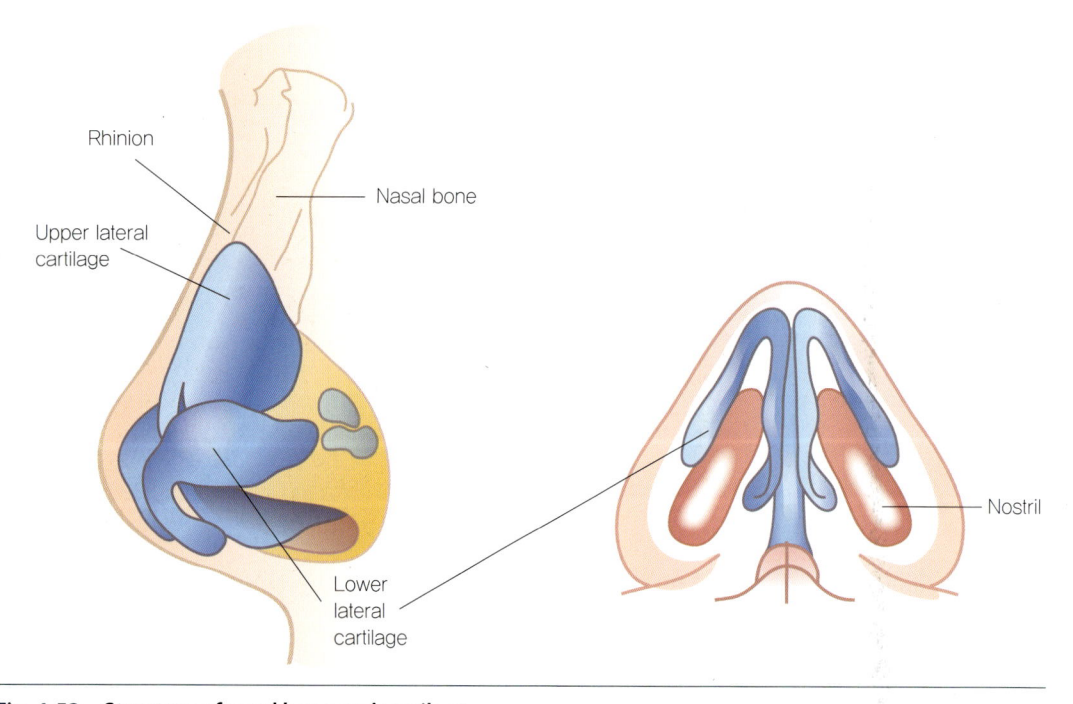

Fig. 4-52 **Structure of nasal bone and cartilage**

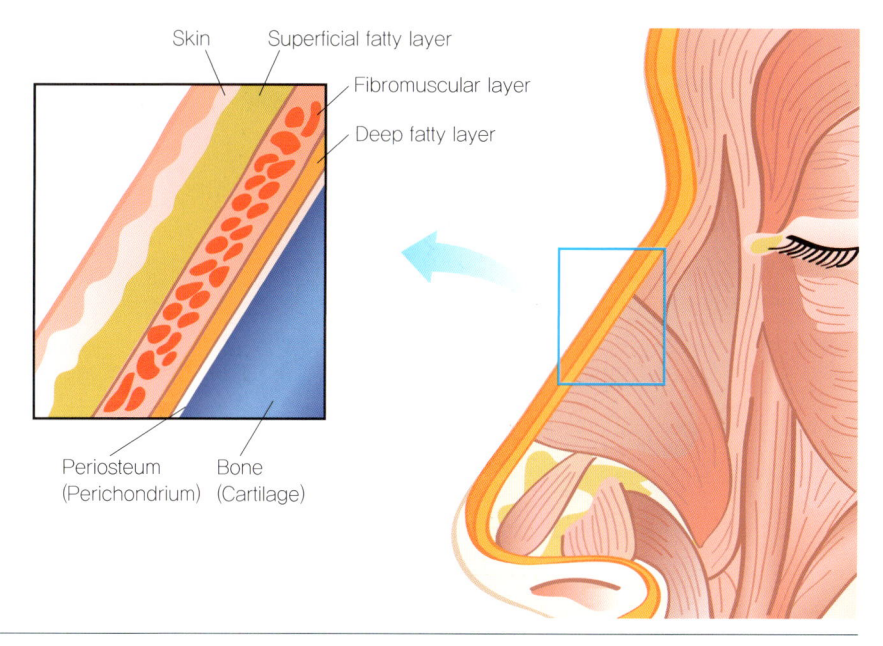

Fig. 4-53　Cross section of the nose skin

Arteries in the nose are located in the fibromuscular layer or in between the fibromuscular layer and the deep fatty layer (Fig. 4-53). As for the glabella and radix, the superficial vein is often developed around the midline as well.

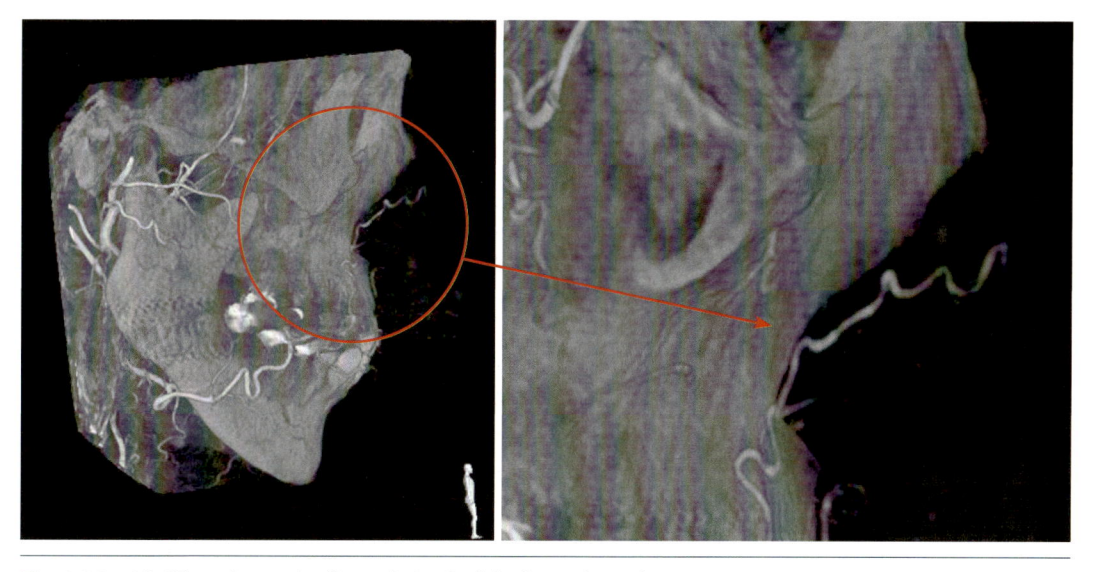

Fig. 4-54　3D CT angiography (lateral view) of the lateral nasal artery

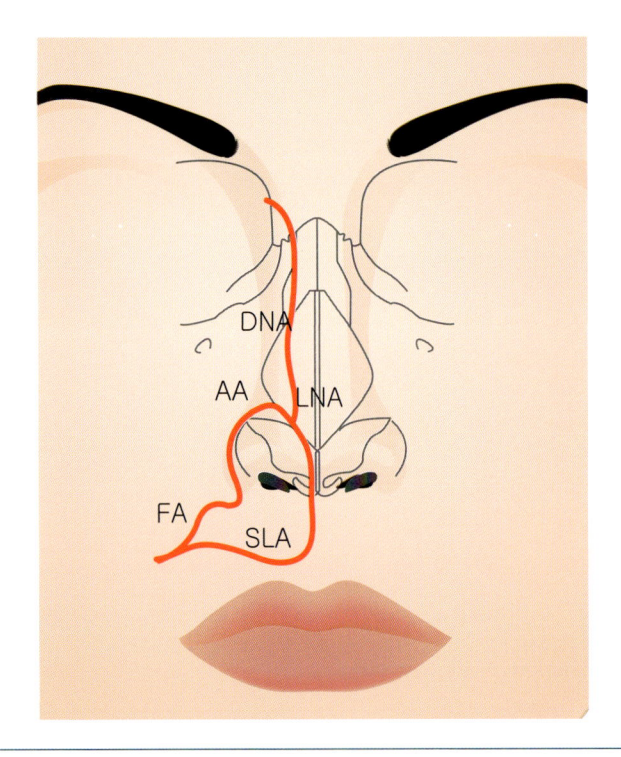

Fig. 4-55 Arterial supply of the nose.
DNA: dorsal nasal artery, AA: angular artery, LNA: lateral nasal artery, SLA: superior labial artery, FA: facial artery

Intercanthal vein

This is the vein that connects the angular veins on both sides of the nose like a bridge. It is located in the subcutanous layer on top of the procerus muscle.

When filler substance is injected intravenously by an accident, it is expected to flow via one of the following two routes:

1) Supratrochlear vein → supra-ophthalmic vein → cavernous sinus → int. jugular vein
2) Angular vein → facial vein → ext. jugular vein

Both 1) and 2) can result in embolism by venous drainage.

During procedures, use the opposite hand to pinch the treatment area and make sure the vessel is lifted before injection in order to prevent injecting into the blood vessel.

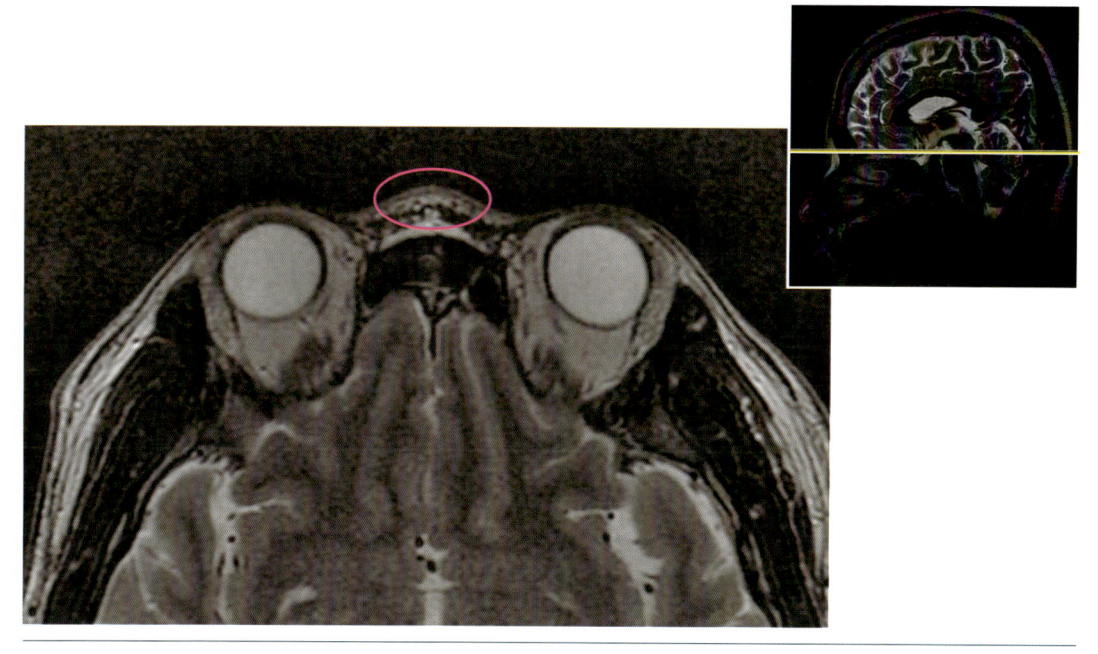

Fig. 4-56 MRI of the nose (1)

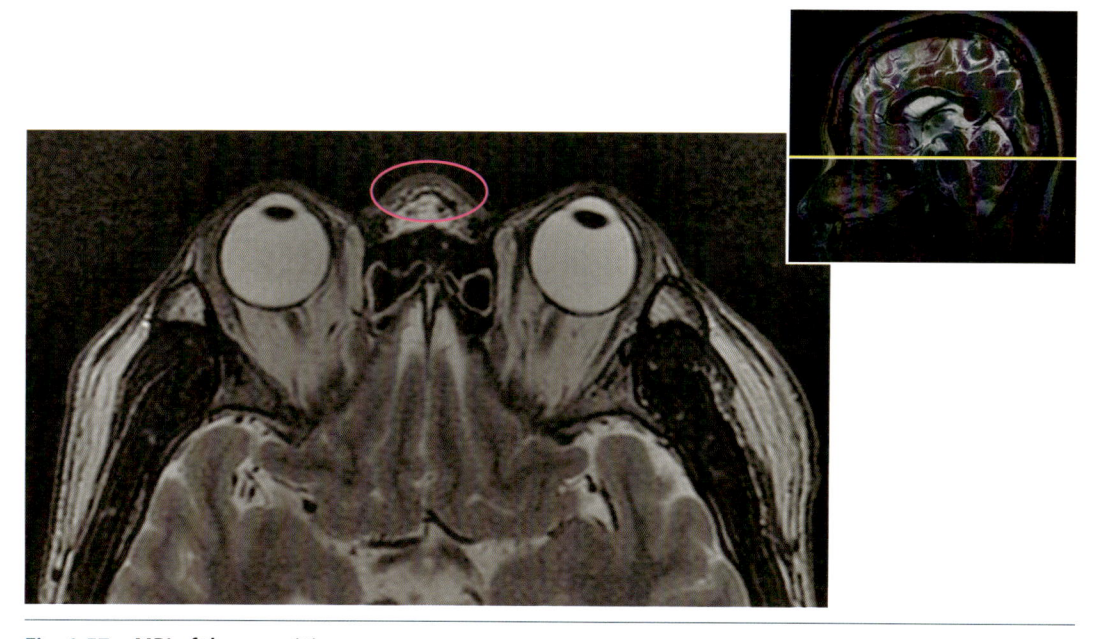

Fig. 4-57 MRI of the nose (2)
This clearly shows that blood vasculature lies within the subcutaneous fat layer. For procedures on the bridge of the nose, targeting just above the periosteum of the deep layer would be safe.

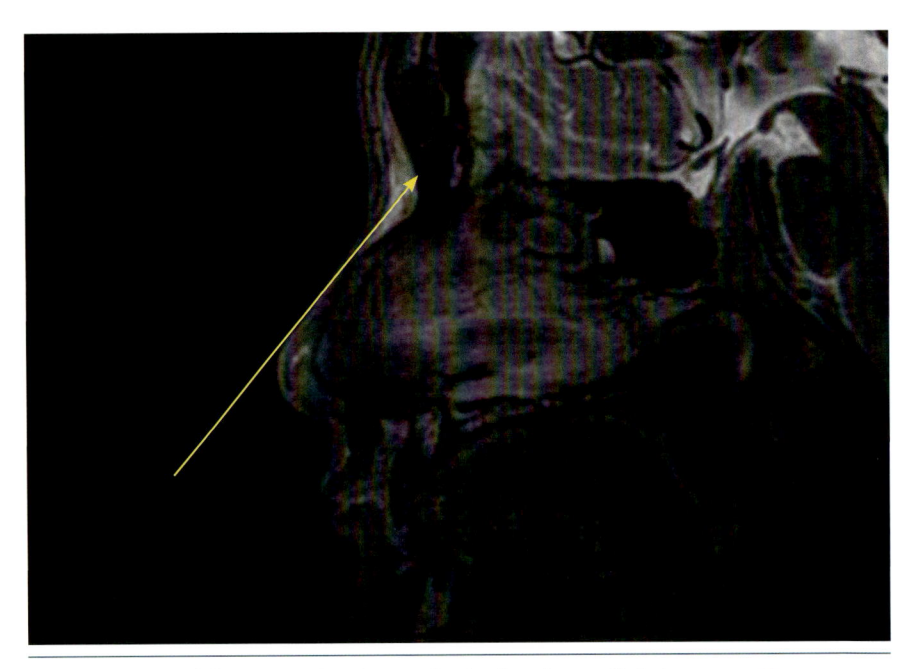

Safe Filler Injection Technique Demonstration – using live imaging tools

Fig. 4-58   MRI of the nose. Injection method using the sagital view-cannula

3 Choice of Filler

- Calcium fillers are advantageous for relatively high durability and ability to maintain their original shape. However, due to these characteristics that are quite difficult to reverses, caution must be taken not to cause malpractice or consequent complications.
- It is best to choose HA fillers with hard physical characteristics. For instance, biphasic fillers with large particles and high viscoelasticity would be appropriate to use. As for monophasic fillers, fillers with high viscoelasticity and concentration are anticipated to bring better results.
- If the procedure is performed on the bridge of the nose without causing significant bleeding, the finished shape will likely be maintained for a long period of time even with monophasic fillers. In fact, for the bridge of the nose or the tip of the nose, it is best to use biphasic or monophasic fillers with high viscoelasticity.
- For the best result, it is crucial to choose the most appropriate filler after carefully analyzing the shape of the patient's nose.

4 Demonstration of Technique

1) Augmentation of the Dorsum and Radix

Depending on the method of the procedure, there are different approaches for using a needle or a cannula.

Moreover, the injection method can be also varied by the location of the entry point. Here, we introduce two different injection techniques that the authors commonly use, each using a cannula or a needle.

Firstly, the method for using a cannula involves making an entry point at the tip of the nose or between the tip of the nose and the nose bridge. In this method, the cannula is inserted to reach the space between the lower lateral cartilage and the supra-pericondrium, which is right above the upper lateral cartilage – or the supra-periosteum, right above the nasal bone – radix, as seen in Fig. 4-60. After that, injection slowly take place while pulling out the cannula cautiously.

For needle use, the same method can be used (Fig. 4-60). Additionally, injections can be performed at multiple points that are relevant to each division of the entire nose. By entering each point perpendicularly or at a slope, injection can be proceeded after touching the cartilage or the bone (Fig. 4-59).

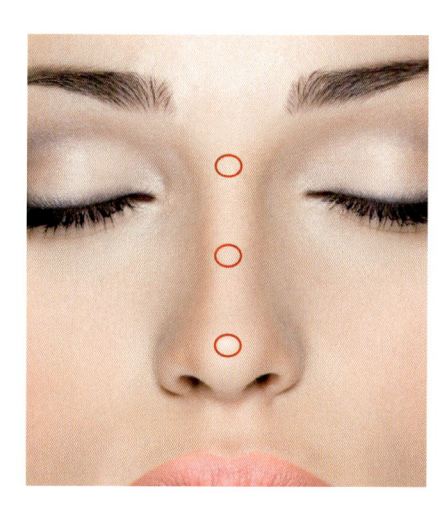

Fig. 4-59 Injection method for the nose

Safe Filler Injection Technique Demonstration – using live imaging tools

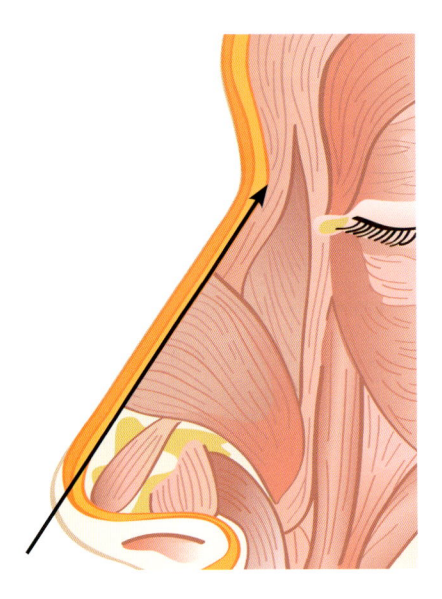

Fig. 4-60 Nose filler injection method using a cannula

2) Collumella Augmentation

- The method of the procedure depends on the equipment used, a needle or cannula.
- The tip of the nose can be lifted by injecting a small amount of toxin into the Depresso septi nasi. This effect of toxin can be enhanced if it is injected together with filler.

3) Cautions to be Taken during Nose Filler Procedures

- The direction of injection should conform the midline.
- The injection plane must be the supra-periosteum/pericondrium in order to reduce the risk of puncturing and pressuring the blood vessels.
- An excessive amount should not be injected. It is advisable to be especially cautious with the tip of the nose.
  - During not only the first procedure, but also during the second (a touch-up) procedure, the injection amount should be adjusted appropriately.

- Even though the filler has dissolved, newly formed collagen around the filler is remained. so, the newly constructed tissues will be denser than before and the mobility of the blood vessels within that region will decrease, increasing the possibility of pressuring the blood vessels even if the same amount filler is injected. Thus, it is advisable to perform the second procedure more gently.
- After a surgery is performed, the thickness and the hardness of the subcutaneous fatty layer should be checked. Filler procedures are not recommended and only the minimum amount is to be injected if it is necessary (occasionally, patients do not disclose that they had a nasal surgery).
• In order to increase satisfaction after the procedure, communication with the patient about what s/he desires is to be made in advance.

5 Complications

1) Skin Necrosis

- After nasal filler procedures, slight skin necrosis may occur.
- Within the nosal area, the distance between the bone (cartilage) and the epidermis is relatively small compared to other facial areas. Moreover, the dermal layer constitutes a great fraction of the skin compared to other facial areas, which consequently suggests that there is insufficient space for fillers to expand the nasal skin. Therefore, when filler is injected into the nose area, there is a high possibility that the blood vessels will be pressed by the filler lumps.
- It is best to inject fillers after confirming the bone (or cartilage) touch.
- Thick nasal tip is commonly seen in many patients. For this particular feature, it is advisable to avoid injecting an excessive amount of filler with a high lifting capacity around the nasal tip (see Blood Vessel Complications, 1-8, Part 5).

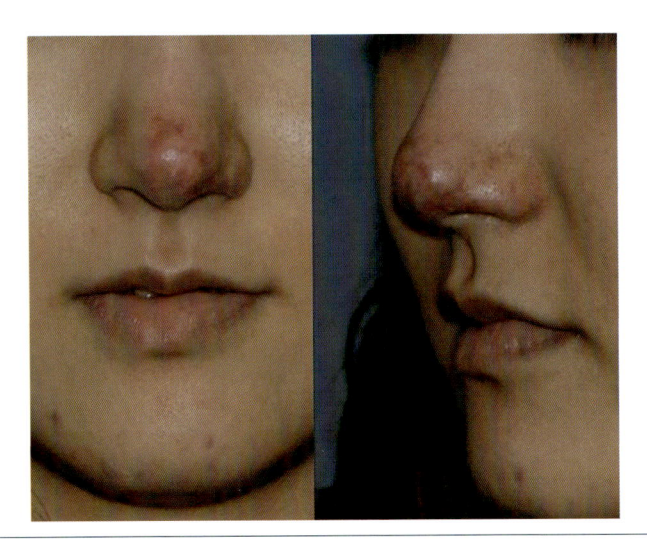

Safe Filler Injection Technique Demonstration – using live imaging tools

Fig. 4-61 Impending necrosis after filler injection

2) Blindness

In the event that the filler substance was injected into the artery, fillers can move backward toward the ophthalmic artery through the dorsal nasal artery, and then block the retinal artery leading to blindness. In case of a treatment around the radix area, injections must be made into the supraperiosteum of midline in order to avoid the blockage of dorsal nasal artery.

3) Hematoma

Around the radix, the intercanthal veins are complexly intertwined in the subQ layer, so caution must be taken when using a needle during the procedure. After pinching it with the thumb and the index finger of the opposite hand and lifting the blood vessels residing in the subQ layer, an injection can be made into the supraperiosteum layer.

SUMMARY of Nose

A
- Understanding of the cross section of the radix, dorsum, nasal tip and columella
- Study on the movements of main arteries, the LNA and the DNA and the veins, and the ICV

B
- Standards of an ideal nose shape
- Ratio, angle, nasal tip, nasal bridge, etc.

C
- Calcium fillers are renowned for highdurability and ability to maintain the original shape
- HA fillers with hard physical properties should be chosen.

D
- Cannula injection: parallel to cartilage/bone, on the suprapericondrium/ supraperiosteum
  Needle injection: perpendicular injection on the suprapericondrium/supraperi-osteum
- In case of a hooked nose, a cannula should not cross the middle part of the nose.

X
- Procedures must be performed only on the middle of the nose. Procedures on the sides are dangerous.
- Caution must be taken for performing a needle procedure on the nose bridge due to the danger of injecting into the intercanthal vein. Inject fillers on the supraperiosteum layer after pinching
- Procedures must only be performed after a bone touch (excluding the nasal tip area)
- Take a great caution regarding the blood circulation and pressure at the nose tip

5. Nasolabial Folds

••• Treatment of nasolabial folds is different from most other filler procedures which involve correcting dermal atrophy seen as hollowness/depressions on the skin. The nasolabial folds form as a result of atrophy or loss of connective tissue in subcutaneous layer and not so much from atrophy of the dermal layer. The mechanism of nasolabial fold formation also involves changes in the fat compartments associated with skin laxity in the malar area that occurs with aging. Hence, simply injecting a lot of filler will not result in an aesthetically desired appearance. Moreover, there is a lot of activity in the nasolabial area ranging from facial expressions to chewing so there is a risk that the implanted filler migrates from the originally injected site.

Therefore, in the event that procedures are performed without clearly understanding the characteristics of the nasolabial folds, there is a risk of an undesired result or patient dissatisfaction. Accordingly, when consulting the patient concerned about the nasolabial fold area, it is best to check the basics. Making a routine check list to be used during consultation is helpful.

1 Beauty

If patient also presents cheek ptosis
- Loss and descent of cheek fat pad → Treat the upper cheek
- Consider loss of skin elasticity
- Resorption of soft tissues and bony structures must be corrected

The severity of nasolabial folds varies by age and filler volume needs to be adjusted depending on age and severity. Using the MERZ AESTHETIC Scales, the current patient status and the amount of filler required can be explained easily (Fig. 4-62, for a more detailed explanation, see Fig. 4-21)

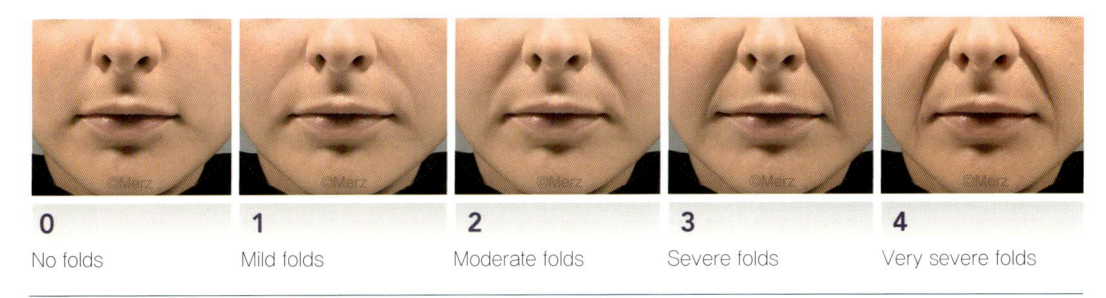

0	1	2	3	4
No folds	Mild folds	Moderate folds	Severe folds	Very severe folds

Fig. 4-62 MERZ AESTHETICS Scales (Nasolabial Folds-at rest)
Copyright© (2009) Merz Pharmaceuticals
Narins, et al. Validated assessment scales for the lower face. Dermatol Surg. 2012;38(2 Spec No.):332-42.

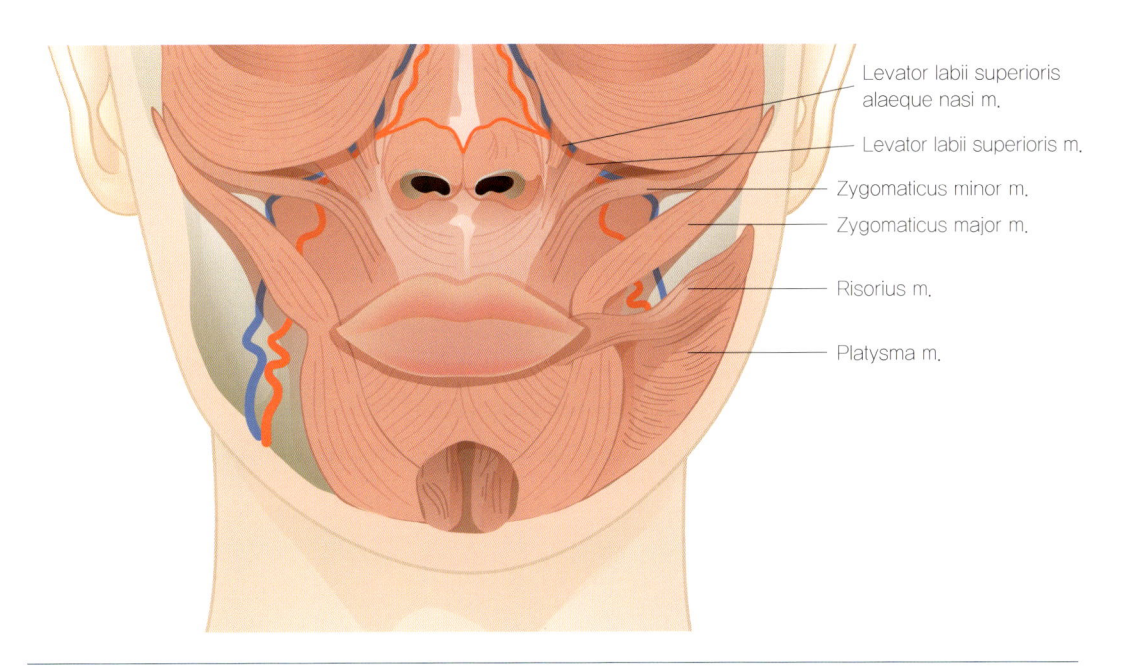

- Levator labii superioris alaeque nasi m.
- Levator labii superioris m.
- Zygomaticus minor m.
- Zygomaticus major m.
- Risorius m.
- Platysma m.

Fig. 4-63 Course of the facial artery and muscles

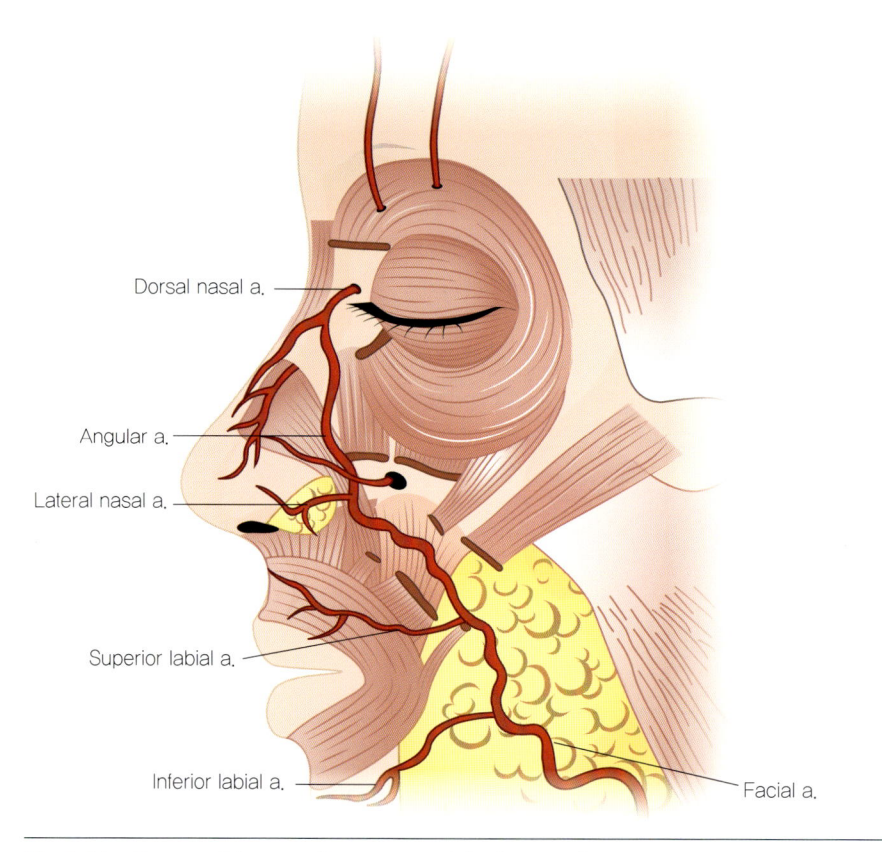

Safe Filler Injection Technique Demonstration – using live imaging tools

Fig. 4-64 Course of the angular artery and the lat. nasal artery

2 Anatomy

Safe treatment of the nasolabial folds requires a detailed understanding of the course of the facial artery and its variations.

- 43% of the time, the facial artery courses within 5 mm of the nasolabial folds

Superficial kinking of facial artery (Fig. 4-66)

- Facial artery becomes tortuous 1.5 cm lateral to the corner of the mouth.
- At the immediate superolateral region to the modiolus.
- Can be confirmed by visual inspection or palpation.

Modiolus (Fig. 4-66)

- Located 20~30 mm lateral and 10 mm inferior to the lateral margin of the lips.
- Chiasma of facial muscles held together by fibrous tissue. Recently being viewed as a tendon.

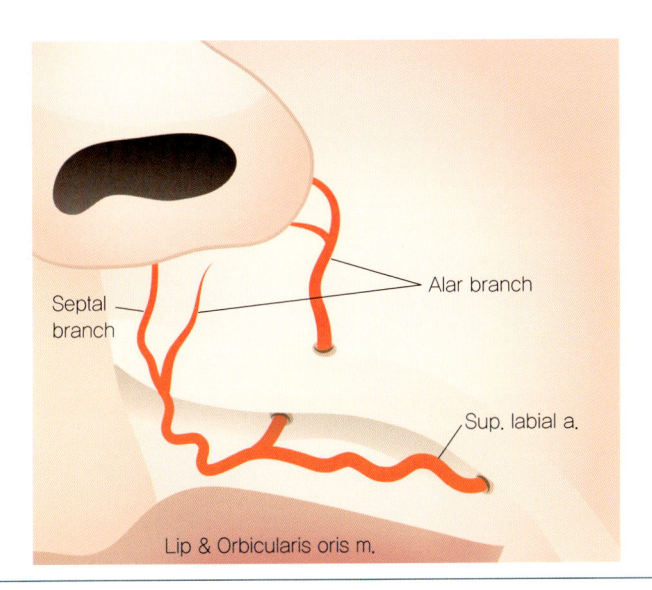

Fig. 4-65 Course of the superior labial artery and the alar branch
The alar branch branches off from the superior labial artery or from a region before the facial artery bifurcates into the lateral nasal artery. It may form a part of the columellar artery and supply the nasal ala area.

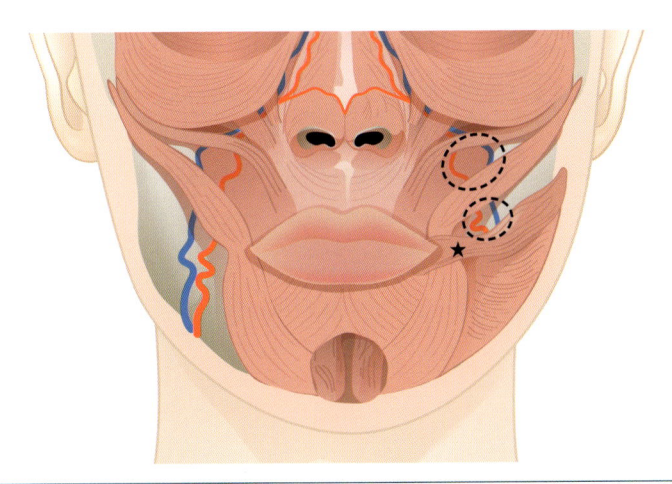

Fig. 4-66 Regions where the vessel kinks superficially (black dotted circle) and modiolus (black star)

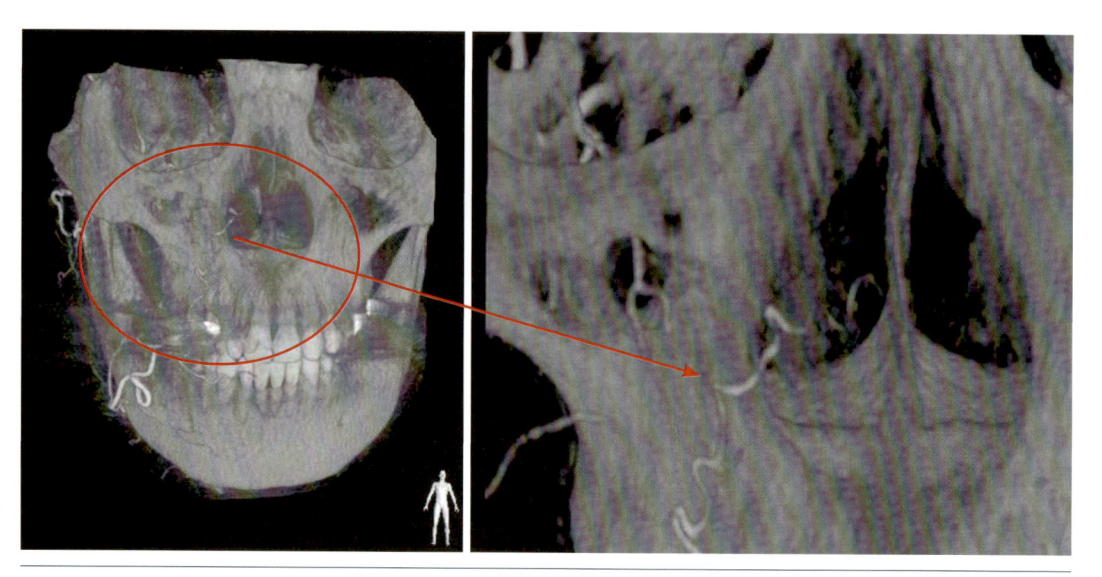

Safe Filler Injection Technique Demonstration – using live imaging tools

Fig. 4-67 3D CT angiography of the facial artery & lateral nasal artery (anterior view)

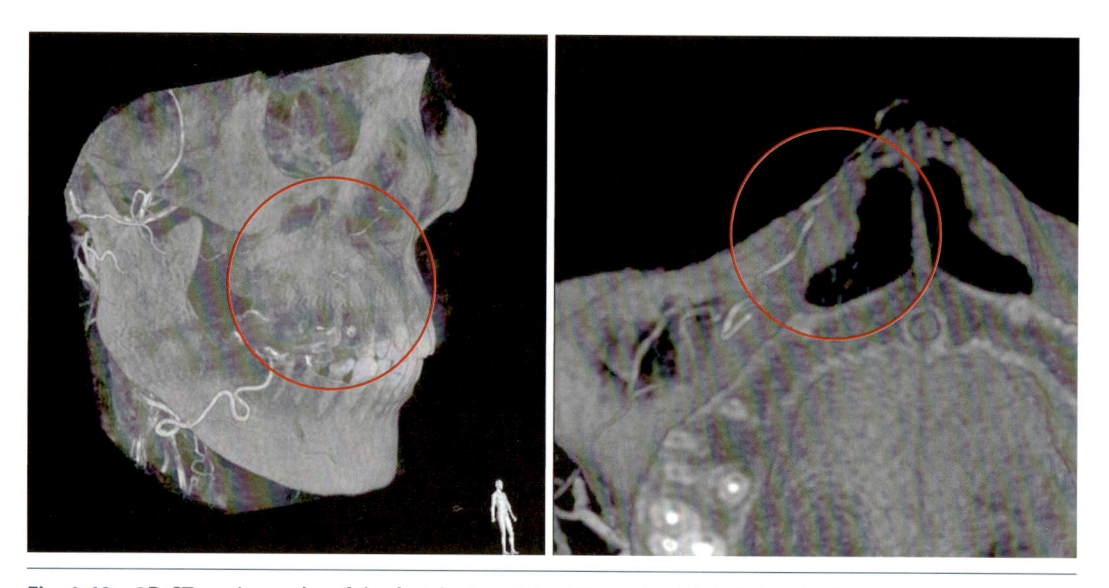

Fig. 4-68 3D CT angiography of the facial artery (Lt: oblique view/Rt: inferior view)

Upper lip elevator (muscle)

- The zygomaticus minor, levator labii superioris (LLS) and levator labii superioris alaeque nasi (LLSAN) muscles attach to the alar recess located in between the nasal ala and the upper lip.

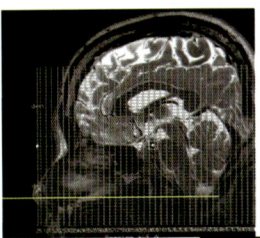

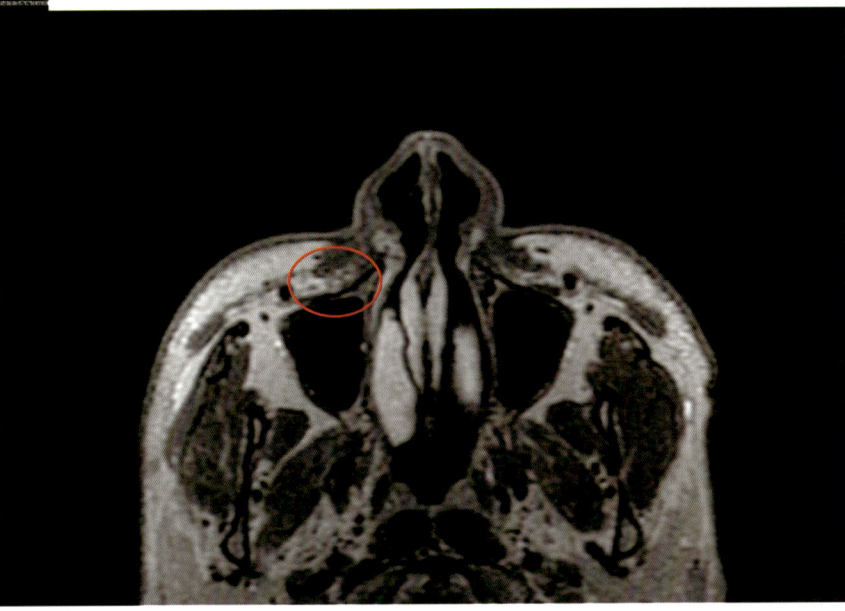

Fig. 4-69 MRI of the nasolabial folds (1). Transverse view

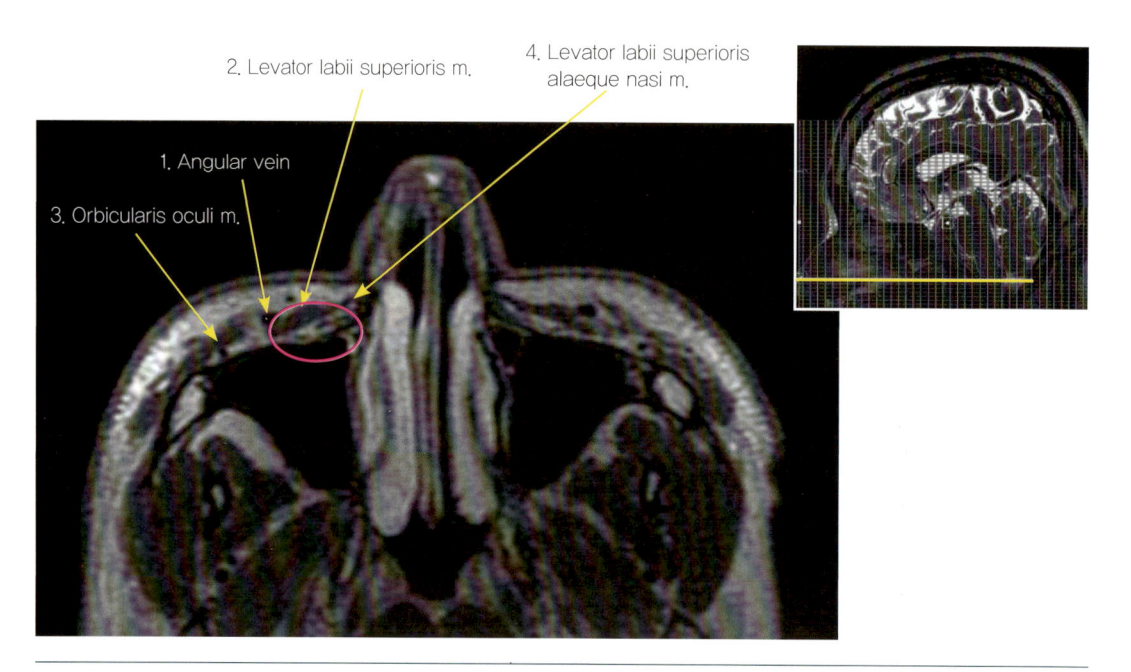

Safe Filler Injection Technique Demonstration – using live imaging tools

Fig. 4-70 MRI of nasolabial folds (2). **1.** Out of the angular artery and the vein, the major vessels of concern, the vein is more visible. The angular a. does not show well on the MRI, but the vein is visible. The size of angular vein is very large and courses superiorly passing through the SOOF layer. **2.** The vessels are located slightly lateral to the infra-orbital foramen so when performing infra-orbital nerve blocks caution must be taken not to injure the vessels. **3.** As the angular artery passes through the subcutaneous fat layer, the fat layer below the muscles is considered safe rather than the subcutaneous fatty layer. Injecting into the angular a. site can lead to blindness. **4.** The area within the red oval is the fat layer below the muscles and is generally the target layer for the treatment of nasolabial folds with fillers. However, there are some blood vessels passing this area.

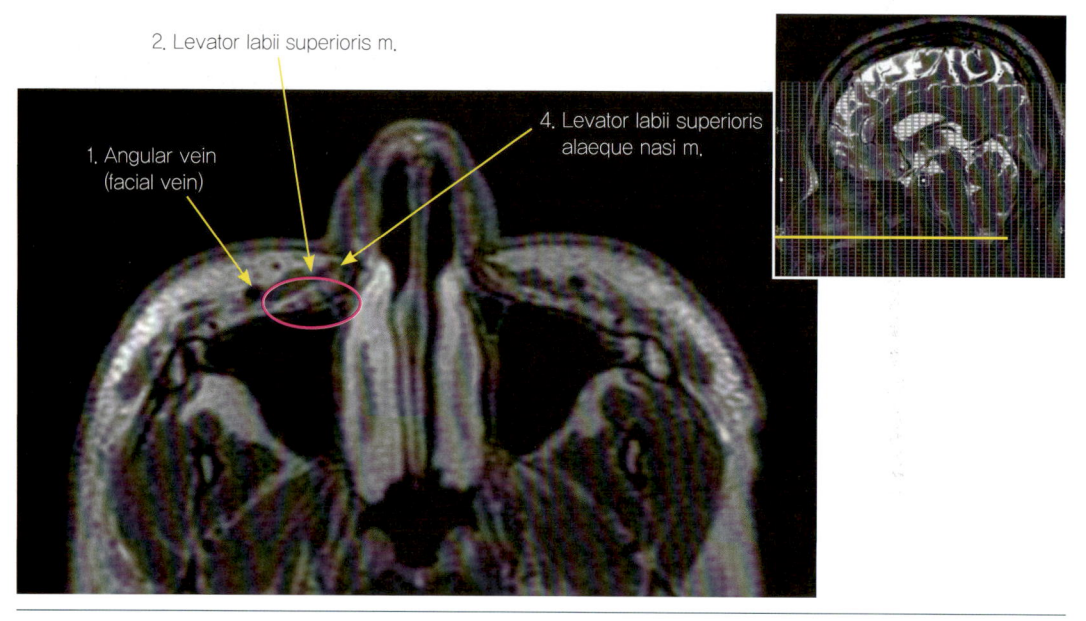

Fig. 4-71 **MRI of the nasolabial folds (3)**

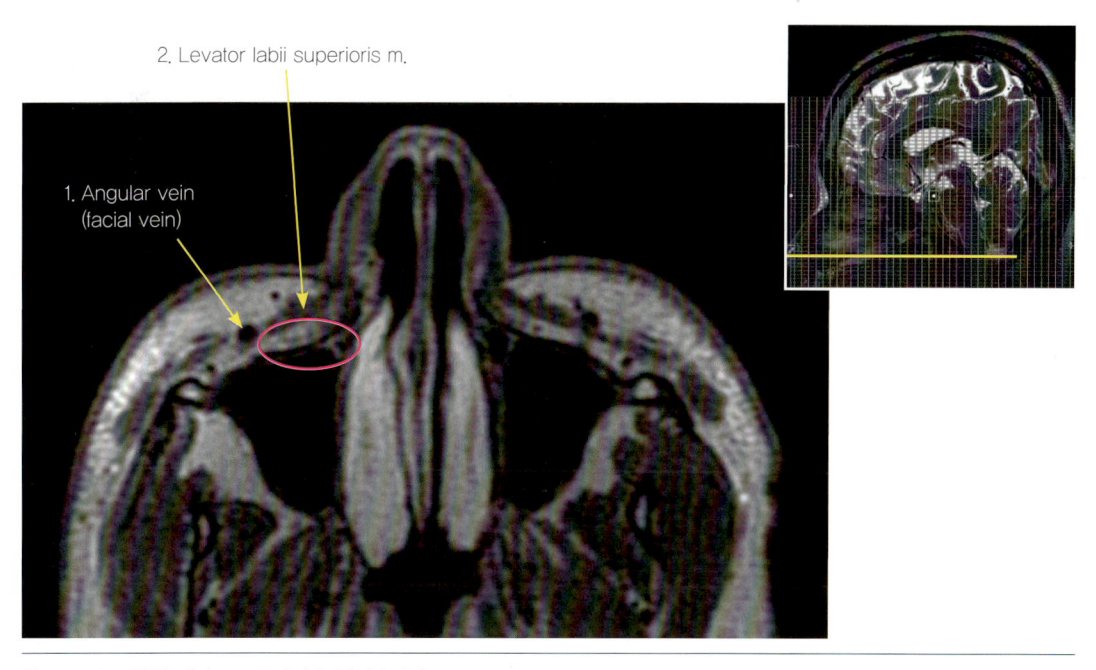

Fig. 4-72　MRI of the nasolabial folds (4)

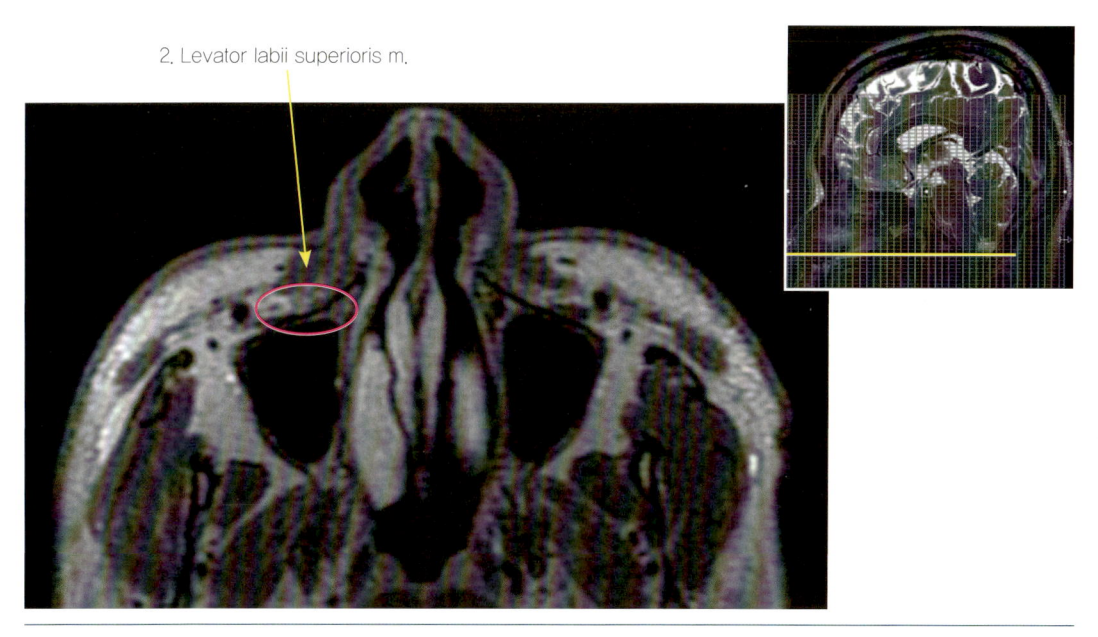

Fig. 4-73　MRI of the nasolabial folds (5)

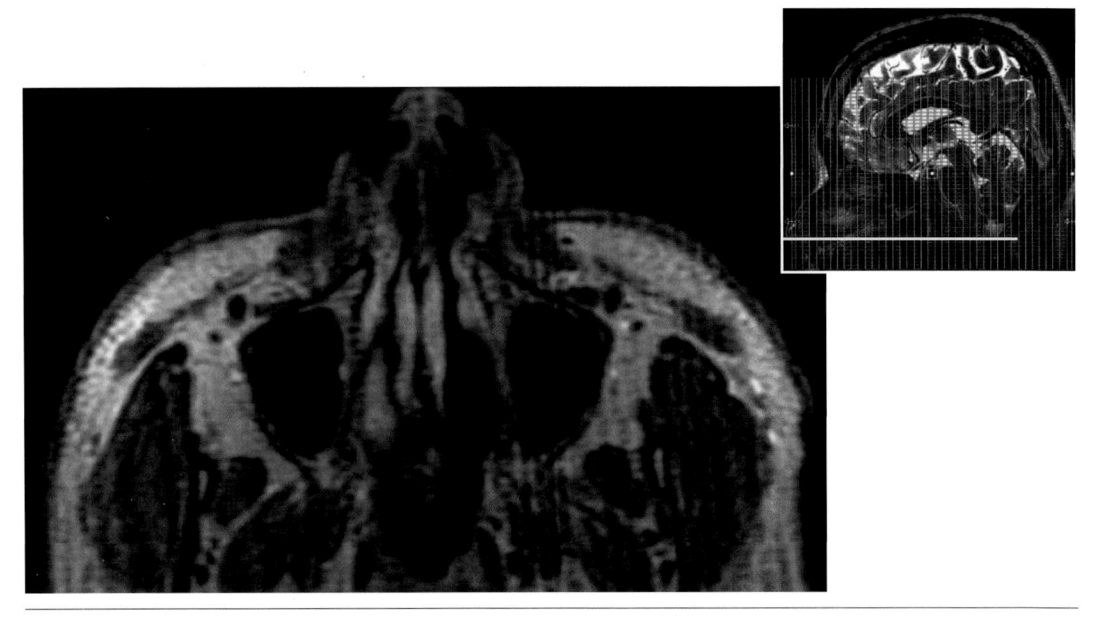

Fig. 4-74 MRI of the nasolabial folds (6)

Imaging explanation

- Inject being cautious not to damage blood vessels in the deep layer.

- When injecting into the superficial layer, separate between dermis layer and the subcutaneous layer and only inject after ensuring that there has been no bleeding. (double layer injection)

- Assess the pressure necessary to push the plunger prior to the procedure. Inject small amounts at a time.

- Review the DPS method. Separate tissue to procure space and then inject carefully.

- When using a needle, do not apply too much pressure and inject carefully into the correct location and depth.

Because the nasolabial fold treatment is associated with a high risk of vascular accidents and blindness, extreme caution is required.

Firstly, in choosing the entry point bear in mind that the region where the facial artery becomes tortuous (approximately 1.5 cm lateral and 1.5 cm superior to the lip margin) is very superficial and occasionally the pulse is visible. In other areas of the face, the vessel variations and difficulty in entry point selection increases the risk of accidental intravascular injection. However, in this region there is a definite and constant danger zone (1.5 cm lateral and 1.5 cm superior to the lip margin) and error must be avoided in making the entry point.

Secondly, 50% of the facial artery is located within 5 mm of the nasolabial folds and branches into the lateral nasal artery at the alar recess. The alar recess is the region that requires the most augmentation during nasolabial fold treatments. In order to prevent intravascular injection, cannula or needle must be inserted gently and filler should be placed right above the bone. Large volumes of filler may compress vessels causing necrosis so large bolus injections should be avoided. This precaution ensures safety and good clinical results even in regions with anatomical variations.

The facial artery is inferior to the lip elevator muscle. The branch of the infraorbital artery that exits the infraorbital foramen is deeper than the facial artery.

Careful and precise injections based on anatomy knowledge and radiology images will prevent filler complications.

3 Choice of Filler

For nasolabial folds, three techniques are used in combination. These include volumizing the deep layer, correcting superficial wrinkles, removing adhesions via separation of dermis and subcutaneous fatty layer if necessary in addition to filler injections. An appropriate combination of the three techniques optimizes results.

For volumizing the deep layer, biphasic fillers with large particles, monophasic fillers with a high concentration, or calcium fillers are recommended. For the upper layer of superficial subcutaneous tissue, monophasic or biphasic fillers with medium-sized particles are recommended. This area is prone to formation of uneven lumps and bumps, so caution must be taken with respect to the injection method and bevel direction.

4 Demonstration of Technique

The following is a summary of items to assess prior to nasolabial fold treatment.

1. Assess if nasolabial fold is simply a depression or aggravated by sagging of soft tissue.
2. Assess if patient will improve from treatment. In patients with malar fat pad descent, filler injections may not significantly improve the appearance of nasolabial folds.
3. Assess if patient has gummy smile. The pressure created by muscle movement may alter the shape of the filler body or cause filler to migrate.
4. Assess for presence of adhesions.
5. Assess vasculature. Caution against serious complications that can arise from compression of the angular artery/lat. nasal artery or filler emboli.

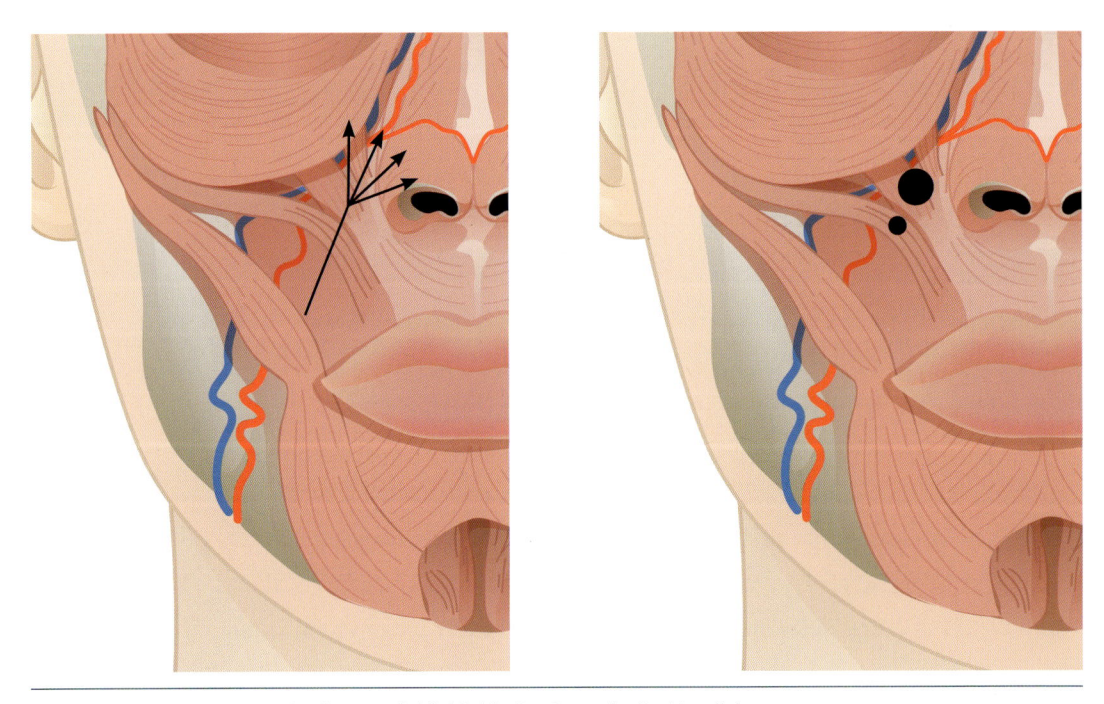

Fig. 4-75 Injection route in the nasolabial folds (Lt: Cannula, Rt: Needle)

Novice injectors may begin their filler injection training with treatment of nasolabial folds, but this is a region that even intermediate and the most advanced physicians pay the greatest attention in terms of safe techniques and review of anatomical structures. Injection techniques such as cannula use, filler selection, location of entry point, and injection layer varies depending on the physician. The authors recommend two techniques for the treatment of nasolabial folds, a technique using a cannula and a technique using a needle.

1) Injection Method - Volumizing a Deep Layer Using a Cannula

A cannula can only be used after carefully studying the DPS injection method. An entry point should be made on a point that lies along the line of the nasolabial fold. The region where the facial artery ascends from the deep layer and begins to course in the subcutaneous layer must be avoided (Fig. 4-77, top figure). In general, the region where the facial artery begins to course in the superficial layer is located 1cm lateral and 1 cm superior (1.5/1.5 cm) to the lateral margin of the lip. Lidocaine is injected where the facial artery pulse is not palpated. Then, make the smallest possible puncture into the dermis using a 23G needle. After this, using either a 21G or 23G cannula, pass through the dermis perpendicularly and enter into the subcutaneous fat layer. Do not begin to the move cannula sideways as soon as there is decreased resistance with entry into the subcutaneous layer. Instead enter more deeply (Fig. 4-77, bottom figure).

The facial artery branches into the angular artery after the facial artery begins to course in the subcutaneous layer. The angular artery courses superiorly towards the eyes passing the side of the nose. Therefore the cannula should be inserted below the muscle layer at puncture site before proceeding toward the nasolabial fold. At the alar recess, separate the soft tissue layer to procure space. When separation is completed, withdraw the cannula completely and check for bleeding. Performing this step is necessary to determine if there was damage to the angular artery or vein. Next, cautiously proceed with the cannula again(no further separation of tissue but rather proceed the cannula through the route already made) and inject fillers gently in the desired area.

Filler placement should be limited to the triangular space made by the alar recess. This is to minimize filler migration into the regions along the tract.

Safe Filler Injection Technique Demonstration – using live imaging tools

In the DPS method, space is procured in the desired layer in advance (subcutaneous layer, muscle layer or the upper periosteal layer) and then filler injected. Due to variations in the course of the angular artery, there are cases in which the angular artery and the treatment region overlap. Prior to injecting, palpate for the pulse along the planned tract and treatment area by the alar recess. It is important not to inject the filler near the angular artery coursing the superficial subcutaneous layer.

This technique involves separation of soft tissue and procuring space prior to filler placement. Some degree of filler migration into undesired areas due to facial muscle activity is inevitable. Especially in regions like the nasolabial area where there is a lot of activity due to speaking and eating, there is a higher risk of significant filler migration. Therefore, physicians can anticipate migration and use this to their advantage. Separating soft tissue and procuring space in the treatment area will guide the movement of the filler body to the desired region.

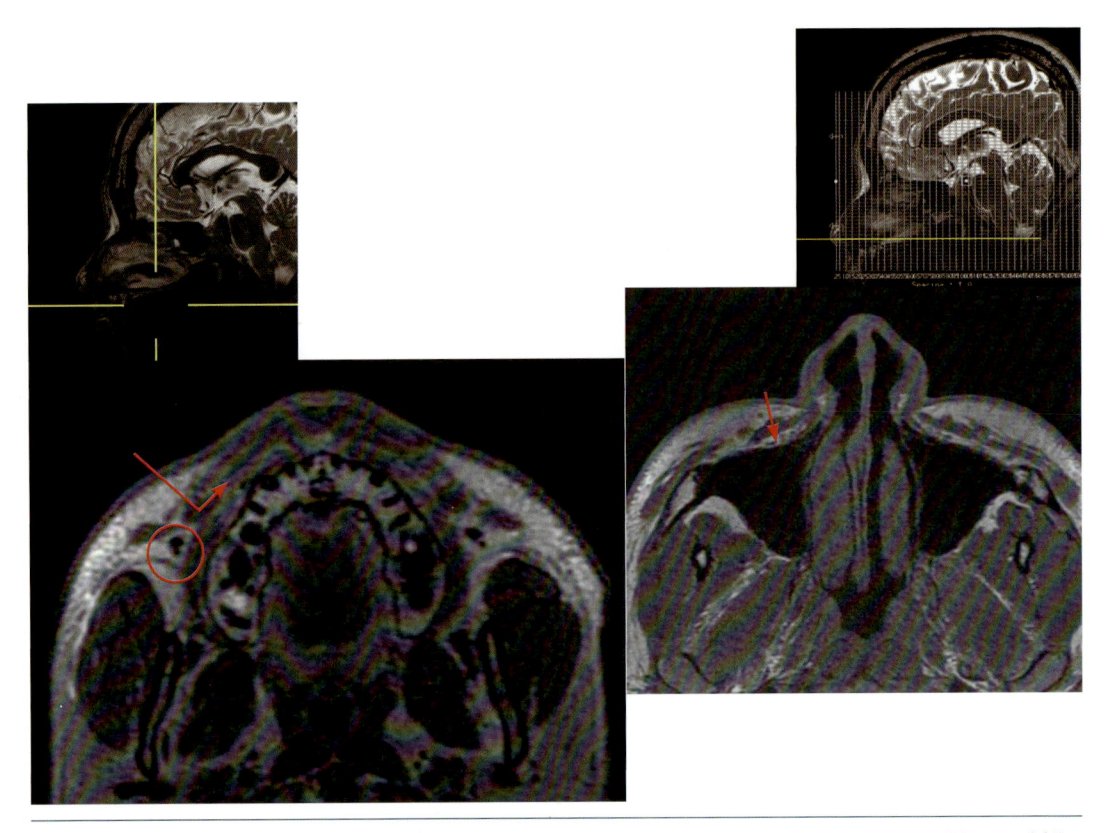

Fig. 4-76 **MRI of the nasolabial fold. Transverse view** (Lt: Entry point, Rt: Cannula entry and layer of filler injection)

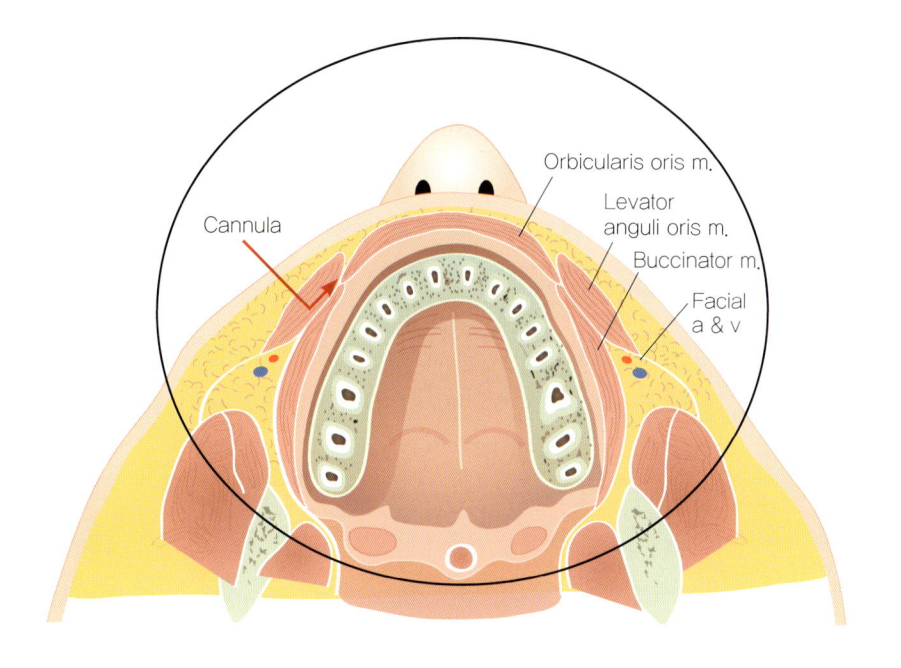

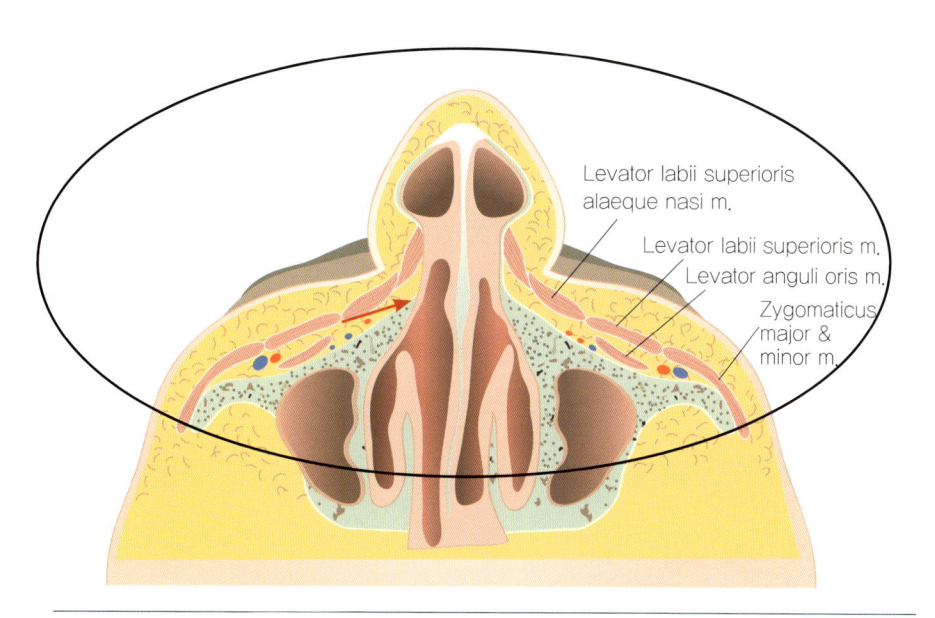

Fig. 4-77 Illustrations of the nasolabial folds (Top: entry point, Bottom: cannula entry and filler injection layers)

In the patient with a gummy smile, it is necessary to weaken the levator labii superioris alaeque nasi muscle with a small amount of botulinum toxin in advance. This reduces excessive elevation of the medial cheek that occurs when smiling, which in turn reduces the risk of the filler lumping.

By the entry point located laterally to the lips, the facial artery is coursing between the superficial and deep layers, so caution is required. After carefully puncturing the skin to minimize bleeding, enter into the deep layer. Then proceed cautiously to the alar recess. By injecting into the fat layer below the muscles, the angular artery can be avoided, but as there are other blood vessels in this area fillers should always be injected with caution.

2) Injection Method - Volumizing the Deep Layer Using a Needle

With needles, the perpendicular pulling method is recommended. As previously mentioned, the angular artery tends to pass the superficial layer of the subcutaneous tissue by the alar recess. Palpate for the angular artery to avoid injury of the vessel before puncture. Puncture and proceed close to the bone. Finally, apply slight pressure on the plunger and make a bolus injection (Fig. 4-78).

Needle injection into the deep layer for treatment of nasolabial folds is generally safe. In the nasolabial fold area, the angular artery course makes a transition from the deep to superficial layer. Moreover this artery is tortuous. Considering these factors, the best practice is to inject into the deep layer, muscle layer, or fat layer below the muscles. However, filler injection into muscle layer is associated with a more rapid resorption of the filler and higher risk of nodule formation.

The optimal layer is the fat layer below the muscles. In this layer, however, there are various blood vessels, so cautious handling is required. Injecting into the deep layers does not guarantee safety.

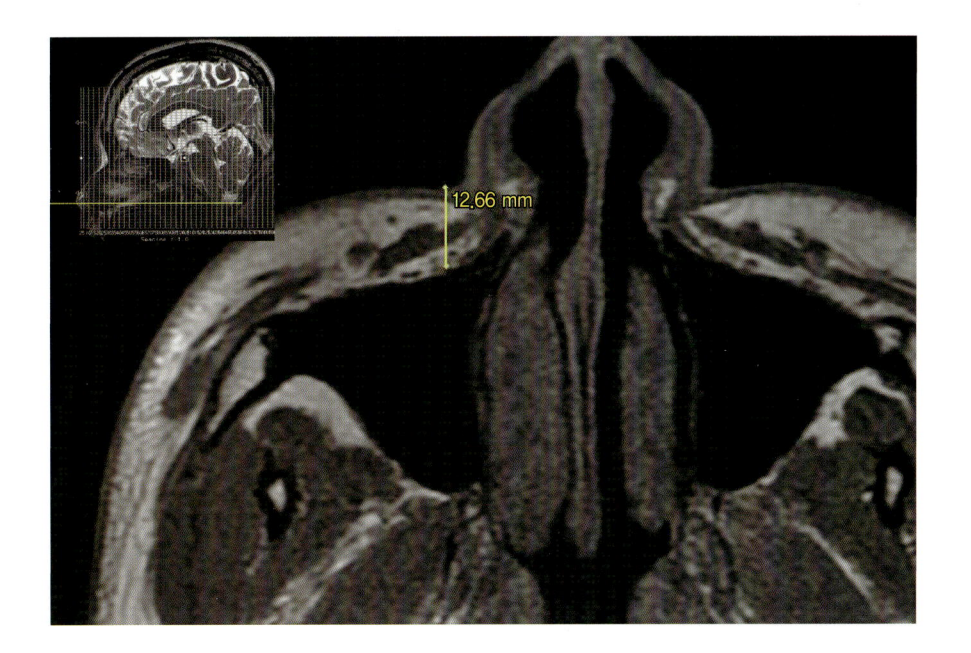

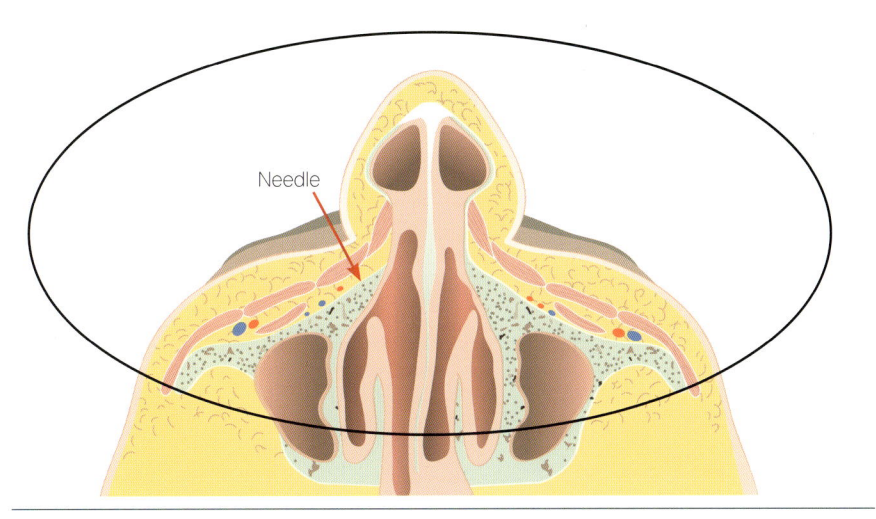

Fig. 4-78 MRI of the nasolabial fold areas - Transverse view and depth of needle injection

3) Massaging after Injection

The DPS injection using a cannula is a filler technique that creates a space for fillers to spread in advance. Therefore, vigorous massaging is not necessary. However, it is recommended to massage the area if asymmetry between the two sides is observed. When massaged, calcium fillers, biphasic fillers, and HA fillers with large particles spread less, whereas monophasic fillers with small particles or low HA concentration spread relatively better. Each filler type has its own unique set of disadvantages and advantages. However, these are intrinsic properties of the fillers and no conclusive statement regarding the superiority of one type of filler over another can be made.

Fillers that spread well can be used in areas where spreading is needed. Fillers that do not spread as well are better suited for regions where the maintenance of the initial shape is needed in creating the aesthetically desired outcome (examples include injecting into the deep layer in the infraorbital area and the deep layer of the nasolabial fold).

4) Injection Method for the Treatment of Fine Wrinkles – Needle and Cannula

This method is similar to the method used in treating the glabellar and forehead lines.

However precaution is needed by the modiolus where angular artery begins to course superficially.

- Fillers with mid to low viscosity is recommended.
- Use the retrograde linear thread technique.
- After injection, massage the procedure area moderately.
- Regardless of filler type, the depressions in the dermis associated with the deep wrinkles do not smoothen out completely to match the adjacent, normal skin.

5) Precautions with Nasolabial Procedures with Fillers

- Inquire about any past procedures. Check for history of autologous fat transfer or filler injections in the nasolabial fold area.

- Check arterial pulse (depth and location)
- Injections into the subdermal and supra-periosteum layers are safe (avoid injections into the subcutaneous layer).
- During touch-ups, do not inject an excessive amount of filler (same precaution needed during nasal procedures).
  - As in the initial treatment, filler amount must be adjusted appropriately in the touch- up procedure.
  - In repeat treatments after a prolonged period after the filler has resorbed bear in mind that there is collagenesis and formation of denser tissue in the treated area. This reduces the mobility of the blood vessels and risk of vessel compression increases. An amount that was tolerated previously may not safe in consequent treatments. Perform these repeat procedures with extreme caution.
  - Concurrent treatment of the nasolabial folds and the nasal tip increases the risk of compressing the lateral nasal artery. Accordingly the procedures should be spread out across two sessions with only a small amount added at each visit.
- Confirm patients' goals for treatment. Inquire whether the patient desires augmentation of the fold or wrinkle correction. Explain treatment plan and expected outcomes as the patient assesses his/her reflection in the mirror.

5 Complication

1) Dermal Necrosis

Excessive amounts of filler injected into the alar triangle can compress the lateral nasal artery, which can ultimately lead to dermal necrosis. Inject conservatively using moderate amounts.

2) Nodule

If filler is injected into the orbicularis oris m., there is a risk of nodule formation. Avoid intramuscular injection.

SUMMARY of Nasolabial Folds

A
- Know the anatomy and variations of the facial artery
- Remember that the facial artery becomes tortuous by the modiolus (superficial kinking)

B
- Nasolabial fold correction is essential to create soft, peaceful appearance
- Consider concurrent correction of the marionette lines
- Significant augmentation may not be aesthetically pleasing (chimpanzee-like face)
- There should be small difference between the face at rest and the face when smiling

C
- Select fillers with larger particles and less prone to migration

D
- Injection plane
  → Dermal plane (fine line): needle
  → Subdermal plane: Needle or cannula
  → Supra-periosteum (folds): Cannula or needle (perpendicular)
- Selection of injection layer is most important in treating the folds
- DPS Method
  → After skin puncture, proceed to the alar recess region that is deep to the muscle layer below the subcutaneous fat layer.
  → At the alar recess area, procure space using the fan technique and then withdraw the cannula. Check for bleeding
  → Once it is confirmed that there is no bleeding, inject filler into the space
- Perpendicular pulling method
  → After palpating the pulse in the alar recess area, insert needle in the center of the recess. After bone touch, inject as bolus injection.

X
- Avoid the angular artery
- It is important to inject into the deep layer above the periosteum plane

4

Filler Treatment for Each Facial Area

6. Cheek (Upper Cheek and Lower Cheek)

••• In the past, filler procedures that replace surgeries in areas such as the nose and the nasolabial folds were popular. Recently, procedures that trim the contour of a face have become a huge trend. The cheeks, which comprise almost a half of the mid-face, are critical determinants of a beauty that a beautifully rounded face outline adds fullness and loveliness to the face.

Normally, beginners learn filler procedures starting from the basic areas such as the nose and the nasolabial folds. Next, they move on to procedures for the cheeks. Without any concrete aesthetic standards, moderate cheek augmentation performed similarly with the nose or nasolabial folds treatment can bring counterproductive results. Thus, the amount of consideration put on aesthetic standards would significantly affect the adjustment of cheeks relative to the whole face, or the whole image of the person.

With aging, the cheeks experience three types of changes, changes within the skin, the fat, and the bone. The procedures to be performed must consider all these factors.

1 Beauty

The standards of beauty change according to the era. Recently in Korea, faces, so-called "The Gangnam Beauty", with excessively augmented cheeks due to fat transplant or filler procedures have become prevalent. It is necessary that doctors who devote themselves to upward-leveling of beauty better understand not only the procedure techniques but also the essence of beauty.

Of course, we cannot make Asian faces that are the same as the Caucasians'. This is because the cheek bone structure is substantially different between the two ethnic groups. The line from the nasal border of the maxilla connecting to the zygomatic arch makes a natural curve for Caucasians (Fig. 4-80). Compared to Asians, Caucasians tend to be more concerned about the volume of the cheek bones and more obsessed with the inverted S-line (or Ogee curve) portrayed from the side. In Korea, surgery for reducing the cheek bones is popular, whereas augmentation of cheek bones using silicon prostheses is favored by Caucasians.

In Asians' faces, cheek bones that are excessively developed do not make a good impression. However, too little volume in the cheek makes it appear barren, so it is good to have a moderate amount of volume. In case where the zygoma are excessively developed, augmentation of the temples connected thereto or volumization of the side cheeks can be done to make the cheek bones look smaller and softer.

1) Ideal Cheek of Caucasians

- Caucasians differ from Asians in the area that highlights the cheek bones. The highlighted area has the following characteristics:
- It is in an oval shape.
- The most highlighted or augmented area is located above the center of the oval and on the outer region of the lateral canthus.

Ogee curve

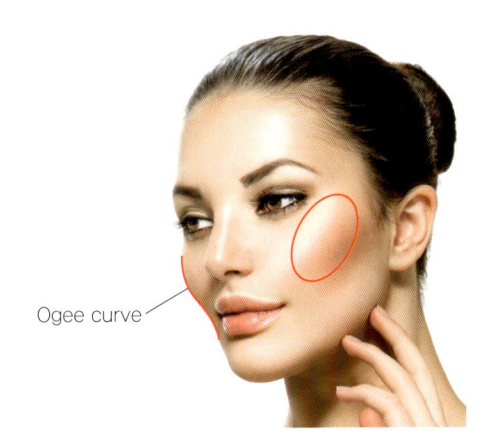

Fig. 4-79　Ideal line of Caucasian's cheek (Ogee curve)

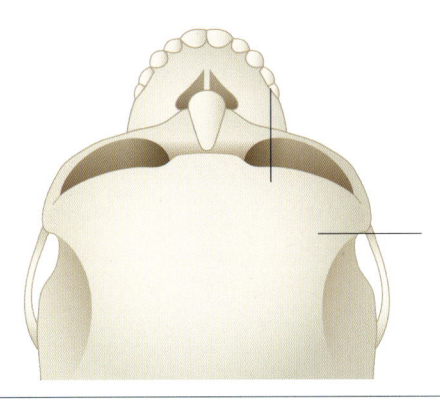

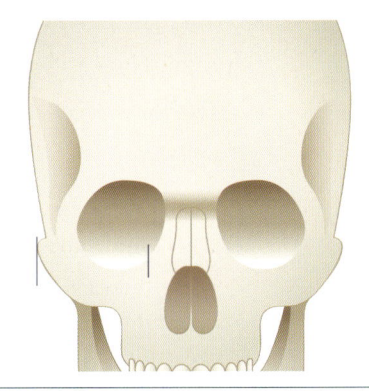

Fig. 4-80　Structure of Caucasian's cheek bone

2) Structure of Asian Cheek Bones

The structure of the cheek bone is not the same for all Asians. The authors separate them into two types and perform procedures accordingly.

Firstly, Asian Type I has a curve to the cheek bone, which is connected from the maxilla to the zygomatic arch. This type is similar to that of Caucasians in that it has the Ogee curve visible from the side view. In these cases, the adjustment is made by injecting a small amount of filler slightly on the lateral side rather than the medial of the highlight.

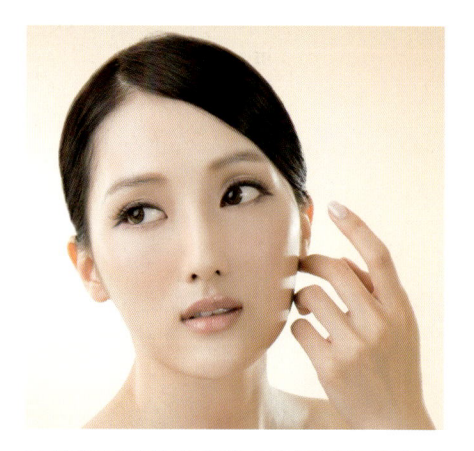

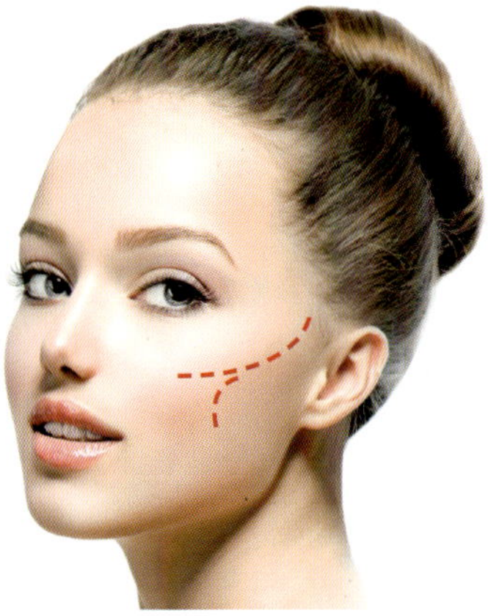

Fig. 4-81   Asian Type I

Fig. 4-82   Asian Type II

Asian Type II does not have a smooth curve. The contour continues as a flat line along the upper cheek and then makes an abrupt curve at the zygomatic arch. In these cases, the Ogee curve in the inverted S-shape is not seen from the side view. Here, it is good to give volume in the medial side of the upper cheek to transform the flat cheeks into curvy and smooth cheeks.

3) Changes in the Cheek from Aging

The shape of cheeks changes noticeably with aging.

In a youthful face, the cheek is full and uniformly rounded like an apple, showing a three-dimensional surface contour of the lid-cheek junction. With aging, the sagging of the skin forms three lines (the nasojugal groove, the palpebro malar groove, and the mid-cheek furrow) and these lines divide the sagging cheek into three segments: the lid-cheek segment, the malar segment, and the nasolabial segment.

Normally the nasojugal groove forms first, and then depending on the person, either the palpebro malar groove or the mid-cheek furrow forms next. As aging progresses further, all three lines appear eventually. (The mid-cheek furrow and malar round are explained in 7. Dark Circles, Part 4. Fig. 4-99)

For explanation on the aging process of the upper and lower cheeks, the Merz Aesthetics Scales are useful. Depending on age, the sagging and depression differ and the amount of filler needed for adjustment differs accordingly. This can be explained easily to patients by showing them Fig. 4-84 and 4-85 during consultation. (See also the explanation in Fig. 4-21 for the method of use.)

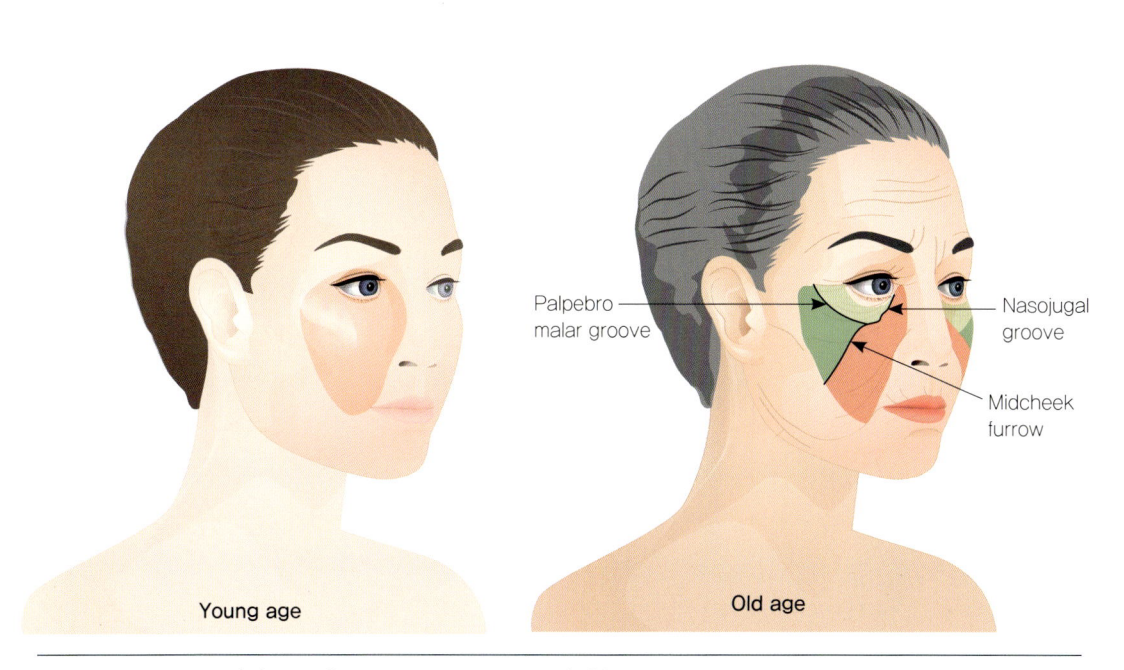

Fig. 4-83   Structural change between young age and old age

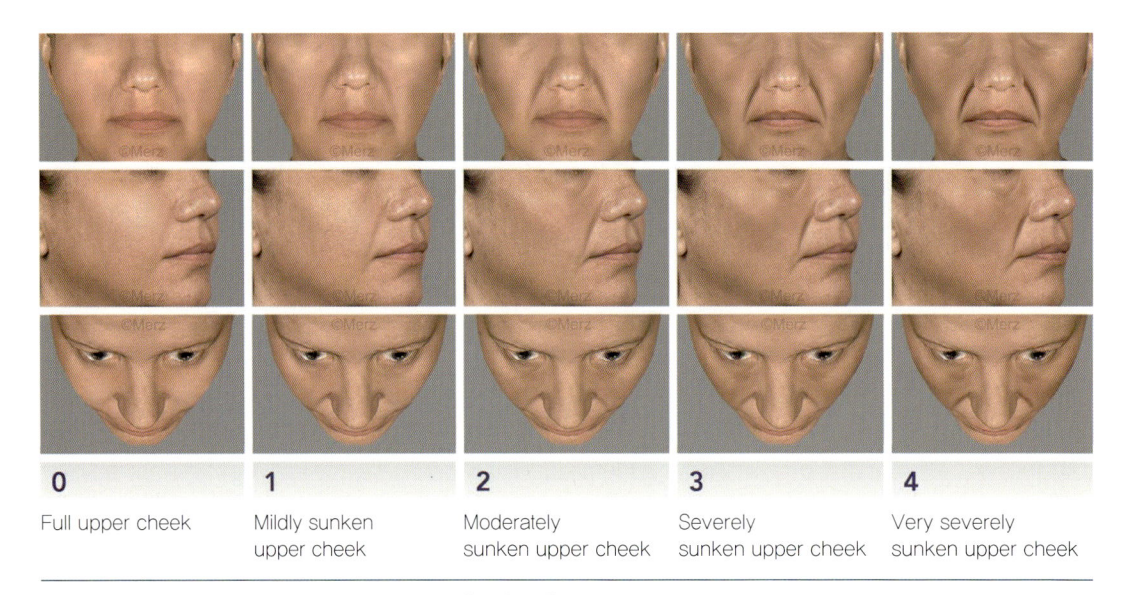

Safe Filler Injection Technique Demonstration – using live imaging tools

0	1	2	3	4
Full upper cheek	Mildly sunken upper cheek	Moderately sunken upper cheek	Severely sunken upper cheek	Very severely sunken upper cheek

Fig. 4-84 Merz Aesthetics Scales (Upper Cheek Fullness - at rest)
Copyright© (2010) Merz Pharmaceuticals
Carruthers, et al. Validated assessment scales for the mid-face. Dermatol Surg. 2012;38(2 Spec No.):320-32.

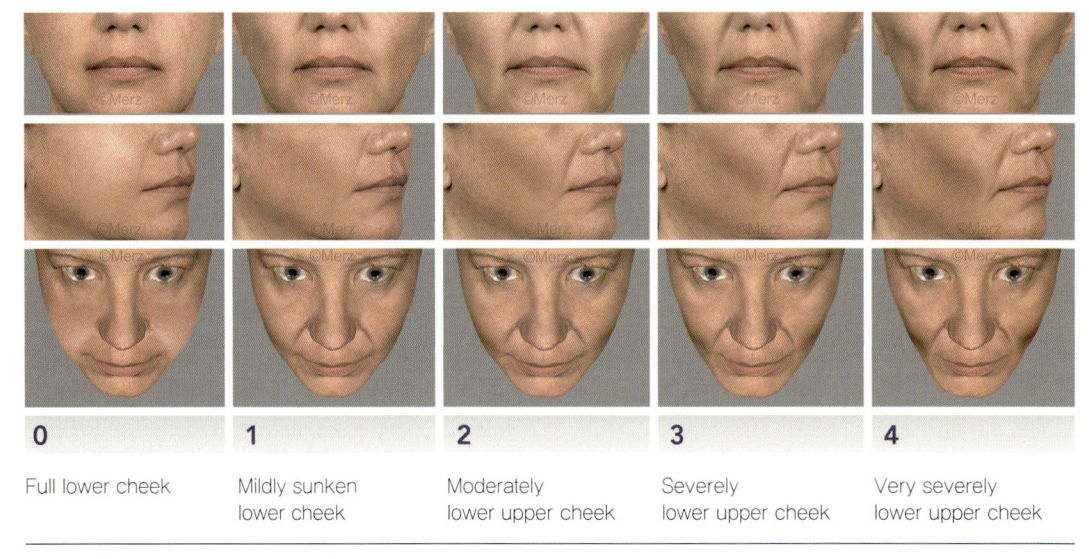

0	1	2	3	4
Full lower cheek	Mildly sunken lower cheek	Moderately lower upper cheek	Severely lower upper cheek	Very severely lower upper cheek

Fig. 4-85 Merz Aesthetics Scales (Lower Cheek Fullness - at rest)
Copyright© (2010) Merz Pharmaceuticals
Carruthers, et al. Validated assessment scales for the mid face. Dermatol Surg. 2012;38(2 Spec No.):320-32.

2 Anatomy

For the cheek, changes derived from atrophy of subcutaneous fat or absorption of the bone in addition to superficial skin changes (sagging of the skin) are important determinants for aging .

1) Fat Compartment

Cheek is a region where any reduction in the fat is easily noticed. This is directly related to formation of the dark circles and deepening of the nasolabial folds.

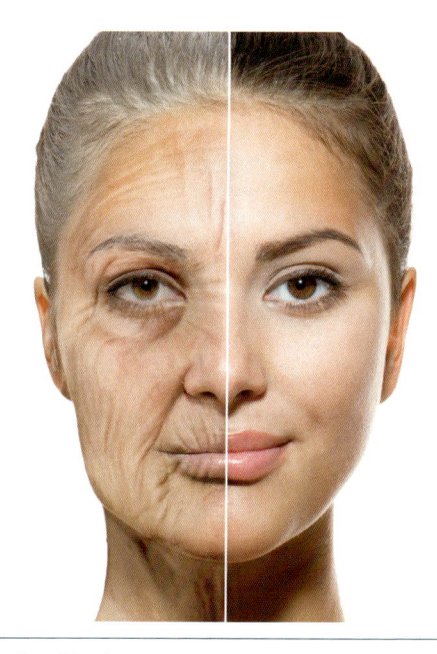

Fig. 4-86 Changes to the skin due to aging

2) Bichat's fat (Buccal fat pad)

- Located in a deeper layer than the risorius muscle

3) Aging and Mobility of Skin Tissues

- Area between the mid-facial line (vertically elongated to edge of the mouth) and the line of the frontal zygomatic region
- This area sags easily due to the sagging of fat and ligaments.
- In areas that are outside this region less sagging and more retaining of structures occur.

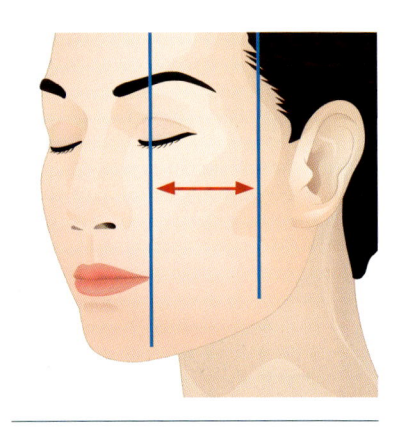

Fig. 4-87   Mobile area of mid-face

4) Muscles of Mid-face

There are various types of muscles existing in the mid-face.

When proceeding a cannula horizontally with a bone touch, it passes the space between the LLS and the LAO, and then meets the infraorbital artery, vein, and nerves at the infraorbital foramen. When passing the region above the LLS, the cannula would meet the border of the orbicularis oculi m.. During the filler procedure, it is crucial to perceive whether the cannula (or the needle) is passing above or below which muscle even though the origin and insertion of muscles are not clearly located.

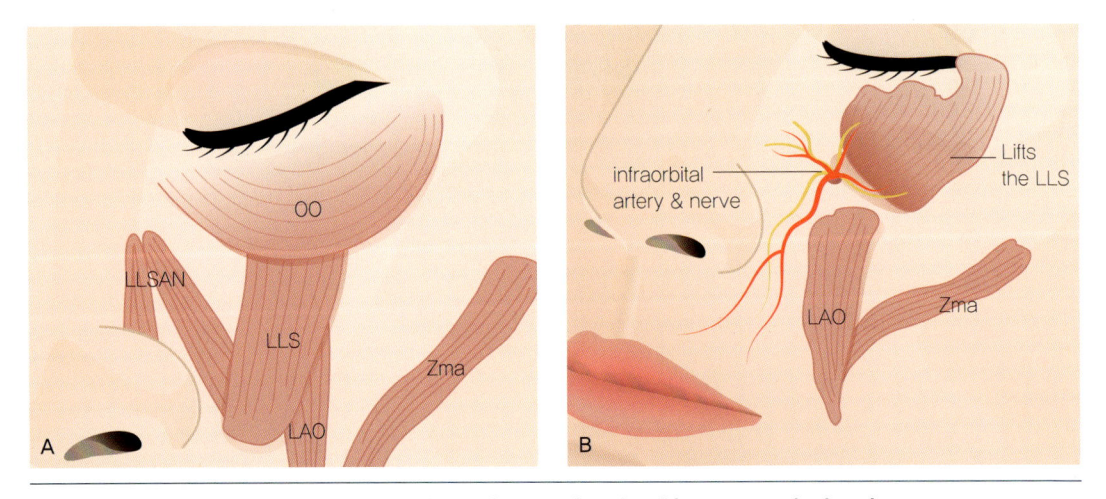

Fig. 4-88   A. Anatomy of the infraorbital muscles, B. Infraorbital foramen and related structures
OO: orbicularis oculi m., LLSAN: levator labii superioris alaeque nasi m., LLS: levator labii superioris m., LAO: levator anguli oris m., Zma: zygomaticus major m.

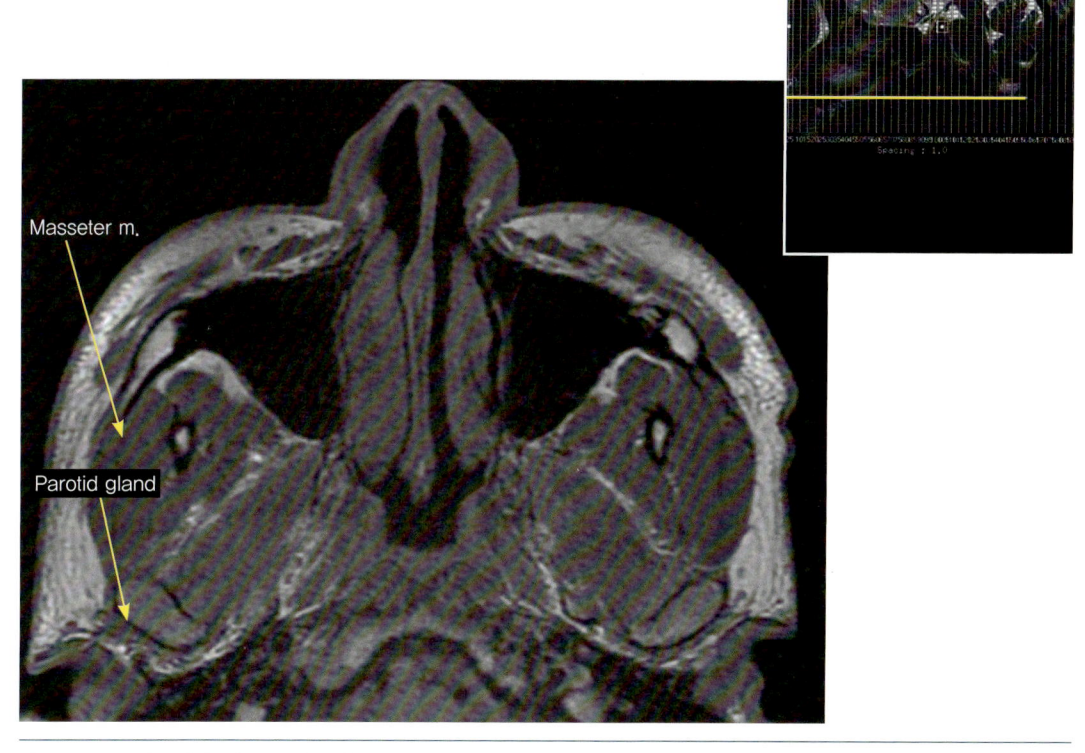

Fig. 4-89 MRI of the lower cheek (1)

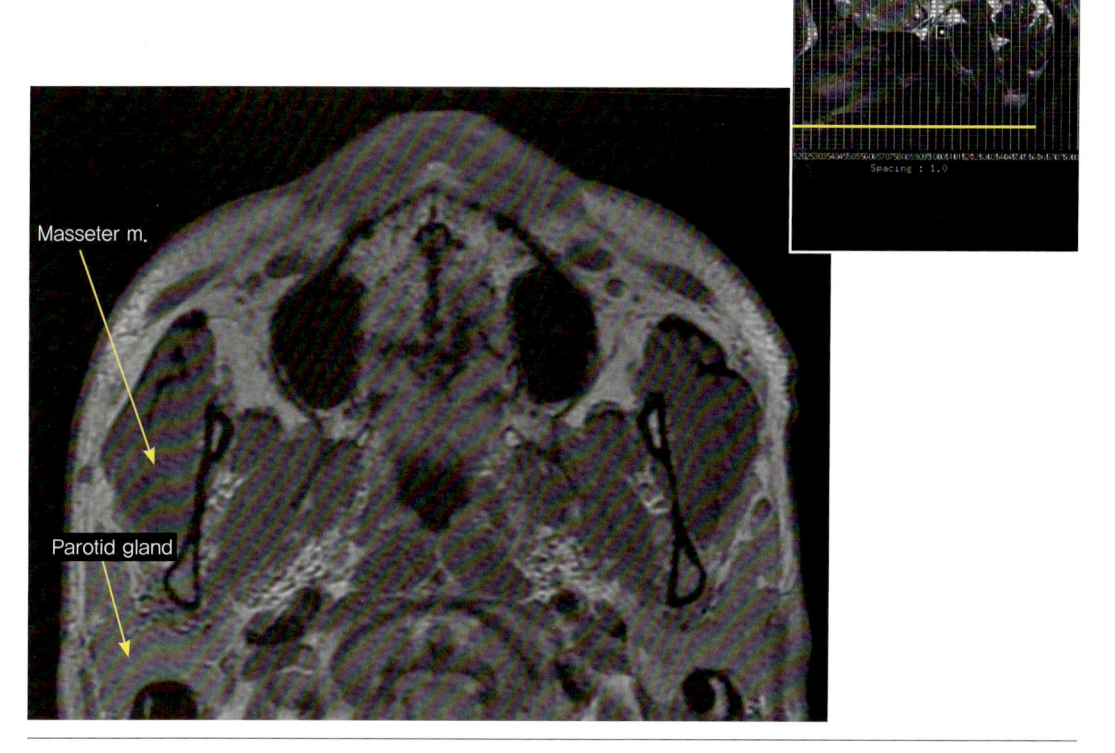

Fig. 4-90 MRI of the lower cheek (2)

217

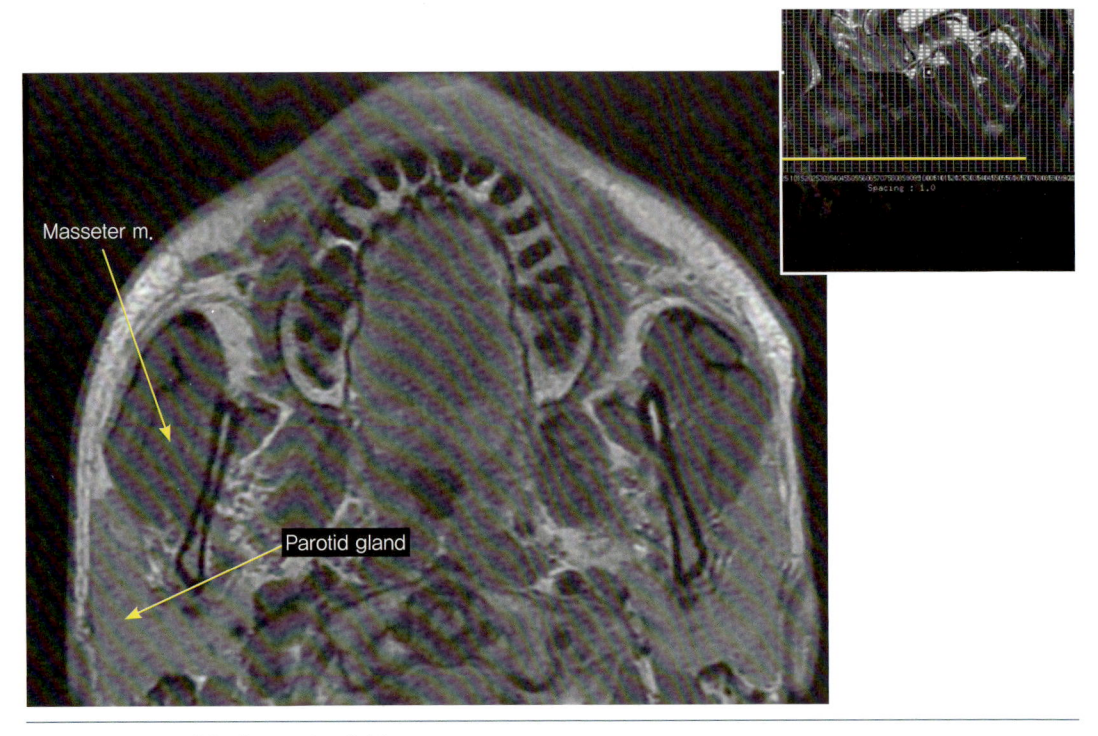

Safe Filler Injection Technique Demonstration – using live imaging tools

Fig. 4-91 MRI of the lower cheek (3)

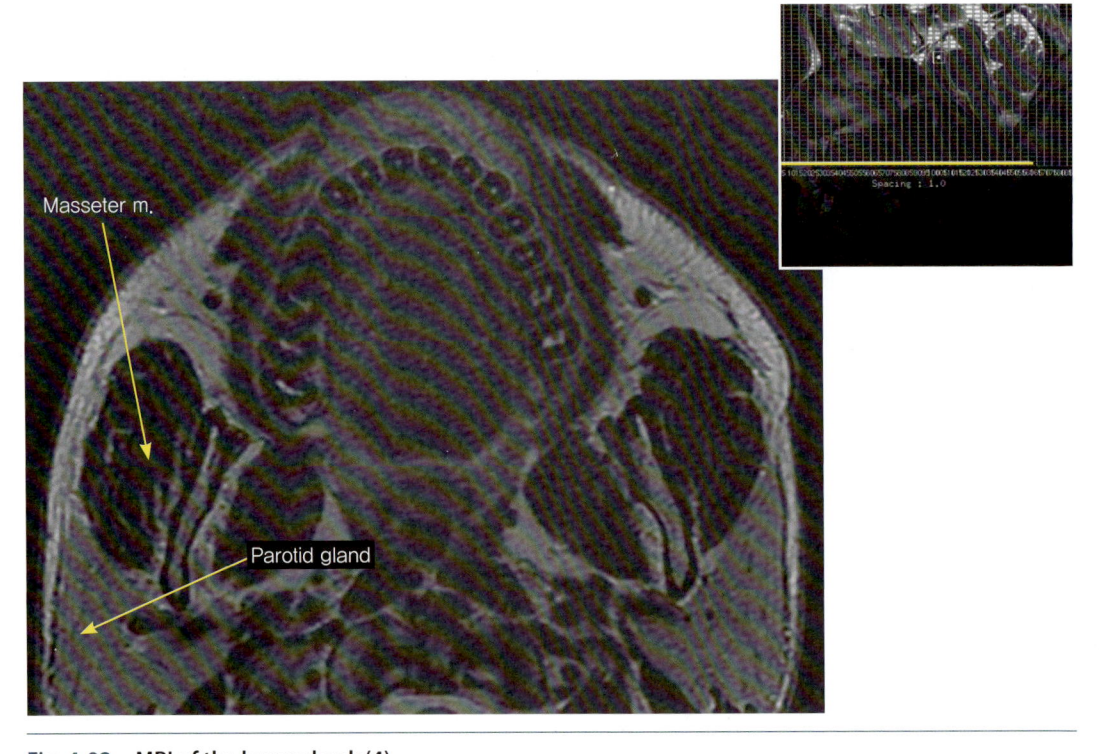

Fig. 4-92 MRI of the lower cheek (4)

> **Imaging explanation**
> - It would be relatively safe to inject alongside the subcutaneous fat layer as long as proceeded with caution. Since there are no large blood vessels present in that layer, the risk of vascular complications would be small.
> - The area that requires caution during treatment is the parotid gland. As injection continues alongside the subcutaneous fat layer, the change in depth must be examined.

3 Choice of Filler

1) Upper Cheek

For upper cheeks, fillers with high viscosity that produce great volumizing effects should be used.

Since the fat compartment in the upper cheek moves upward when smiling the treatment must be designed in a way that both of the static and smiling face of the patient are considered. In most cases, it is effective to use biphasic filler with low mobility and high viscoelasticity or monophasic filler with high concentration. If a procedure is targeting multiple layers, it is recommended to use monophasic filler with mid-concentration that spreads well in the subcutaneous layer. Among the layers, the skin around the upper cheek and just below the eyes is thin and prone to creating lumps caused by filler injection. As treating multiple layers at once could bring an inferior result than volumizing only the deep layer, it is advisable to avoid treating the superficial layer until a significant amount of experience has accumulated.

2) Lower Cheek

In contrast to procedures on the upper cheek, the bottom of the lower cheek is connected to the mucosa of the oral cavity, rather than the bone. Within the lower cheek, procedures can be performed on: 1) the subQ layer; 2) Bichat's fat, and; 3) the subdermis.

1) When volumizing the subQ layer, use fillers with medium to high viscosity. As there is a danger of creating bumps when the face is still or dynamically moving, fillers with great spreadability are to be used. Monophasic fillers of high concentration or biphasic fillers with large particles are recommended.
2) For accurate injection into Bichat's fat, fillers with high viscosity are to be used.

3) For the subdermis, among those fillers with biostimulatory functions, fillers with great moldability are to be used. In the central area of the lower cheek there is a marked tendency to stretching due to aging, and it is an area where facial lifting is often performed. Here, an accurate injection of biostimulator fillers can cause a fine facelift.

4-1 Demonstration of Technique - Upper Cheek

1) Designing Method Prior to Procedures

1. Draw a line connecting the ala to the tragus (inferior cheekbone border; in the event a lower area is punctured perpendicularly, it can enter the oral cavity).
2. Draw a line connecting the lat. canthus to the oral commissure.
3. Mark the infraorbital foramen (IO) and the zygomatico-facial foramen (ZFO). (If injections are made perpendicularly at the IO and ZFO, the risk of injecting into the blood vessels increases.)
4. Mark the infraorbital rim. (If this line is pressed during the procedures, injection of filler substances in upward direction can be prevented.)

The space between the infraorbital foramen (IO) and the zygomatico-facial foramen (ZFO) is the region where intersection of the two lines described above occurs. Here, injection can be made safely.

As explained previously, in the case of an Asian Type I face, the Ogee curve can be created by volumization, adding a small amount filler slightly laterally from the intersection.

In the case of an Asian Type II face, augmentation slightly on the medial side of the intersection can be done. In order to provide volume in the flat cheek, a greater amount of filler should be injected than for lateral augmentation.

There are various methods of designing, and the best among them would use the most convenient and simplest method.

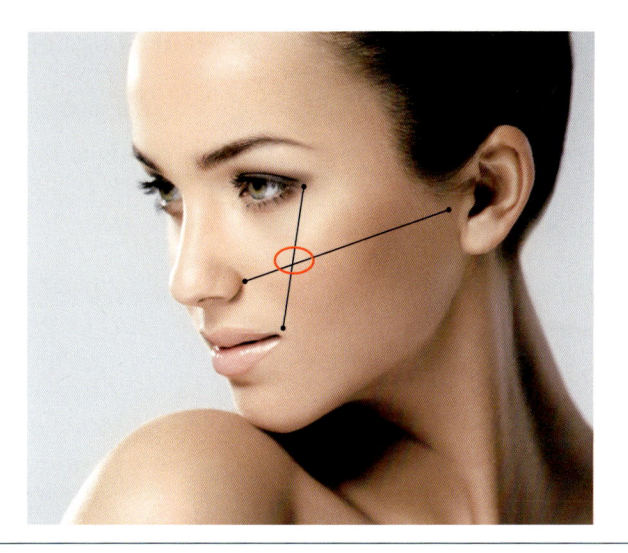

Fig. 4-93 Mapping

2) Injection of Cannula (Upper Cheek)

It is advised to inject at the intersection of the two lines, with the entry point to be made 2~3 cm laterally from there. As the core technique of filler injections guides, at the puncture point, pressure must be applied quickly to minimize bleeding and prevent bruising. Thereafter, a cannula is be injected perpendicularly or at a slope to the point where it touches the bone, and then pushed into the zygomaticus minor (ZMn) or below the LLS. After proceeding to the desired area for injection with fillers, the DPS method would be followed through making space. Once space is procured, the cannula can be removed. After checking that there is no bleeding, the cannula can be reinserted through the same route although this process is not absolutely necessary. Next, a bolus of filler is injected into the desired area and molded into the desired shape. The area underneath the eye becomes pressured especially when the face is smiling. A filler with low viscoelasticity can easily move upward, and this phenomenon may cause the hollowness under the eyes to look more severe and emphasize the cheek bones, which is unwanted. Given this fact, it is not recommended to use monophasic filler with low viscosity. For the under-eye area, monophasic fillers of high concentration and viscoelasticity should be used. If a lesser degree of volumizing is desired, there is a method of injecting into the ZMn or above the LLS. Moreover, if correction of a mid-cheek furrow is desired, injection into the superficial subQ layer can be performed. However in that case, fillers of medium viscosity are to be used in order to avoid forming lumps and spread the filler well. In general, the angular artery is located alongside the outer border of the nose, but in some cases, it is located substantially distant from the nose line, near the center of half face of the face. Therefore, extra caution is necessary when injecting the filler into the subQ layer of the mid- face.

3) Needle Injection (Upper Cheek)

After inserting the needle perpendicularly to the periosteum of the intersection point of the two lines (the safe area), a bolus injection can be made gradually. Next, the injected filler can be molded. Fillers with high viscosity are to be used.

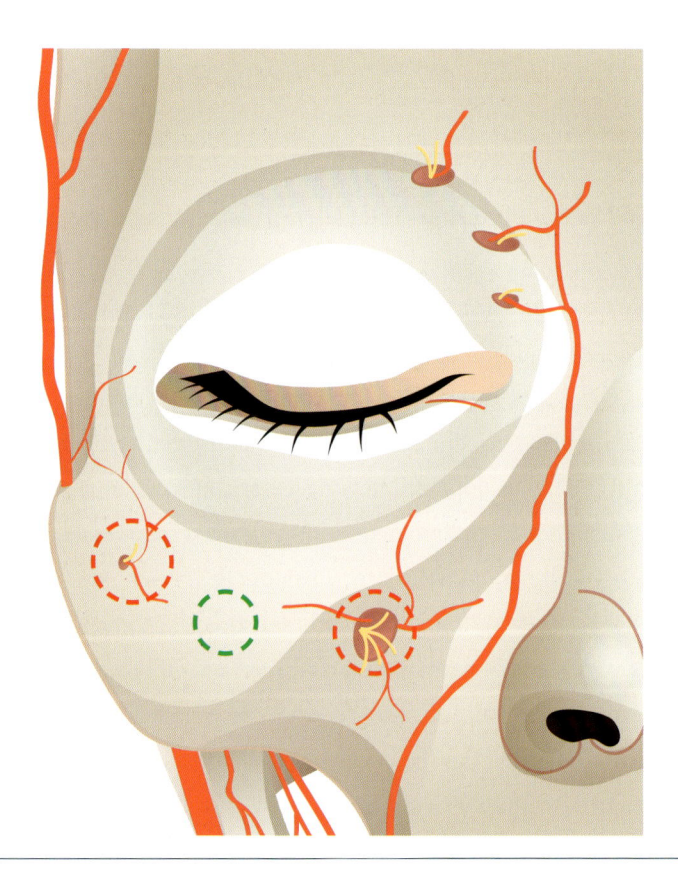

Fig. 4-94 Relatively safe area for procedure (Blood vessels are less dispersed.) and places where perpendicular insertion of needle is convenient.
Green dotted circle: safe injection area. Red dotted circle: dangerous area.

4-2 Demonstration of Technique - Lower Cheek

For lower cheek, a different procedure is applied to that of the upper cheek as the bottom of its skin layer connects to the mucosa of the oral cavity, rather than the bone. Accordingly, the needle is not to be inserted perpendicularly to the very bottom.

1) SubQ Layer Injection (Fig. 4-95)

The easiest method is to adjust the hollowness of the lower cheek through volumization of the subcutaneous fat layer. Fillers with medium to high viscosity are injected mostly with a cannula just because it is easier to use compared to the needle. When injecting into the lower cheek, the subcutaneous layer is safe in terms of preventing any surface unevenness after injection. For that reason, designing is very important. According to the treatment design, the filler should be injected primarily into the area of hollowness that is noticed in both static and smiling faces. In case of the area of hollowness that occurs in either of static or smiling face, DPS method should be used to create space. After withdrawing the cannula, check for any bumps based on changes in facial expression, and then re-insert it to give an additional injection of fillers. Next, evenly spread the filler by massaging. The key here is to avoid prominence in any one area affected by change in facial expression.

As it is an area that dynamically moves by different facial expressions, the hollowness may show up again after some time. Once the filler is fixed to the treatment region quite well, an additional touch-up can finish the treatment.

Safe Filler Injection Technique Demonstration – using live imaging tools

2) Injection into the Bichat's Fat

An accurate injection into the Bichat's fat requires a high level of training. In case of a deep-layer injection, a large amount of high viscosity filler is needed for volumizing. Both needle and cannula can be used for this injection technique.

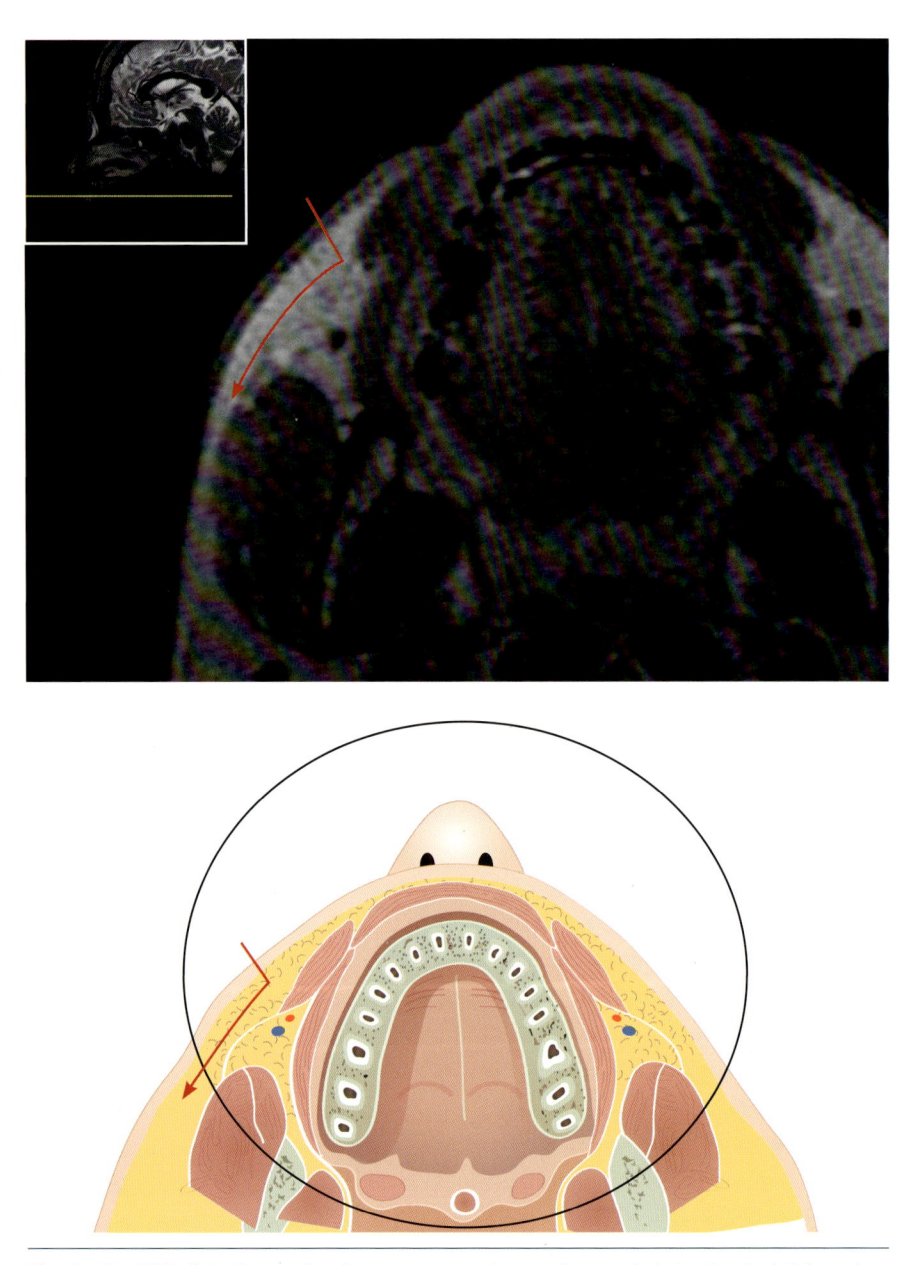

Fig. 4-95   MRI of the lower cheek - transverse view and cannula injection(subQ layer)

3) Injection into the Subdermis (for lifted looking effect) (Fig. 4-96)

Rather than lifting with volumes, this method lifts sagged cheeks by promoting regeneration of collagens in the subdermis, using biostimulator fillers. If a cannula is to be used, carefully design the sunken area, dissect a sufficient space for injecting fillers with a cannula, and then inject fillers using the fan thread technique. If dissection is insufficient or if filler with high viscosity is being injected, caution must be taken not to result in nodules even with molding. Using a needle or a cannula, tiny amount of filler injections can be made through more than two entry points with the fan technique (Fig. 4-97).

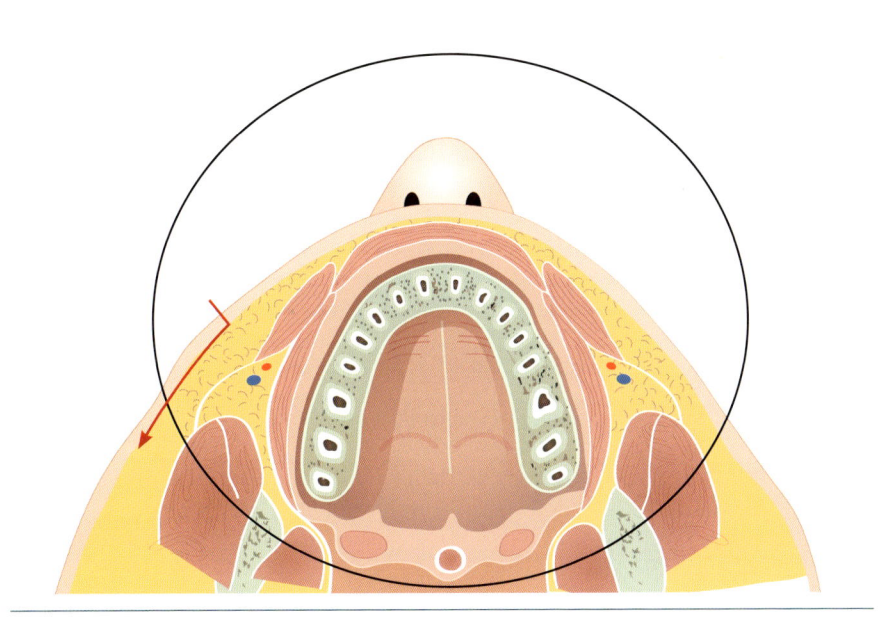

Fig. 4-96 Subdermis injection method

Safe Filler Injection Technique Demonstration – using live imaging tools

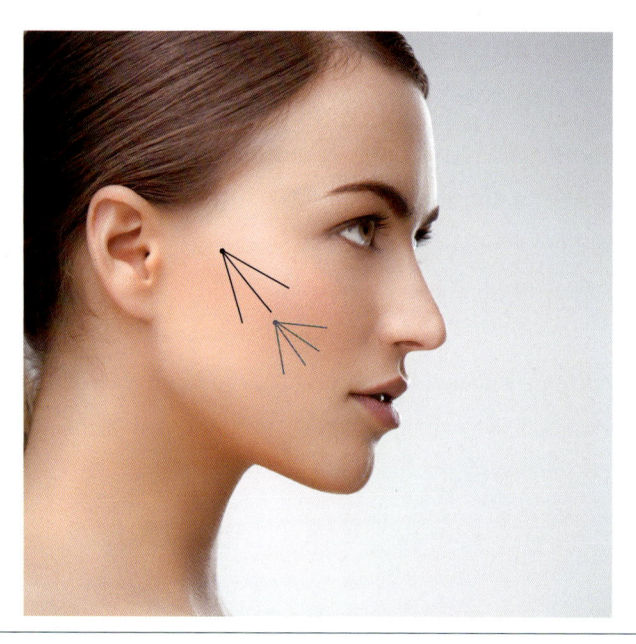

Fig. 4-97 Subdermis layer injection method

5 Complication

1) Over Correction of the Upper Cheek

If an excessive volume is injected into the upper cheek or into either medial or lateral cheek bone, the result can look unnatural. There was a time when injecting a large amount of autologous fat into the upper was a big trend. While there are some people who still desire this style, not so many people prefer it anymore. Prior to the procedure, it is always helpful to have a sufficient discussion with the patient about the areas to be treated and how much of the volume is expected to be added.

2) Nodules of the Lower Cheek

In the procedures for the lower cheek, nodules can occur after injecting into the subdermis layer or the superficial subcutaneous layer. As previously mentioned, this can happen when there is insufficient dissection or when fillers with high viscosity are used. Therefore caution must be taken to decrease the risk of forming nodules.

SUMMARY of Upper Cheek

A
- Understanding of fat compartment.

B
- Key areas of an "Apple Face"
- There must be a smooth curve in the facial contour and natural prominence of the cheeks.

C
- Necessary to inject calcium fillers or HA fillers with large particles into the deep layer immediately above the periosteum.

D
- Perpendicular pulling injection method: Injection is performed after safety check.
- DPS Method: After making a route from the spot, 2 cm below the lateral canthus, to the zygoma, reach the area just above the periosteum with a cannula, make space, and then inject fillers.
- The area for filler injection coincides with that around the infraorbital n.. Hence, the method of anesthesia must be carefully considered.

X
- Be cautious when injecting a needle into the infraorbital foramen, and be cautious of the zygomatico-facial n. a. v. (Nerve/Artery/Vein)
- Remember the average amount of pressure applied during injection; if pressure higher than normal is required, the procedure must be discontinued for safety check up.

SUMMARY of Lower Cheek

A
- The area below the ala-tragus line is the oral cavity space. Given this, no bone touch and perpendicular entry should take place.

B
- Type 1   Western type – Ogee curve is visible from the side view.
- Type 2   Asian type – A convex curve is visible from all sides.

C
- Product with large and long-lasting particles and good viscoelasticity.

D
- Lateral cheek
  - After making space with a cannula, inject filler into the subdermis/subQ.
  - Prior to injection, check bleeding and the shape of the cheeks.
- Volumize the cheek area by injecting a small amount of filler on the supra-periosteum plane in the upper cheek, and also injecting into subdermis/subQ layer with a fan technique in the lower cheek.

X
- Be cautious of the facial/infraorbital/transverse facial a.

4

Filler Treatment for Each Facial Area

7. Dark Circles

Definition

Dark circles are defined as a darkening or difference in color of the skin in periorbital region.

Causes and Treatments

Causes of dark circles can generally be divided into three: color, contour, and skin laxity (wrinkles). Treatments differ completely depending on the cause. Contour changes around the eyes, a change that everyone is subject to with aging, can be treated with fillers. As aging progresses, the infraorbital fat becomes prominent, the volume of malar fat decreases and sags, and there are changes in the bone structure with bone resorption. Amongst these treatment methods, filler injections are suitable for problems that can be solved with volume augmentation. Structures and landmarks relating to dark circles have varying terminology and definitions across the different fields, but an understanding of basic anatomy is necessary for appropriate treatment.

1 Beauty

Table 4-1 Causes and treatments for dark circles

Causes		Treatments
Color	Pigmentation (PIH)	Pigment laser, brightening
	Vascular (hypervasculature, thin/translucent lower eyelid skin)	Blood vessel laser, fat transplant
Contour	Herniation of infraorbital fat	(Trans-conjunctival) Fat removal
	Malar fat change	Filler, fat transplant
	Tear trough	Fat removal, filler
	Bone (orbital, malar) change	Filler, fat transplant
Skin laxity	Wrinkle	HIFU, radiofrequency, lower blepharoplasty

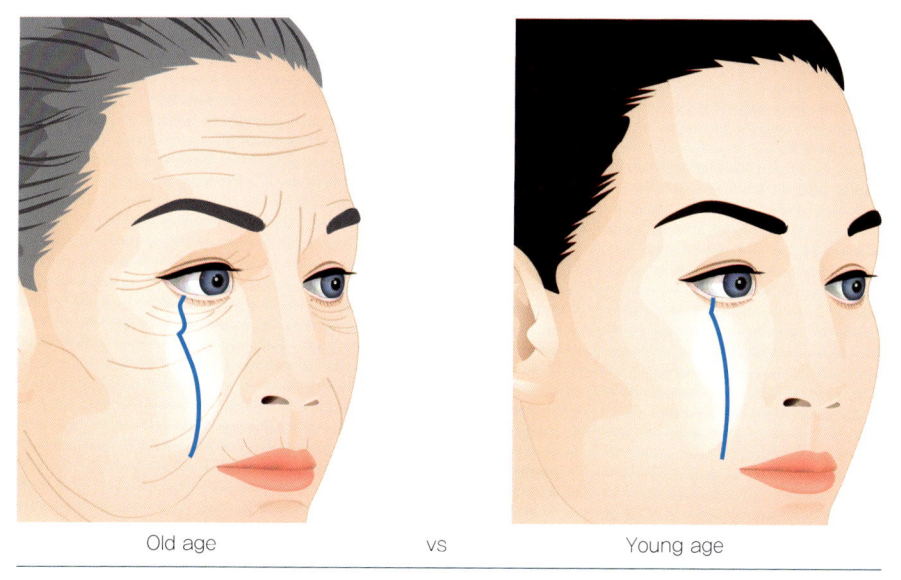

Fig. 4-98 Changes in the under-eye contour that occur with aging

When dark circles are viewed directly from the front, they can be mistaken as a mere change in color or formation of lines. However, when changes in contour or skin laxity, are viewed from the side, concave surface as seen in Fig. 4-98 is observed. The contour changes that occur with aging should be replaced with the smooth curve or arc that is associated with youth. Various treatments, such as augmentation, lifting, or removal of infraorbital fat, may be necessary.

2 Anatomy

Currently, there is no uniform terminology regarding the structures relating to dark circles, so the authors have provided definitions of the most commonly used terminology. When young, the space from below the eyes to the medial cheek (anterior cheek) is an oval shape (or apple shape), without any concavity. However, with aging, lines or grooves form. The nasojugal groove forms first, and then depending on the individual, it is followed by the formation of either the palpebromalar groove or the mid-cheek furrow. The medial cheek is divided into three compartments by these three lines/grooves.

Safe Filler Injection Technique Demonstration – using live imaging tools

3 segments
A: Lid-cheek segment
B: Malar segment (malar mound)
C: Nasolabial segment

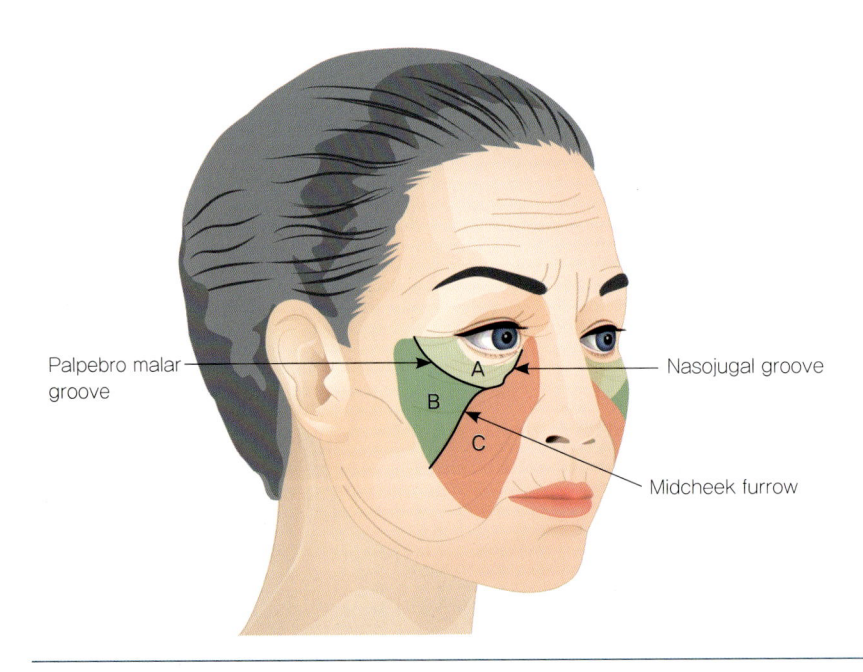

Fig. 4-99 Three compartments that form due to lines/grooves with aging

- Nasojugal groove (tear trough or tear trough deformity)
- Palpebromalar groove (lid-cheek junction)
- Mid-cheek furrow

1) Tear Trough (Nasojugal Groove)

Tear trough is defined as a region of concavity that starts from the medial canthus and descends inferolaterally to the mid-pupillary line. It is also called the nasojugal groove. A "trough" is a large receptacle that holds water or food for animals, and this word is used as the shape of a trough is similar to that of the lacrimal groove. If the concavity of the trough is severe, it is called the tear trough deformity.

2) Palpebromalar Groove

The palpebromalar groove starts from the mid-pupillary line at the point where the nasojugal groove ends and runs superolaterally. It runs parallel to and below the infraorbital rim. The palpebromalar groove appears with aging and forms after the nasojugal groove.

3) Orbital Retaining Ligament (ORL)

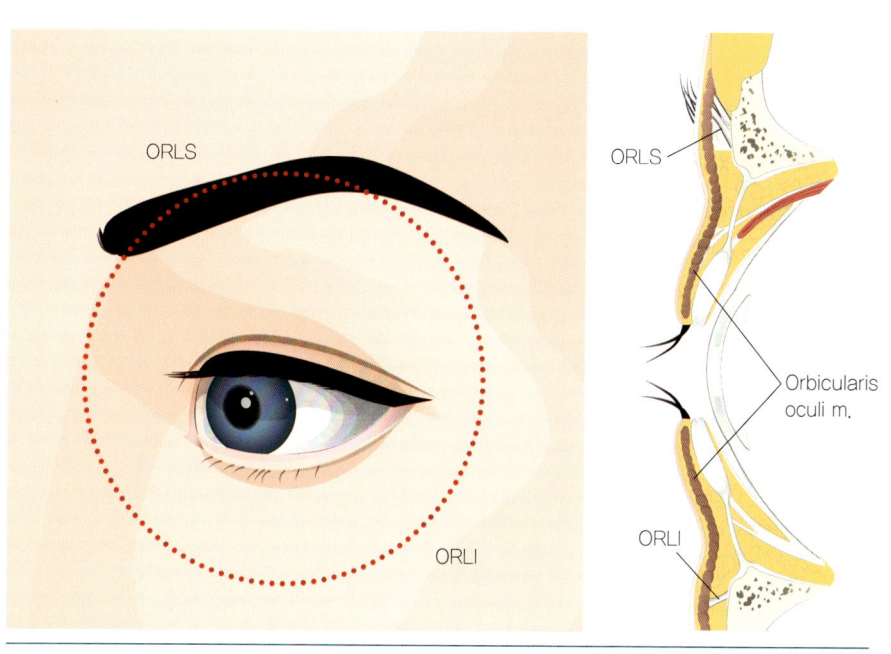

Fig. 4-100 Orbital Retaining Ligament
ORLS: Orbital Retaining Ligament, Superior. ORLI: Orbital Retaining Ligament, Inferior.

Safe Filler Injection Technique Demonstration – using live imaging tools

The orbital retaining ligament (ORL) which encircles the periorbital area is similar to a diaphragm. This structure is not uniform in shape and there is slight variation in thickness and length by region (Figs. 4-102 and 103). Especially, the structure of the ORL in the infraorbital area is significantly different from the structure in the medial and lateral parts. Recently, the medial part is being referred to as the tear trough or tear trough ligament, and some academic branches limit the ORL to the lateral parts only. (The author's opinion is that the term tear trough is more suitable as the medial part functions only partially as a ligament).

Medial part (tear trough)
- Palpebral portion of the orbicularis oculi muscle is solidly attached to the bone. It is a dense and tight fibrotic attachment (does not have the length of a ligament)

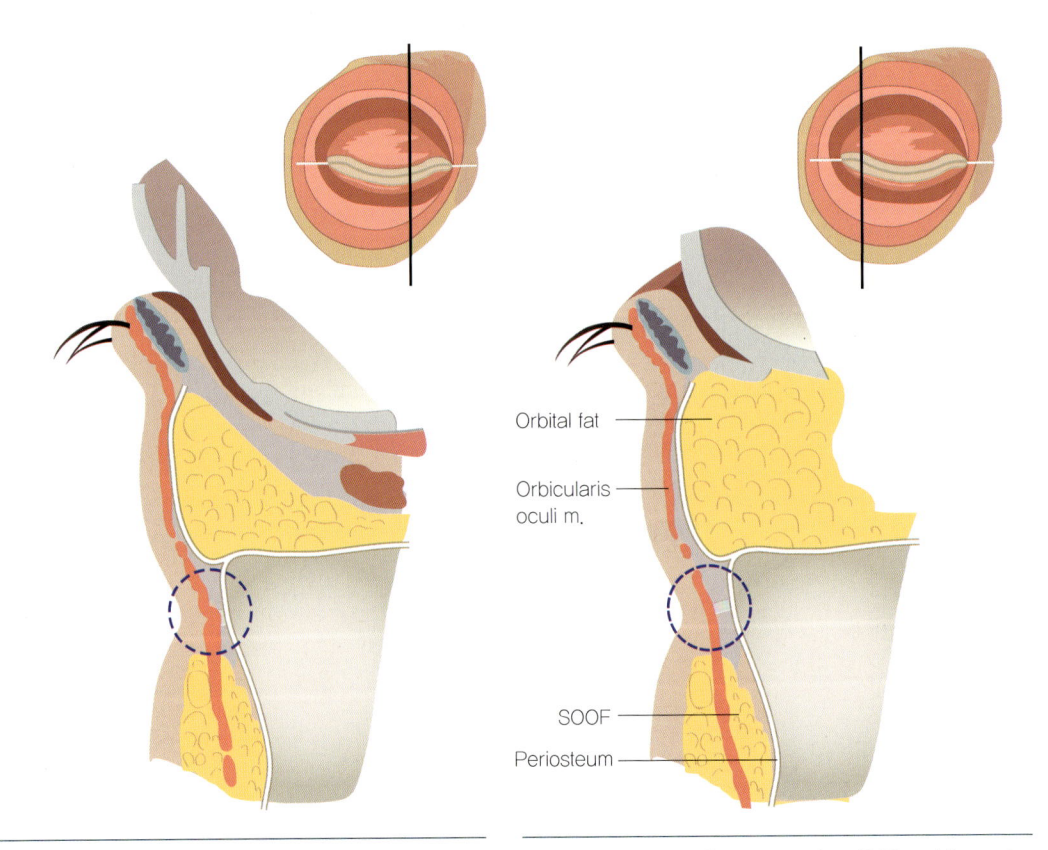

Fig. 4-101   Medial cross-section (tear trough)

Fig. 4-102   Lateral cross-section (ORL, orbitomalar ligament)

Lateral part (ORL, orbitomalar ligament)

- Ligamentous attachment/loose/mobile
- Connected to the tendon. There is sufficient space between the orbital bone and the orbicularis oculi m., and by injecting fillers into this area, hollowness is corrected.
- Dissected more easily compared to the medial part; useful in procuring more space for filler administration.

4) Mid-Cheek Furrow & Zygomatico-Cutaneous Ligament

This structure begins from where the tear trough and the palpebro malar groove meet, and descends inferolaterally. Although the zygomatico-cutaneous ligament looks as though it is connected to the tear trough, it is located inferior to the tear trough. It is because of this structure that the furrow forms (attached to the maxilla~zygomatic bone).

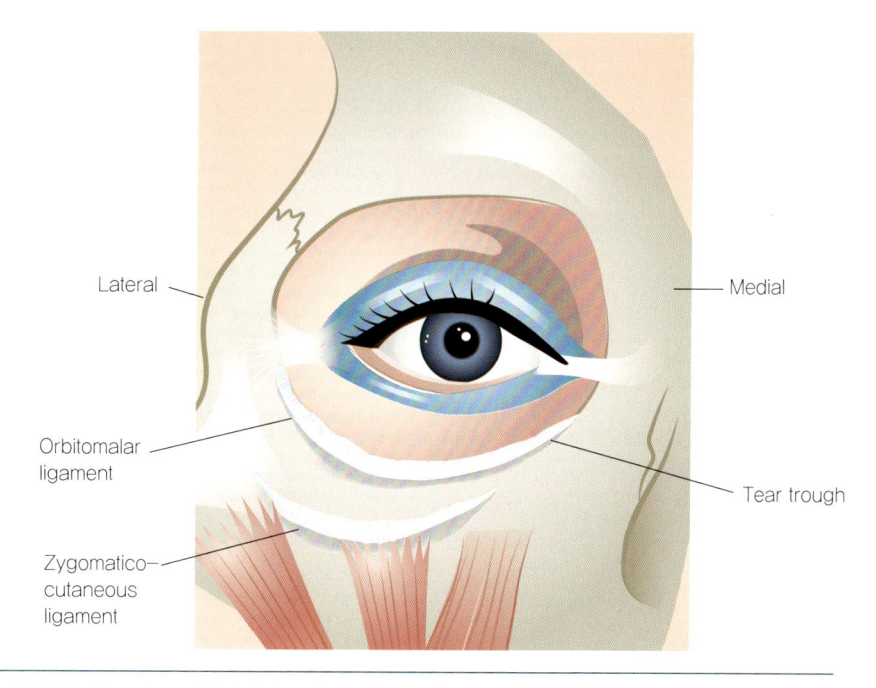

Fig. 4-103 Structures that determines the under eye contour

The bulge that forms due to the malar fat located in between the mid-cheek furrow and the palpebro malar groove is called the malar mound.

Both the tear trough (nasojugal groove) and the lid-cheek junction (palpebro malar groove) coincide with the superior border of the malar fat pad.

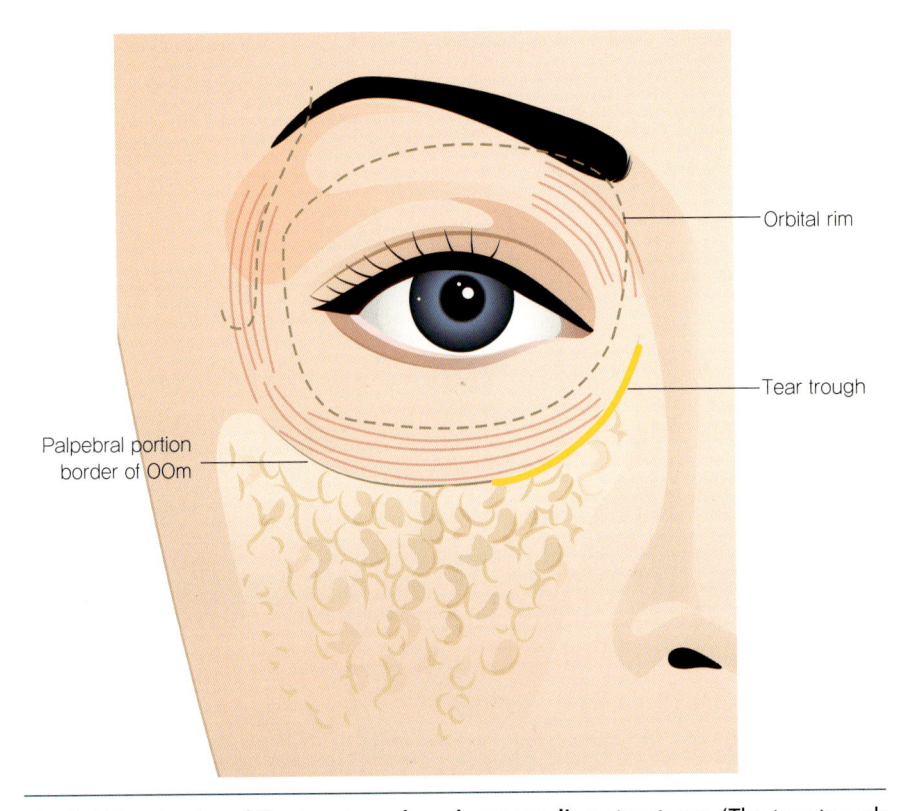

Fig. 4-104 **Border of the tear trough and surrounding structures** (The tear trough divides the palpebral and orbital portions of the orbicularis oculi m., and coincides with the superior border of the malar fat.)

5) Orbital Fat

Orbital fat is seen in both the infraorbital and supraorbital areas. The depressions in the tear trough and lid-cheek junction become more severe with the herniation of the orbital fat.

6) SOOF (Sub-Orbicularis Oculi Fat)

- Angular vein is located in the SOOF.
- The layer deep to the SOOF is the prezygomatic space.

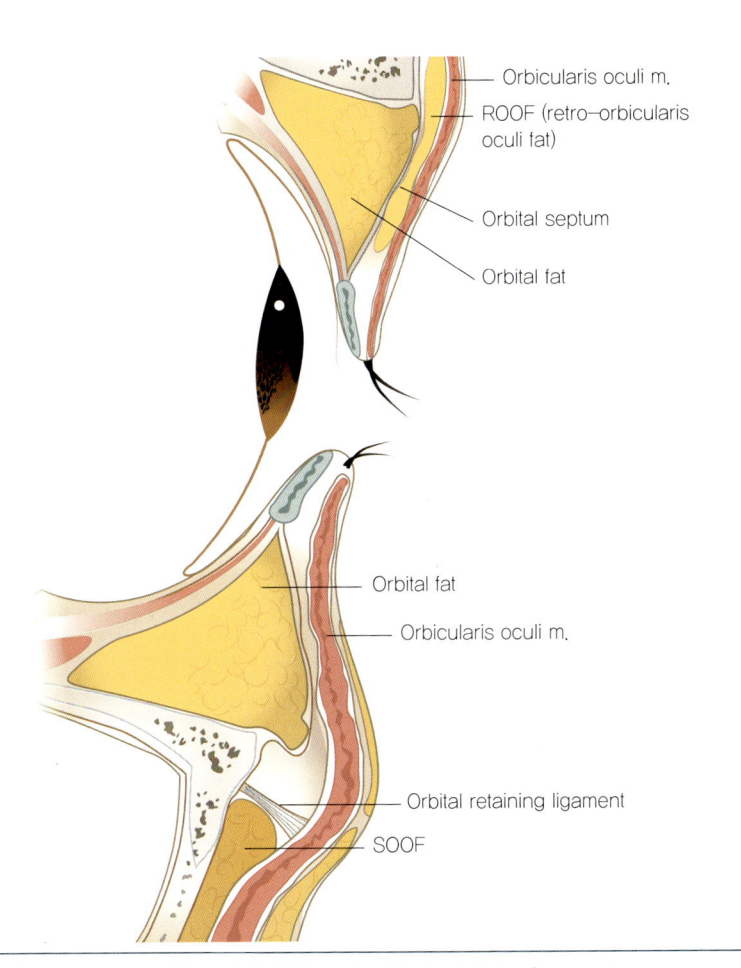

Fig. 4-105 Cross-section of the orbital fat and orbital retaining ligament

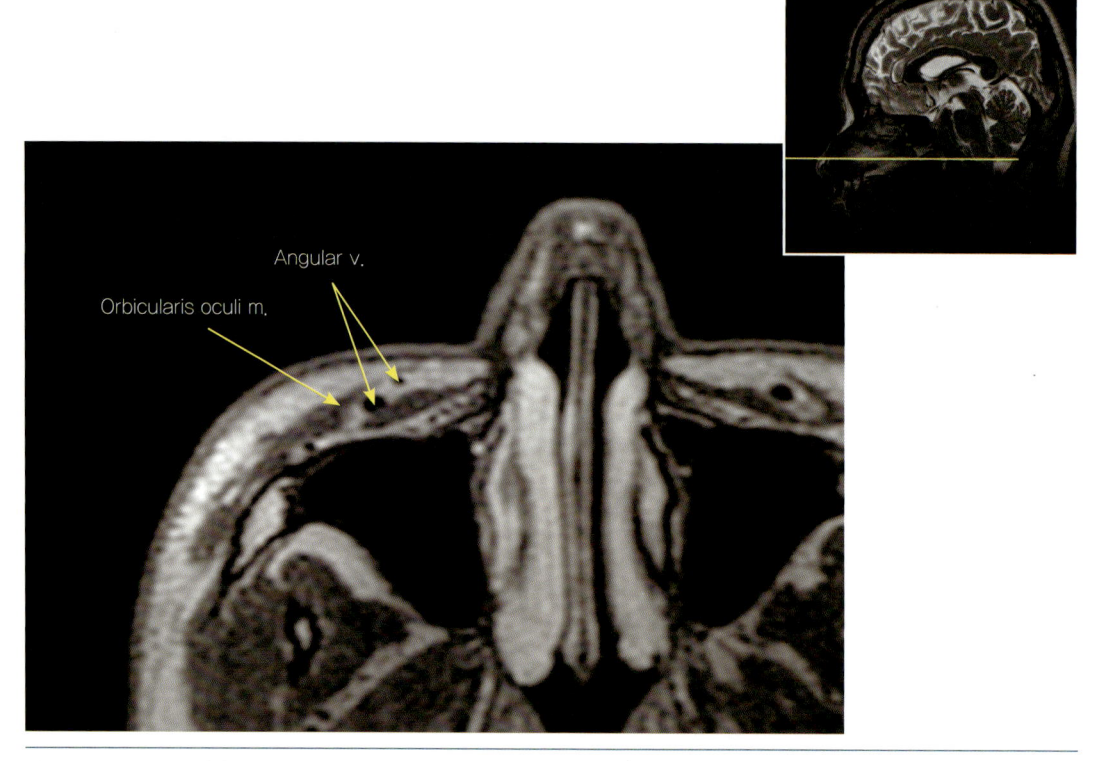

Safe Filler Injection Technique Demonstration – using live imaging tools

Fig. 4-106 MRI of the area under the eyes -transverse view (orbicularis oculi m. and blood vessels)

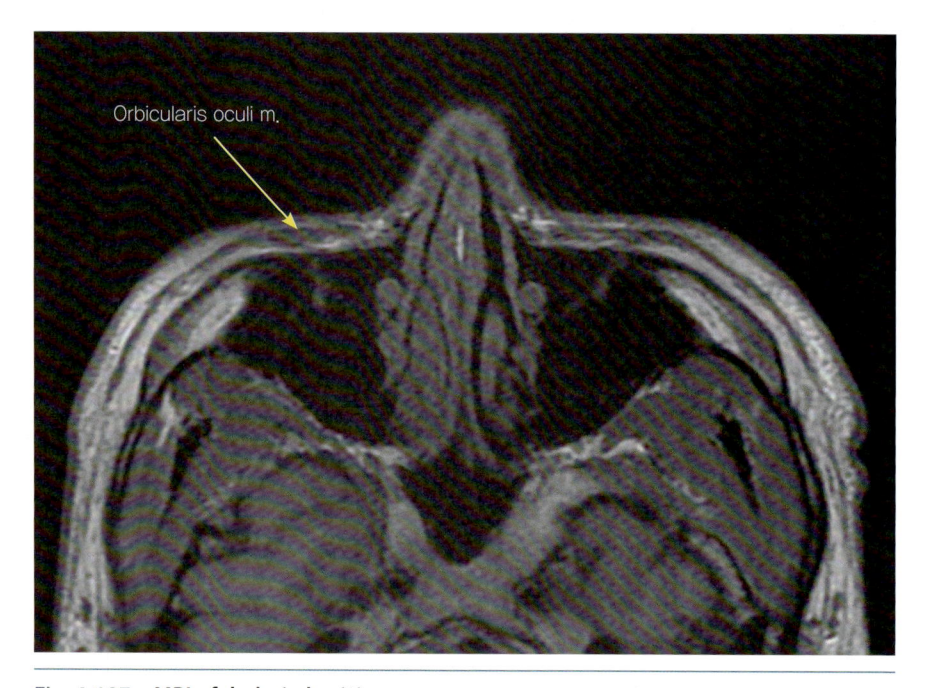

Fig. 4-107 MRI of dark circles (1)

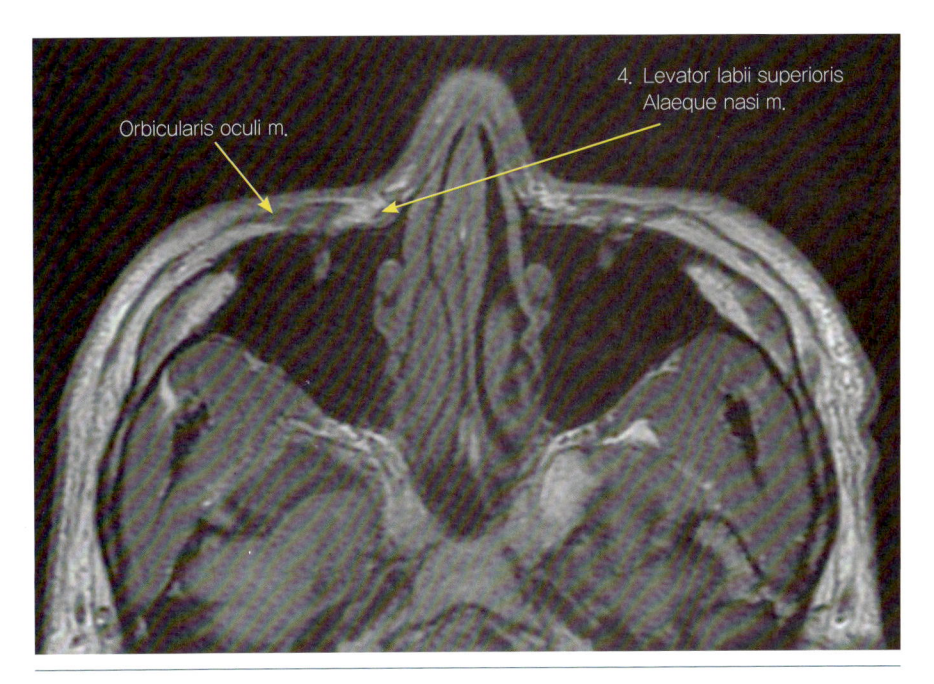

Fig. 4-108　MRI of dark circles (2)

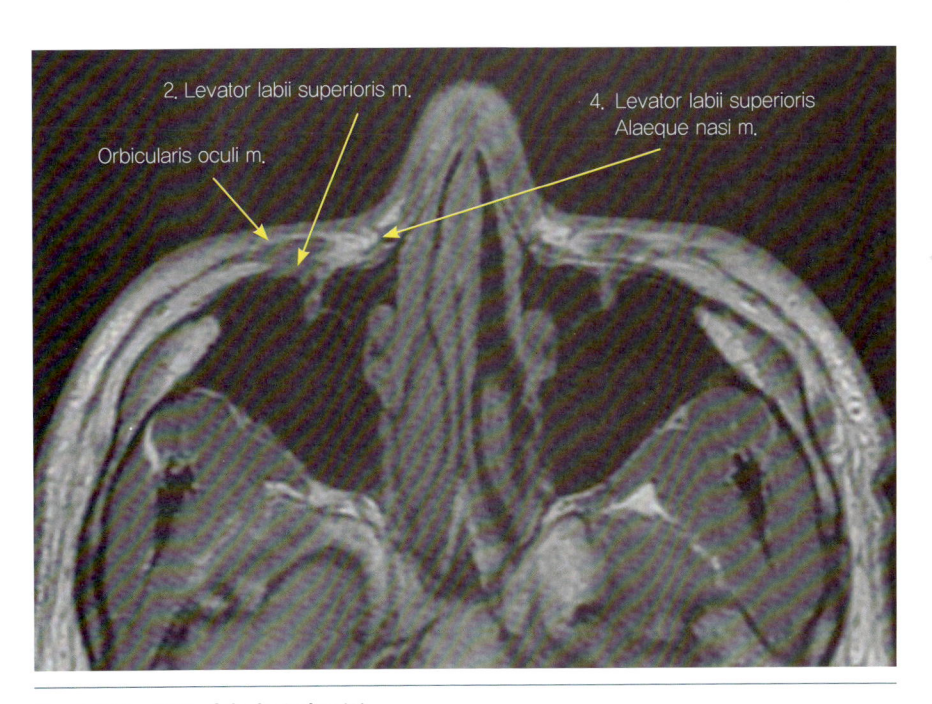

Fig. 4-109　MRI of dark circles (3)

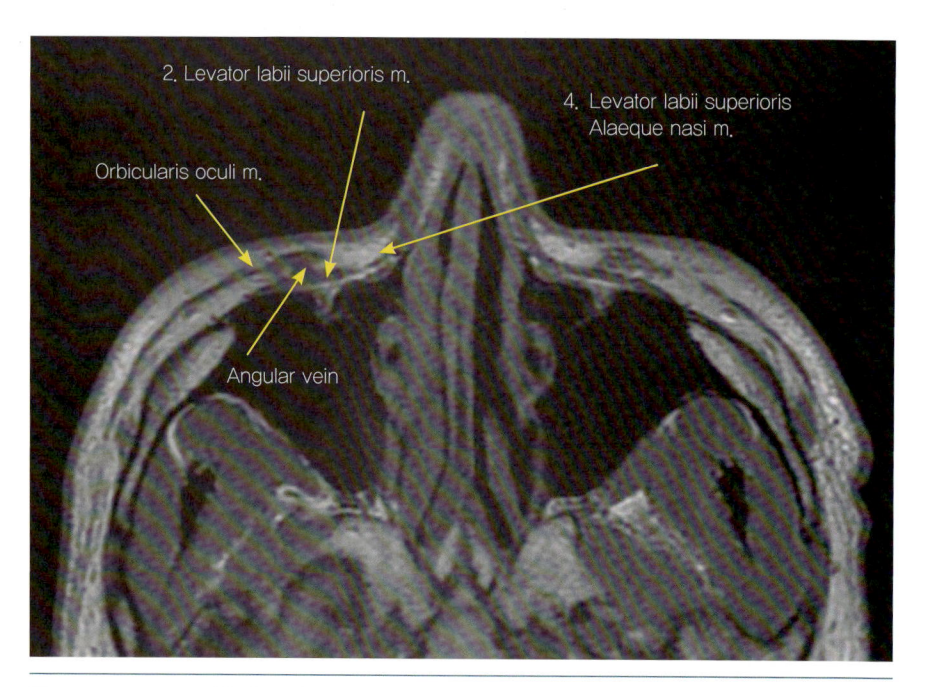

Safe Filler Injection Technique Demonstration – using live imaging tools

Fig. 4-110 MRI of dark circles (4)

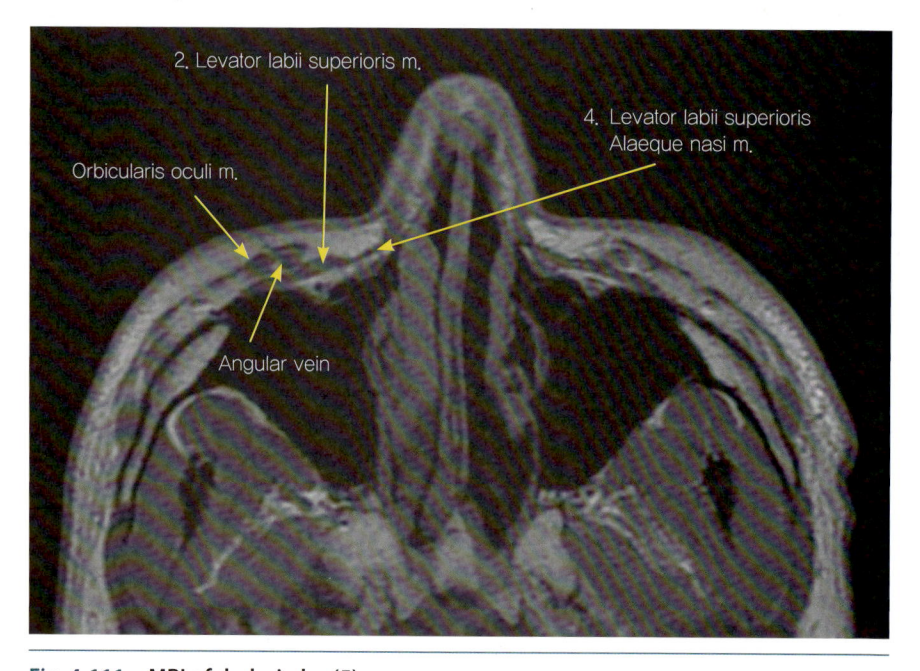

Fig. 4-111 MRI of dark circles (5)

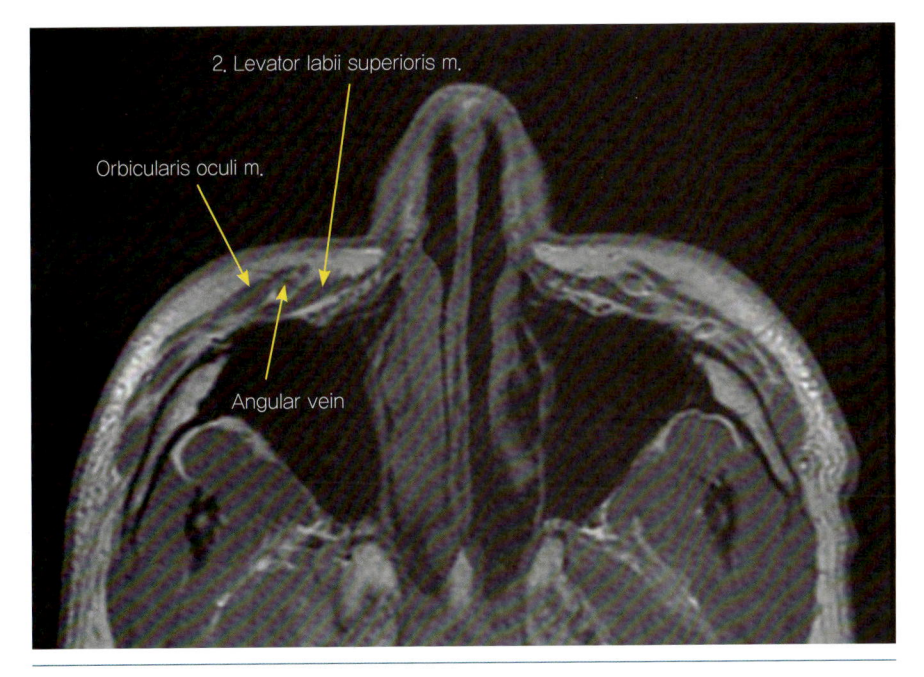

Fig. 4-112 MRI of dark circles (6)

> **Imaging explanation**
>
> - Dark circles usually cannot be treated with fillers alone. In many cases, surgery is necessary to remove fat under the eyes.
>
> - Caution is necessary in order not to damage the angular artery and vein. The vein especially, is a very large in size and courses through a deep layer (SOOF) and ascends via the medial border of the orbicularis oculi muscle. Exercise caution when using cannulas or needles.

3 Choice of Filler

The dark circle area is subject to a lot of movement. Therefore, even if surgery has corrected the aesthetic defect, there are cases in which the results do not look natural at the follow up visit and further correction is needed. Monophasic fillers with low G′ are not recommended in the deep layers. After the surgical procedures, patient satisfaction decreases mostly due to movement. Biphasic fillers with small to medium sized particles or the harder monophasic fillers are recommended.

If the filler is to be injected into the superficial layer, movement of the eyes must be considered. Assess the eye movements when the patient is looking up and down. Also, have the patient be aware of his/her eye movements.

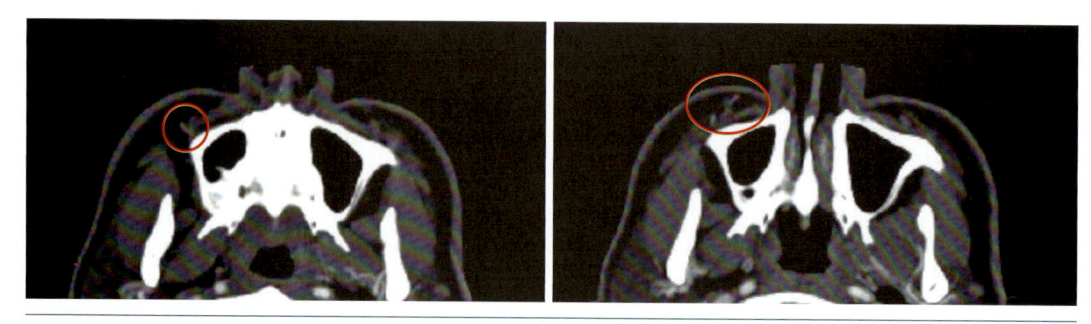

Fig. 4-113 CT cross-section of the infraorbital area (Course of the angular artery)

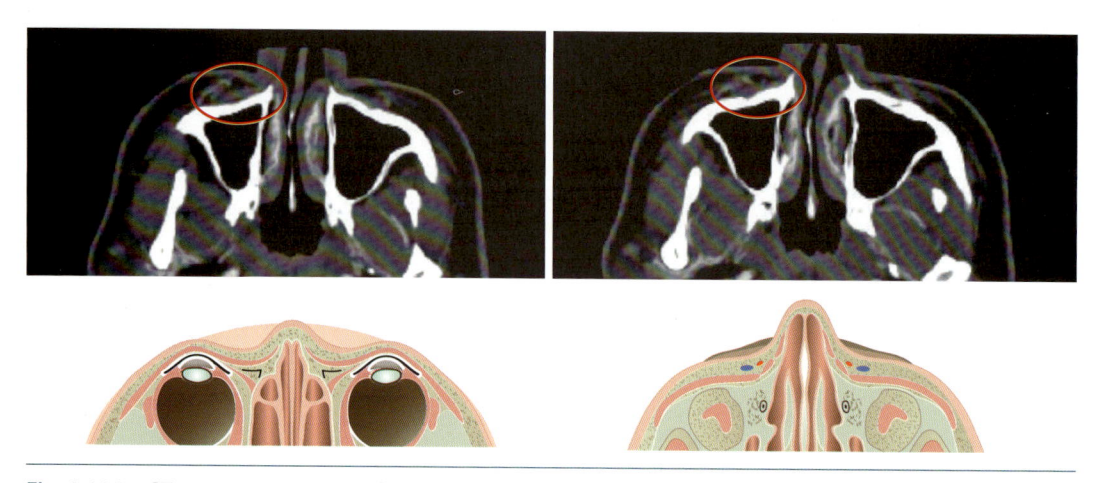

Fig. 4-114 CT cross-section view of the infraorbital area (Course of the angular artery)

Inject so that the dark circles are the least visible when the patient is looking straight ahead. If improvement of dark circles is evident only when the patient is looking up or down, patient satisfaction may decrease. Take into consideration that there is not as much flexibility in terms of molding the filler in this area.

4 Demonstration of Technique

The lines/grooves that form under the eyes, namely the tear trough and the lid-cheek junction, refer to the signs of aging that are seen on the surface of the skin. However, the cause is due to structural differences in the sub-muscular plane. Therefore improvement of the tear trough deformity and lid-cheek junction requires correction of the layer below the muscles.

1) Anesthesia

Infraorbital nerve blocks can provide comfort for both the patient and physician. Even with the local anesthetics, ice packs pre-treatment, or administration of fillers containing lidocaine, some pain may be experienced.

2) Design

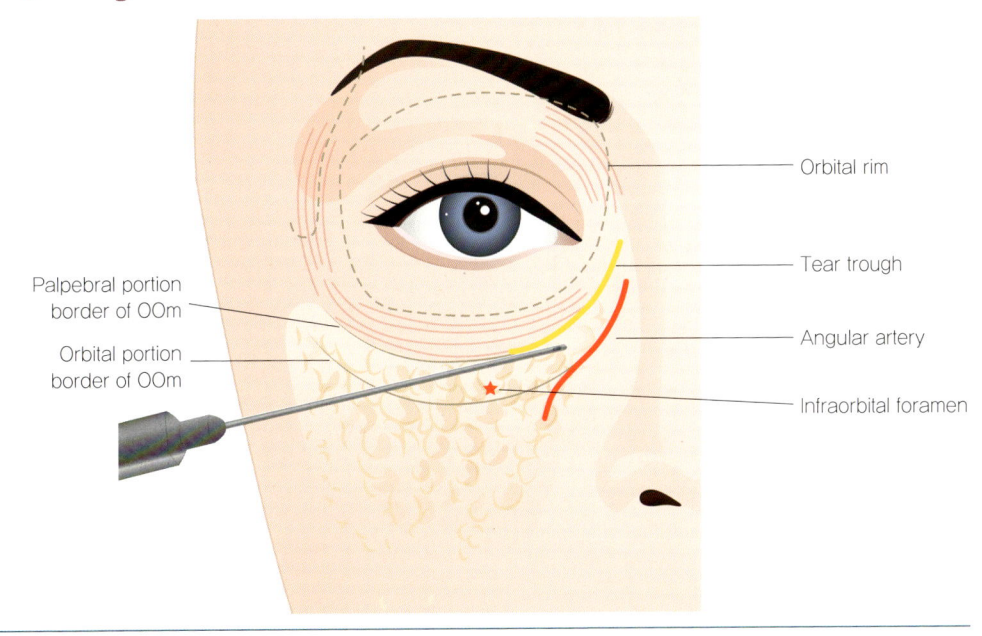

Fig. 4-115 Cannula injection method and surrounding structures

3) Injection of Cannula

The entry point should be slightly above the point where the nasojugal groove and the Indian band meet to form a continuous line. After the cannula touches the bone, follow along the prezygomatic space and inject immediately inferior to the tear trough. Inject gradually using the retrograde linear technique. As most of the tear trough is dense and short, injection into this plane may not provide sufficient correction. If this is the case, insert the cannula in the layer superficial to the orbicularis oculi muscle and inject gradually using the retrograde linear technique. If the tear trough is long enough or has been released, injecting into just the deep layer provides sufficient correction.

Treating the Indian band is easier than treating the tear trough. Improvement of the Indian band will be achieved with simultaneous filler administration in to the deep and superficial fat layers.

With the correction of the nasojugal groove and Indian band, improvement in the palpebromalar is observed due to the volumizing effects. If additional treatment is necessary, filler administration can be made deep to the orbicularis oculi muscle as the orbital retaining ligament in this area is on the loose side. If further correction is needed, filler can be administered superficially to the orbicularis oculi muscle.

4) Cross-Section of the Entry Site Area and Care to be Taken

After the facial artery branches into the lateral nasal artery, it branches into the angular artery. The facial artery is tortuous and courses along the side of the nose ascending to the eyes (see Fig. 4-113). As the facial artery courses in the fat layers above and below the muscle layer, exercise caution when injecting. For infraorbital filler treatments, the angular artery is avoided and the injection is made into the fat layer deep to the muscles, which is the space right above the periosteum. However, because branches of the infraorbital arteries and veins spread out in a complex netlike system in this layer, caution is still required.

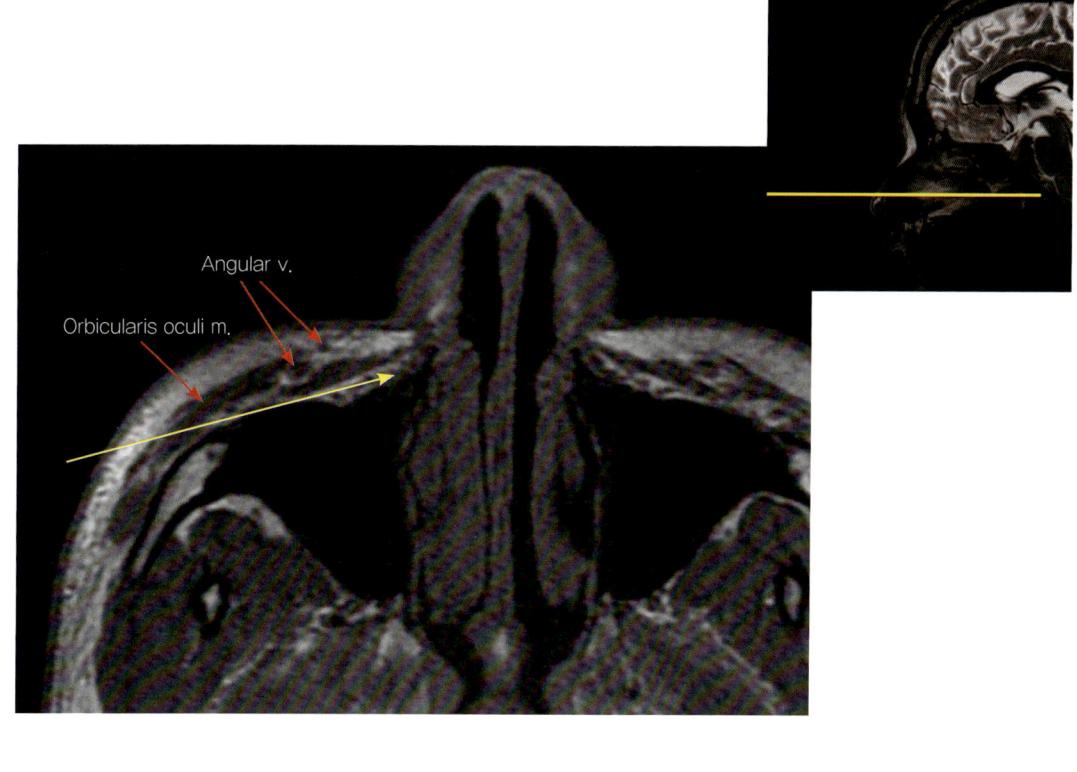

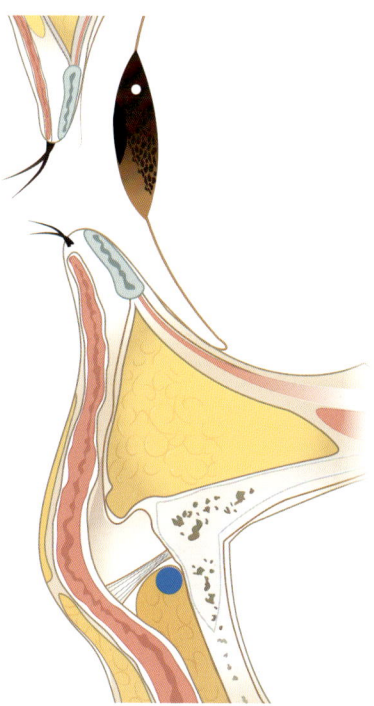

Fig. 4-116 MRI - Transverse view of infraorbital region (cannula injection route) and cross-sectional illustration of the filler injection plane(supraperiosteum level - blue dot)

5 Complications

1) Nodule

Risk of nodule formation increases with injection into the layer superficial to the orbicularis oculi muscle, uneven administration, and administration of fillers with high viscoelasticity.

2) Over-Correction

If an excessive amount is injected, the border along the lower eyelid pretarsal becomes less definite, possibly causing the lower eyelid pretarsal to look smaller.

As the tear trough consists of dense tissue, without sufficient release, concentrating the filler into this area alone can make the dark circles appear more prominent. Accordingly, when injecting in the tear trough area, superficial injections above the muscle layer must be considered.

SUMMARY of Dark Circles

A
- Structures that determine the infraorbital contour
  : tear trough, orbitomalar ligament, zygomatico-cutaneous ligament
- Infraorbital fat
  Orbital fat (surrounded by the septum)
  SOOF (deep to the orbicularis oculi m.)
  Malar fat (superficial to the orbicularis oculi m.)
- Angular artery

B
- The under eye contour is flat and smooth, without curves and bumps
- Both concavity and convexity are not aesthetically ideal

C
- HA products with smaller particles that spread well are recommended for the superficial layer. For the deep layer, fillers with higher viscoelasticity are recommended.

D
- Dense fibrotic attachment is the cause
- In many cases dual injection is helpful
- Above the orbicularis oculi m.: Fillers with finer particles Below the orbicularis oculi m.: Fillers with larger particles
- No injections into the dermis: High risk of lump and bump formation

X
- Nodule formation
- Over-correction
- Bleeding

8. Lower Eyelid Pretarsal Augmentation

Recently it has become popular to perform filler procedures to thicken the tarsal plates of the lower lid. This area, commonly called the lower eyelid pretarsal, is especially prominent when smiling and plays a supplementary role in making the eyes look more attractive.

Although the lower eyelid pretarsal is not desired amongst Westerners, Koreans consider it a symbol of liveliness and youthfulness.

1 Beauty

The preferred shape of the area immediately below the eyelashes of the lower eyelid is a curve, like a banana. The criteria for an aesthetically ideal eyelid pretarsal are:

- Must be symmetrical on the right and the left
- Must not droop
- Must be even from beginning to end
- Must be continuous, without any lumps or bumps
- Young people with elasticity in the lower eyelids are ideal candidates.

As patients have different aesthetic perceptions and goals, it is important to sufficiently discuss these matters prior to performing the procedures. Consult with the patient during and after the procedure by showing the patient's reflection in the mirror.

2 Anatomy

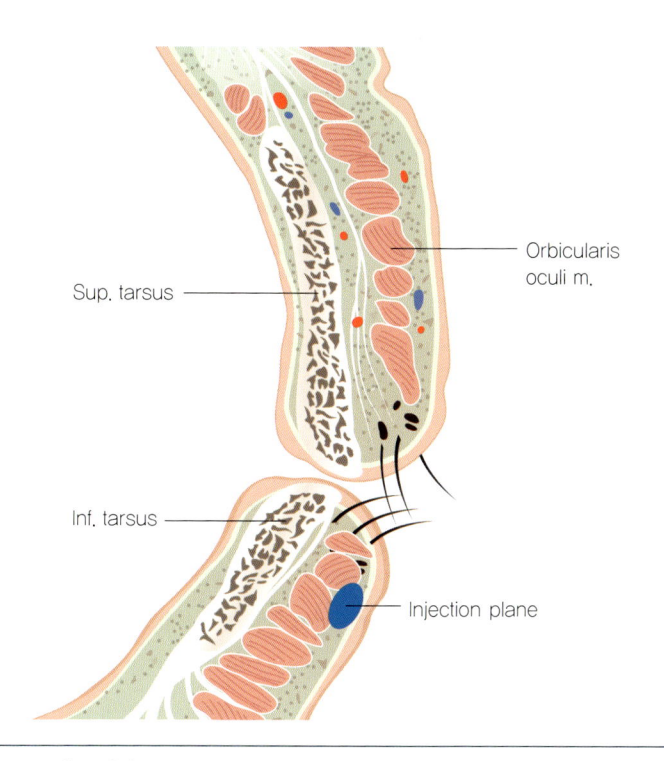

Fig. 4-117 **Anatomy of eyelid**

3 Choice of Filler

Fillers with smaller particles can reduce the risk of bump formation. Also, a moderate degree of cohesiveness is required so that the filler does not disperse or flow inferiorly. This is an area where perfect shaping is not easy.

Initially, it is easiest to use a needle and monophasic filler with low concentration. By creating a tunnel from the beginning to the end with consistent depth in about three stages, a natural and aesthetically pleasing shape can be made by spreading after injection.

With experience, fillers with larger particles or higher concentrations can be used. With the use of a cannula, filler injection can be made into the same layer without resistance, and it will spread evenly.

4 Demonstration of Technique

1) Anesthesia

- Apply anesthetic ointment to the lower eyelid and cover with a vinyl wrap. Ensure that the ointment does not get into the eyes.
- Infraorbital nerve block is also possible.

2) Injection Amount

- 0.2~0.3 cc on each side
- The injection amount differs depending on the depth and desired volume of the lower lid pretarsal.

3) Molding after the Procedures

Regardless of whether a needle or a cannula is used, after the procedure, apply lubricant or eye ointment with a cotton bud. While rolling, push the bud from the bottom to upwards, and then fix the shape.

Patients who have a thin and feeble skin around the eye may experience a slightly drooping lower eyelid in the pretarsal area. Since it is not very attractive to have a droopy lower eyelid, it is necessary to continuously lift it up. If lifting up is done continuously for a number of days, upward movement of filler would be possible.

In cases where the lower eyelid pretarsal shows only when smiling, continuous lifting of filler toward the lower inner eyelids as much as possible for a number of days can possibly improve the look.

4) Injection Route - Needle

- Inject in three installments.
- All the entries must have the same depths at beginning and end in order to connect evenly. Otherwise, layers will be formed.
- The entry site must target the upper third of the area between the eyelashes and the tarsal crease (close to the eyelashes).
- Injection should be performed just above the orbicularis oculi m.
- The whole front view of the tarsus is target areas.

- Make a channel with a needle and distribute the filler evenly along the channel. Use fillers with small particles and low viscoelasticity.
- The innermost side of the eye should not be injected too thick.
- Injection should be completed at once by the first entry. If entered twice, the possibility of bruising increases.
- Hold the filler in place by putting a tape just below the area of injection so that the space containing filler does not expand downward.

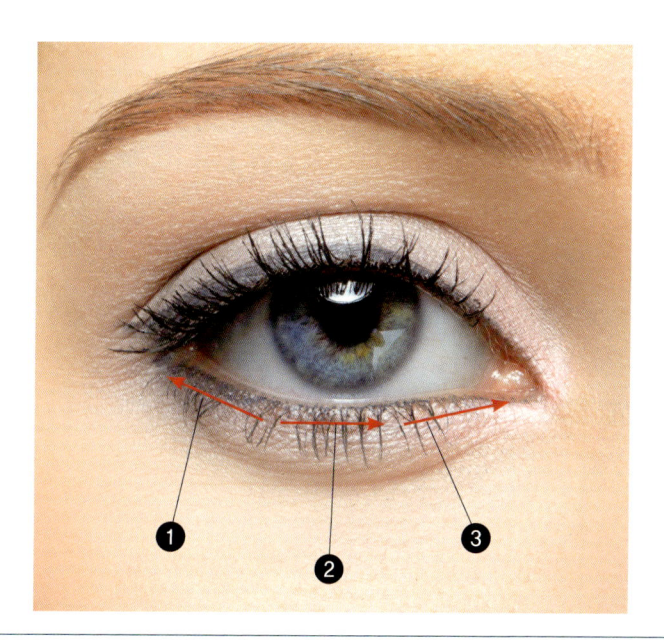

Fig. 4-118　Injection route- needle

5) Injection Route - Cannula

- Puncture at a point slightly below the pretarsal line of the outer lower eyelid. In order to be able to easily apply pressure during hemostasis, the cannula should be punctured at an angle, and entered up to the lower eyelid pretarsal line. From there, a route along the lower eyelid pretarsal line should be created for filler injection.
- By pulling backward, inject the filler along the route.
- The route must not become wider and must not move downward.
- Form the route at the uppermost part of the lower eyelid (right before the tarsus) at a mid-depth.

- Prevent the route from expanding downward.
- Prevent the filler from spreading downward.

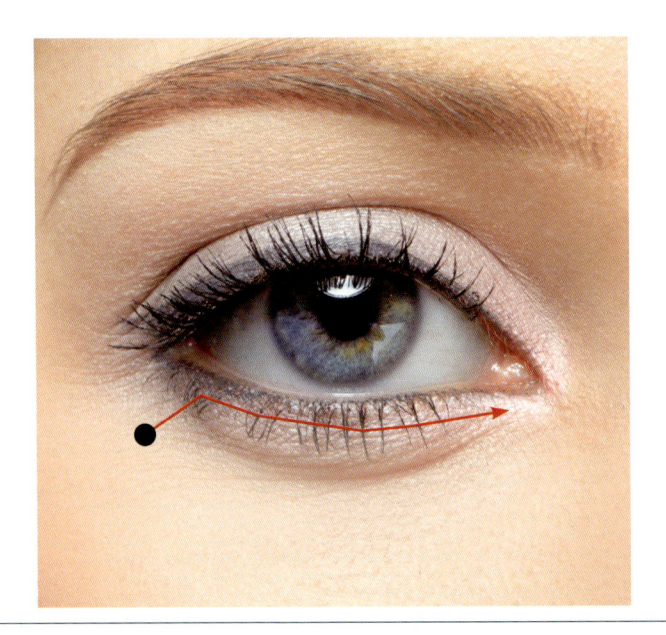

Fig. 4-119　Injection Route - cannula

5　Complications

1) Bruising

- It is important to inject at once to avoid bruising.
- In the event of bruising, a dark circle around the eye so-called the "raccoon eye" could occur. It is difficult to perform hemostasis in this area.
  - It is important to inject a small amount. A touch-up is necessary in the follow-up visit.
  - Fillers with large particles are prohibited in this area.
  - Absorbable filler substances must be used in this area.
  - Overcorrection makes the shape look unnatural, or lead to Tyndall effects.
  - Injection closer to the tarsal crease than the eyelashes can cause the lower eyelid pretarsal to look too thick and dull.

SUMMARY of Lower Eyelid Pretarsal Augmentation

A
- Layers of the lower eyelid
  : skin – subQ – orbicularis oculi m.

B
- The lower eyelid pretarsal should not become droopy.
- Injection must be consistent from beginning to end.
- Injection must be performed continuously without the feeling of crumpling.

C
- HA with small particles should be used.

D
- Needle: linear pulling method, Cannula: linear pulling method

X
- It is important to inject only once not to cause bruising.
- Bruising results in raccoon eyes. Hemostasis via pressuring is difficult in this area.
- During injection, the physician must observe and avoid the blood vessels.
- It is important to inject a small amount. The treatment is followed by a touch-up.

9. Sunken Eyes

• • •   Hollow upper eyelids give the impression of tiredness.

Causes of sunken eyes ≫	• Reduction of fat due to aging • Excessive fat removal during double eyelid surgery • Genetic factor

The former treatment method for the upper eyelid, which is the micro-autologous fat transplantation, likely results in surface irregularity. However, this can be prevented by using fillers with small particles instead.

1 Beauty

In the past, there was a time when hollow-looking upper eyelids without fat were popular and considered attractive. However, since that trend no longer exists nowadays middle-aged women visit the clinic to have their sunken upper eyelids corrected. Most of young Caucasian adults have mildly sunken eyes that look rather charming, but as they grow older and reach middle age, the skin around their eyes become too thin and deeply sunken. It makes them want to recover their eyes to their youthful look. Overcorrection may lead to swollen-looking eyelids, so only a moderate amount of filler must be injected. It is important to make the eyelids look natural even when the eyes are closed.

2 Anatomy

ROOF (retro orbicularis oculi fat) exists in the space between the orbicularis oculi m. and the orbital septum.

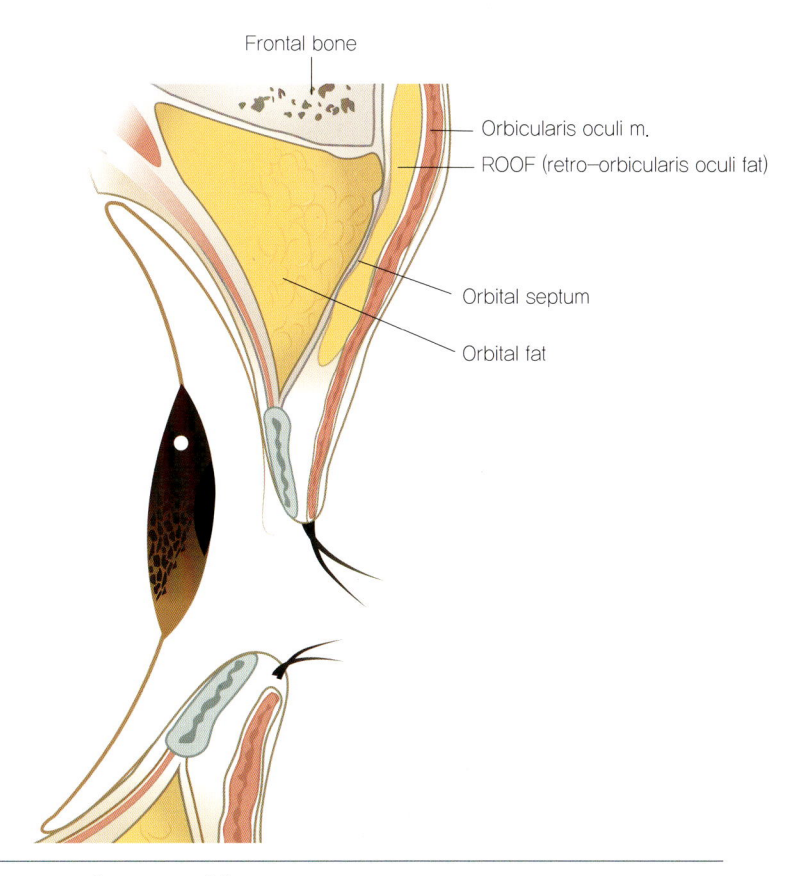

Fig. 4-120 **Anatomy of upper eyelid**

3 Choice of Filler

The upper eyelid and the orbicularis oculi m. are thin. Accordingly, fillers with small particles are to be used.

Molding is not easy in this area, so monophasic fillers with minimum levels of concentration that easily spread out in the skin are preferred. Hard fillers are not recommended.

4 Demonstration of Technique

1) Design

Draw the shape of a crescent moon along the outline of the sunken area.

2) Anesthesia

Apply anesthetic ointment to the upper eyelids and cover with a vinyl wrap. Ensure that no ointment enters the eyes.

3) Puncture Point

The puncture point is at the intersection of a line connecting the lateral canthus and the end of the eyebrow and the orbital rim.

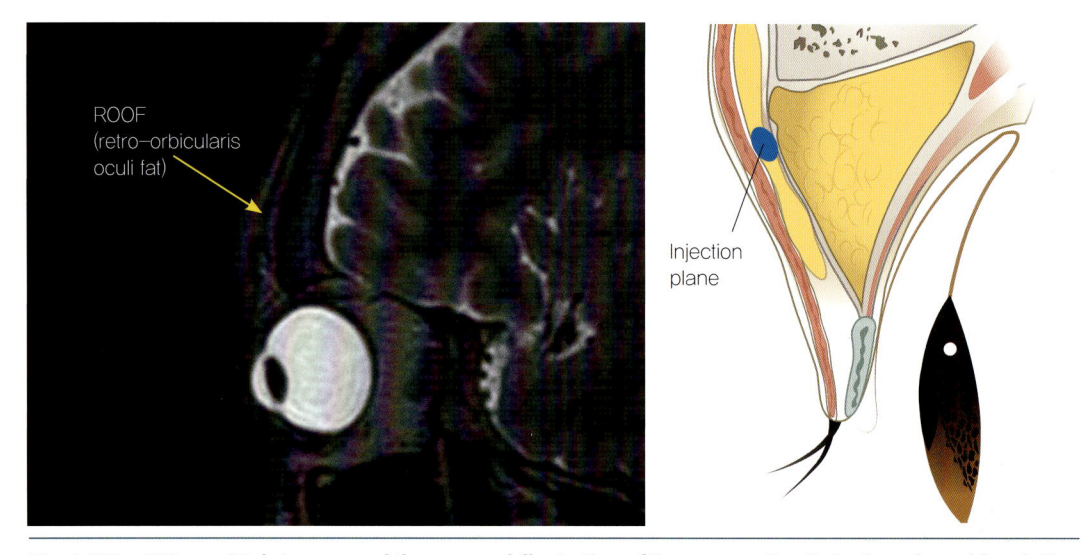

Fig. 4-121   MRI - sagittal view around the eyes and illustration of its cross-section (injection plane- blue dot)

4) Injection Method

- Using a repetitive puncture method, inject via the retrograde technique.
- The ROOF is shown to be located behind the orbicularis oculi m. in the dark area in the MRI image (Fig. 4-121). As molding is difficult in this area, soft filler must be injected and then flattened softly through spreading.

5) Depth

Inject into the ROOF (retro orbicuoculi oculi fat), the space between the orbicularis oculi m. and the orbital septum.

6) Injection Amount

- 0.2~0.4 cc/each side

5 Complications

- Procedures are carried out with the patient's eyes open. Surface irregularity can be seen when patient's eyes are closing.
- Be cautious not to create any nodules when injecting into the subcutaneous layer above the orbicularis oculi m..
- Excessive correction can make the eyes look unnatural or heavy.
- When using a filler with thick particles, be cautious of nodularity.
- Absorbable filler substances must be used.

SUMMARY of Sunken Eyes

A
- Understanding of the ROOF

B
- Supplementing areas with insufficient fat

C
- Soft HA

D
- Using a cannula, inject into the ROOF, a space deeper than the orbicularis oculi m.

X
- Be aware of the risk of forming lumps.

4

Filler Treatment for Each Facial Area

Lower Face

10. Chin

••• According to some old sayings in Korea, face with an under-developed chin gives an impression of less fortune and weakness. In the event that a severe degree of malocclusion is accompanied by uneven teeth, dental treatment would be required. However, in the case of a mere micrognathia, commonly called "having no chin", excellent results can be obtained through a simple aesthetic procedure. In the past, silicon prostheses insertion surgery was performed, but this procedure can be adequately replaced by the use of filler. As the vasculature is not complex in the chin, complications are rare, which encourages the beginners to easily attempt the treatment.

1 Beauty

1) In case the Sideline is not Pretty

When viewed from the side, the curve from the lips to the chin must form an inverted S to fulfill the standard of beauty (Fig. 4-122).

2) In the case of a Round Face

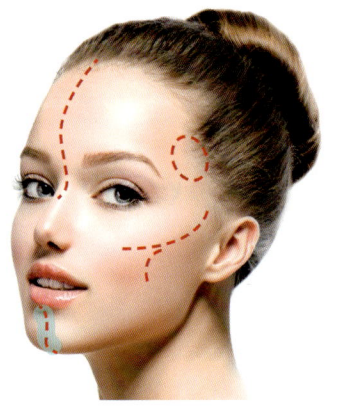

Fig. 4-122 Inverted S line from the lips to the chin

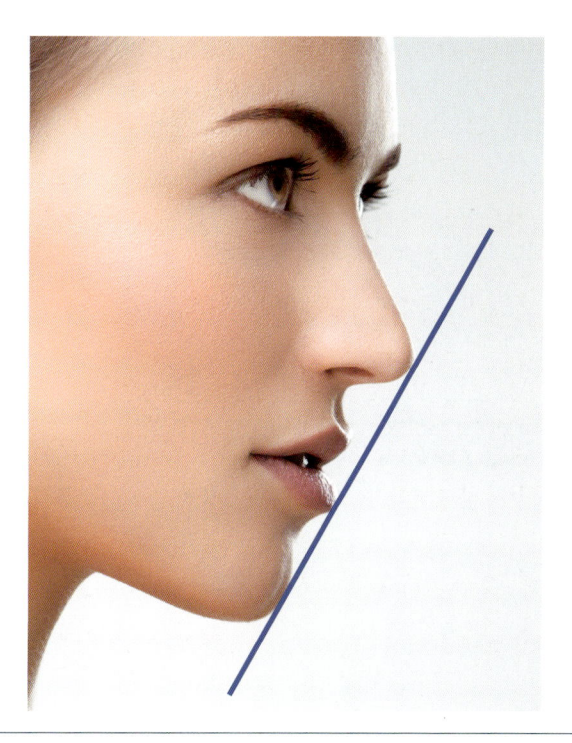

Fig. 4-123   Aesthetic Lines
The lips must not protrude beyond a line drawn from the nose tip to the mentum.

If the face looks round when viewed from the front due to big cheeks, making the chin slightly pointy can change the overall outline of the face to look slimmer forming the V-line.

From the side, the retracted chin can be augmented so it could protrude more (Fig. 4-123). If the jaw line looks flat as a horizontal line or the cheeks are relatively big when viewed from the front, augmentation is to be done slightly downward for elongation of the face in general.

2   Anatomy

1) Mentalis Muscle

Origin of the muscles and insertion

Safe Filler Injection Technique Demonstration – using live imaging tools

Fig. 4-124 Mentalis muscle and orbicularis oris muscle

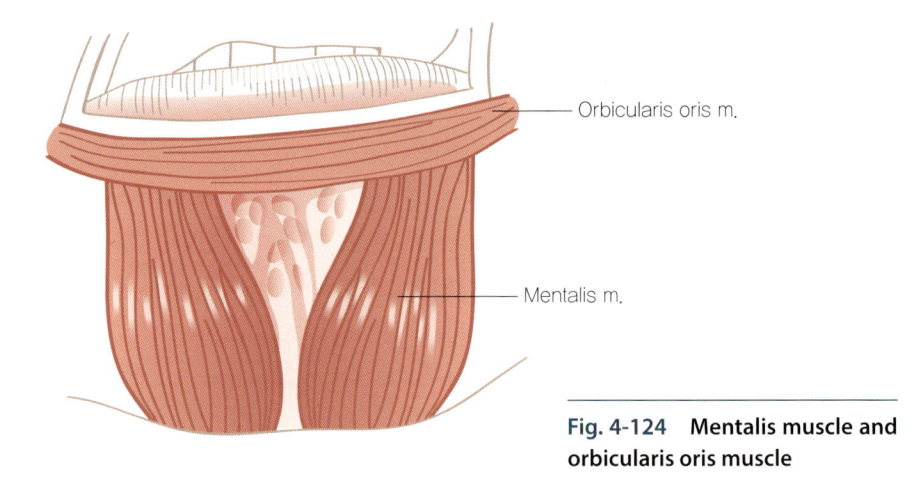

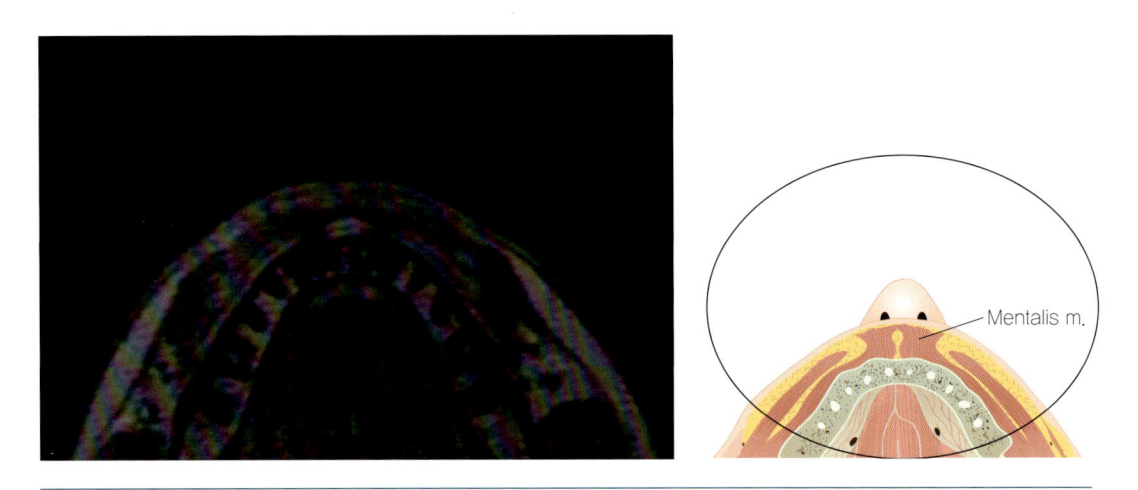

Fig. 4-125 MRI of the chin (transverse view)

3 Choice of Filler

- Products with large and durable particles and good viscoelasticity should be used.
- Due to the simplicity of the procedure, beginners can perform the procedures with assuarance. But to make a perfect chin, still needs good technique.
- Soft monophasic filler is not recommended. Biphasic filler or calcium filler is recommended at the beginning of the procedure.
- For people with a severely cobbled chin, pre-treatment with botulinum toxin is recommended in advance, which could bring a more satisfactory result.

4 Demonstration of Technique

1) Evaluation Prior to the Procedure

Prior to the procedure, ascertain whether the chin is to be projected forward or elongated downward.

- Use a needle (27G±) or a cannula (22G±).
- Inject below the muscle layer, called the supraperiosteum. (Injection above the muscle layer is also possible.)
- Mold after injection.

2) Needle (Fig. 4-126, (a) point injection)

For the chin, handling a needle can be relatively easy and comfortable as there is only a minimal risk of vascular complications. At the midline, the needle should puncture perpendicularly, touch the bone, and then inject immediately. (Due to the increase in volume, slight pain could be felt from the increase in the intramuscular pressure.)

3) Cannula (Fig. 4-126, (b) point injection)

If a cannula is used, approach from both sides or from the center if possible. With accumulation of many clinical experiences, the physician will eventually learn how to make a pretty symmetric chin by approaching from only one side. Immediately after the procedure, the chin might appear as evenly rounded due to swelling, but unless it has been checked carefully by hand, uneven areas are difficult to identify just with naked eyes. While performing palpation, additional fillers must be injected into wherever a bump or a depression is felt. This way, bumpiness in the chin can be prevented after the swelling subsides.

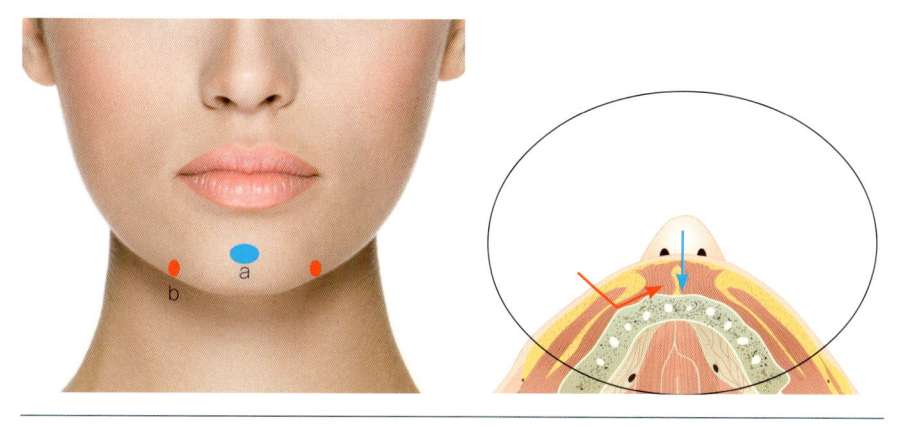

Fig. 4-126 Cross-section of injection depth for chin augmentation

4) Injection of Botulinum Toxin into the Mentalis m.

- A significant number of people with lower face macrosomia show mentalis hypertrophy, or the consequent skin dimples. If botulinum toxin is injected into the mentalis m. the dimple not only disappears, but tensed muscles are relieved, thereby allowing the shape to maintain well after filler injection and molding below the muscles.
- 2~4 U of botulinum toxin per each side.
- 0.5 cm from the midline (center) of the chin on both sides, below the halfway point from the lower lip borderline and the tip of the chin borderline.
- IM (Intramuscular Injection/ The suitable injection point is when the cannula is withdrawn slightly, rather than touching the bone.)

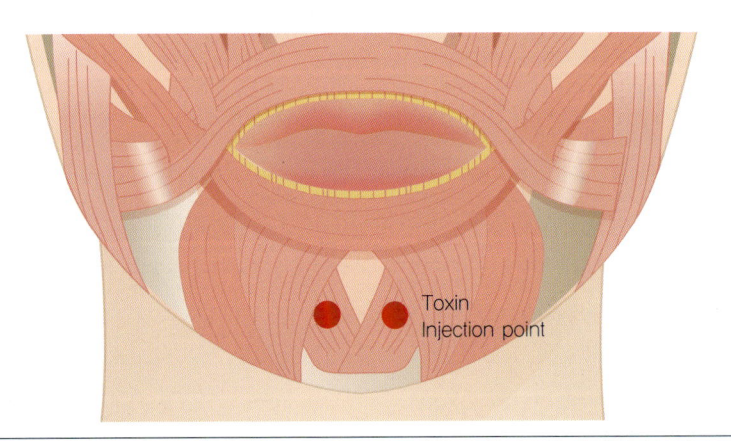

Fig. 4-127   Botulinum toxin injection point

5 Complications

- This is an area relatively safe from blood vessel complications, for procedures using both a needle and a cannula.
- If the injection site is too close to the lips, care must be taken as it can go into the oral cavity rather than the mental protuberance.

1) Nodule

If the skin is too thin due to too little subcutaneous fat, nodules can form when injecting into the subQ. In order to prevent such cases, the amount injected into the subQ must be minimized, and if possible the injection must be made into the space above the bone.

2) Migration

During a procedure for elongation downward, if the direction is too far downward or if the amount is excessive, care must be taken as the filler can move to the platysma muscle in the neck.

SUMMARY of Chin

A
- Origin of the mentalis m. and insertion
- Inferior labial artery course (injecting with a needle perpendicularly into the midline reduces concern)

B
- The lips must be inside a line drawn from the mentum to the nose tip.

C
- Product with long-lasting particles and good viscoelasticity

D
- Method of injecting from the center
    - Needle: perpendicular, supra-periosteum plane
- Inject by needle/cannula from both sides

X
- A relatively safe area for procedures, both with needle and cannula, with the usual care to be taken

4

Filler Treatment for Each Facial Area

11. Marionette Line

••• Marionette lines give the impression of a grumpy, cantankerous person. These lines are also called "grumpy wrinkles". Even with attractive features, wrinkles can make a person look older. If these wrinkles can be improved with intradermal fillers, a youthful face can be obtained without the high costs associated with lifting procedures.

1 Beauty

There is a scale for evaluating marionette lines. This can be utilized for convenient explanation to patients.

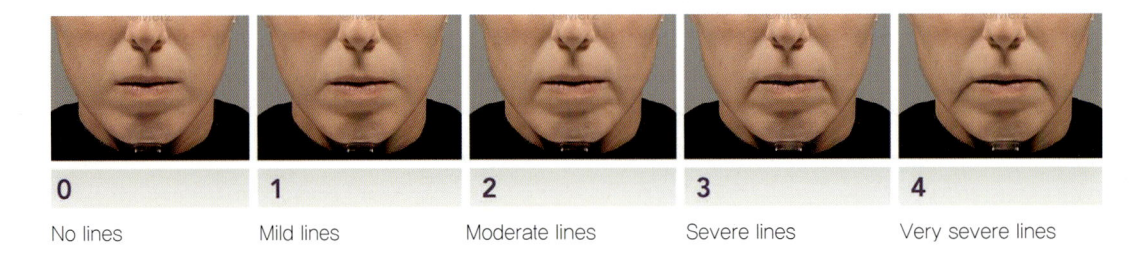

0	1	2	3	4
No lines	Mild lines	Moderate lines	Severe lines	Very severe lines

Fig. 4-128   Merz Aesthetics Scales (Marionette Lines - at rest).
Copyright© (2009) Merz Pharmaceuticals
Narins, et al. Validated assessment scales for the lower face. Dermatol Surg. 2012;38(2 Spec No.):332-42.

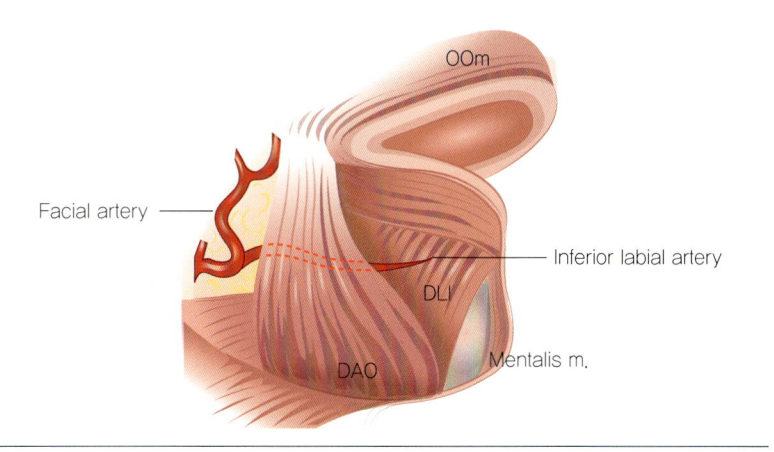

Fig. 4-129 Muscles and blood vessels around the lower lip
OOm: orbicularis oris muscle. DAO: depressor anguli oris muscle. DLI: depressor labii inferioris muscle.

2　Anatomy

The inferior labial artery (ILA) passes approximately midline of the depressor anguli oris (DAO) muscle. (Botulinum toxin injection is usually placed in the lower one third, and this is where the buccal and marginal mandibular branches of the facial artery pass.)

The DAO is more superficial than the depressor labii inferioris (DLI) muscle.

3　Choice of Filler

Any filler can be used without much problem.

When injecting fillers into the marionette lines, the injection amount should not be determined based on the convex area.

As marionette lines are emphasized by the sagging of fat due to gravity, if the fillers are simply injected into the marionette area, an unnecessarily large amount will be used, resulting in an unsatisfactory outcome.

Consider the degree of depression once the skin ptosis and sagging have been resolved prior to filler administration. Better outcomes are observed with the correction of skin ptosis and as opposed to the filler injection itself.

4 Demonstration of Technique (Fig. 4-130)

- Entry point: the lateral point of the marionette line – Point (a).
- From the entry point, direct cannula/needle to the mouth, designing in the shape of a triangle or rhombus.
- Using a cannula of 24~25G, separate tissue along the designed area (subdermal layer or superficial subcutaneous).
- Inject using the retrograde linear thread (fanning technique) method.
- Mold gently.
- Do not inject into the intramuscular space (there is increased risk of nodule formation due to migration and movement of the lips).
- If additional correction is required, inject using the same method at point (b).
- 0.1~0.2 cc for each side.
- Injection can be made using the same method described above at points (c) and (d).

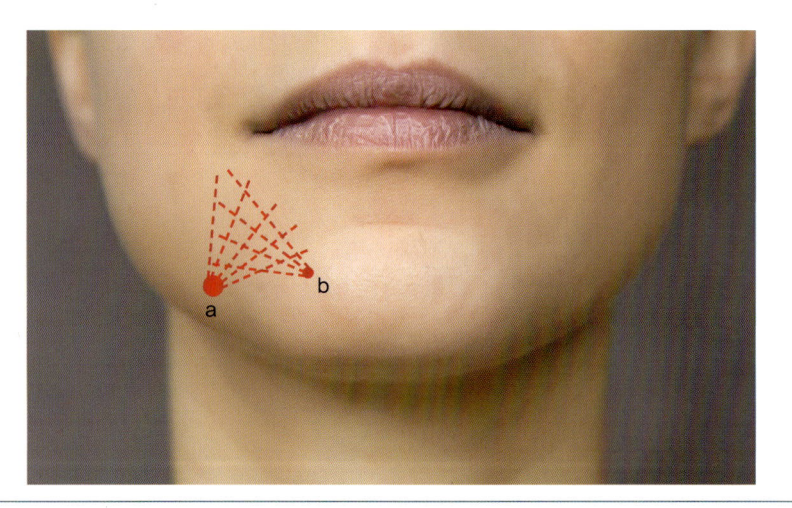

Fig. 4-130 Procedure method (injection point) I

Mentalis m.

a

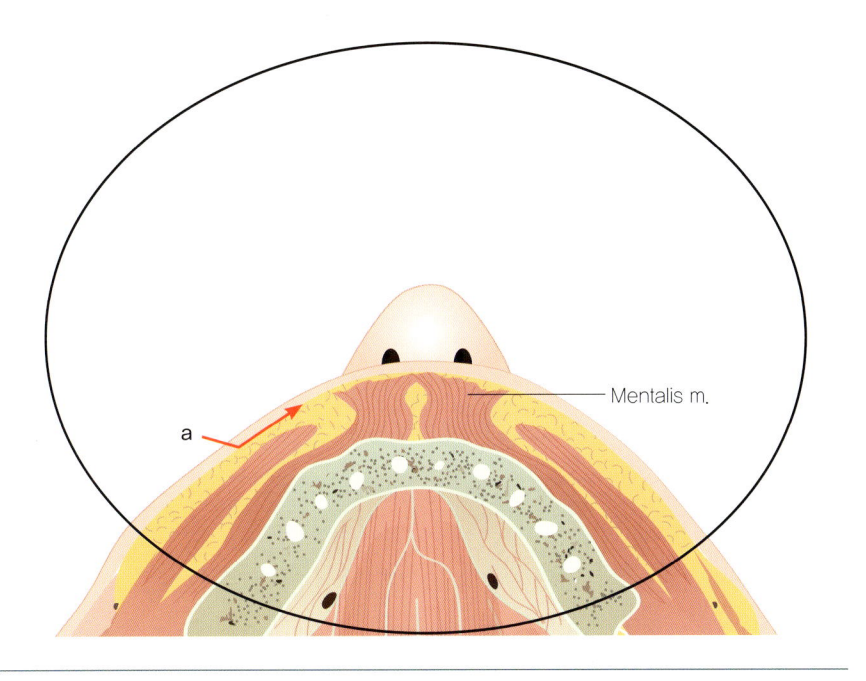

Fig. 4-131 Cross-section for procedure depth

c

d

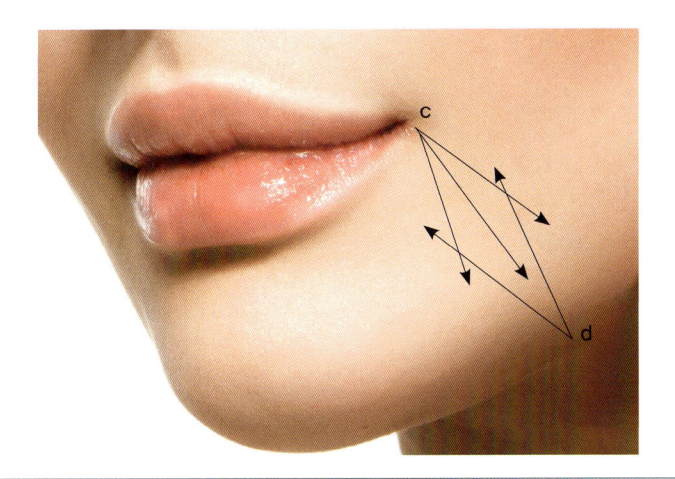

Fig. 4-132 Procedure method (injection point) II

1) Injection of Botulinum Toxin into the DAO

Injecting botulinum toxin into the DAO muscle may improve the marionette line to some extent due to the decreasing of tension. If the toxin is injected together with filler procedure, better results may be obtained.

- 2~4 U for each side.
- Injection point: 1.0 cm lateral and 1.0 cm inferior to the mouth corner
- As the DAO is a very superficial muscle, the injection must not be made deeply and must be made subcutaneously.

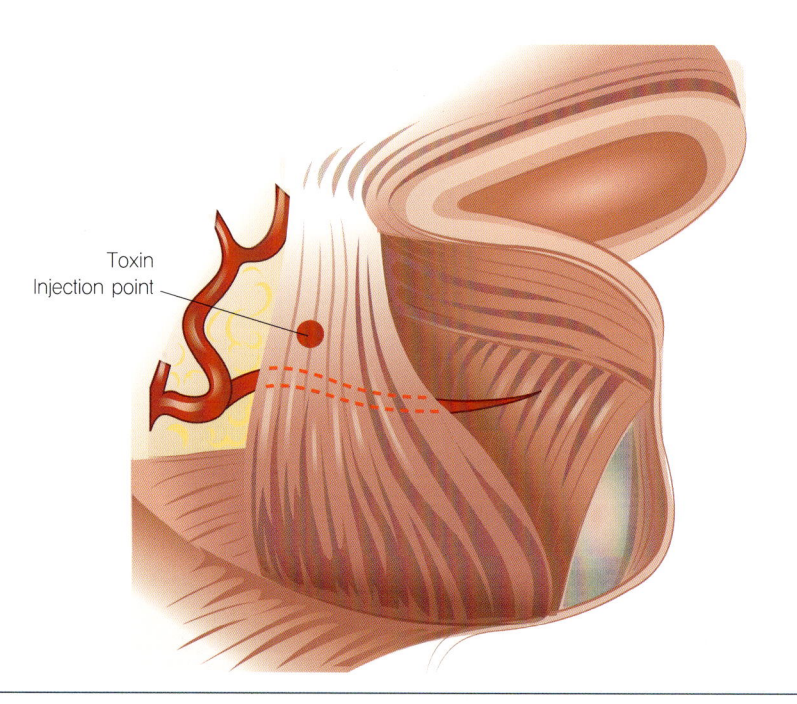

Fig. 4-133 DAO toxin injection

5 Complications

- For both injections in to the subcutaneous and deep layers, be cautious of the mental and inferior labial arteries.
- Risk of nodule formation: Avoid intramuscular injections into the orbicularis oris muscle.

SUMMARY of Marionette Line

A
- Insertion/origin and depth of the DAO.
- Course and depth of the inferior labial artery.

B
- Even with attractive facial features (eyes, nose etc.), wrinkles make a person look older.
- With improvement of this wrinkle, a youthful face can be achieved without the need of a high-cost lifting procedure.
- Rather than injecting a lot of fillers without consideration, evaluate first for presence of excessive fat and sagging of the skin.

C
- Fillers with small particles; fillers that mold well; fillers with low viscoelasticity.

D
- Using a cannula (24G or higher), separate underlying tissue in a triangular shape (subdermis) and then inject HA with small particles or CaHA (0.1–0.2 cc each side).
- Fill finely, using a cannula rather than a needle.
- When using a needle, inject superficially as possible.

X
- Whether injecting subcutaneously or into the deep layer with a needle, be cautious of the mental and inferior labial arteries.
- Risk of nodule formation: Avoid intramuscular injections into the orbicularis oris muscle.

12. Lips

1 Beauty

- The ideal ratio of the upper lip to the lower lip is from 1:1.5 to 1:1.618 (the golden ratio).
- Make the lower lip fuller and add definition to the ridges of the upper lips.
- Koreans prefer the shape of a cherry for the lower lips (fullness in center of the lower lip, like two beads).

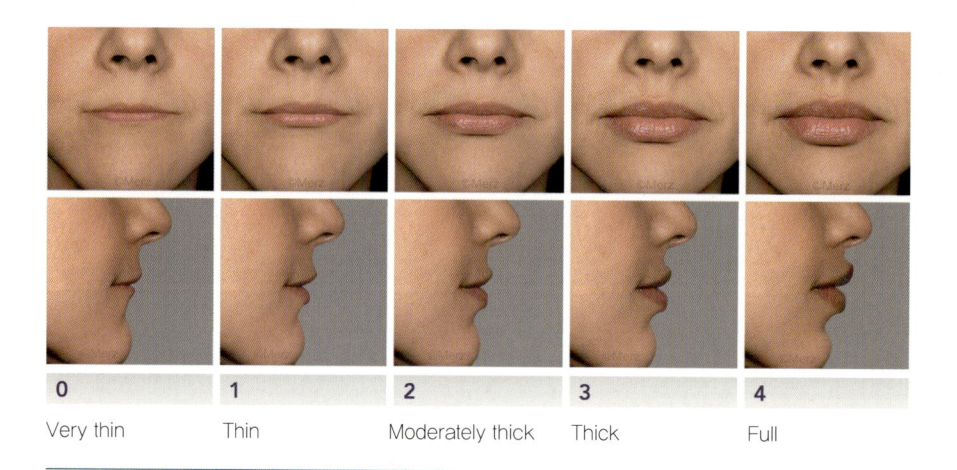

0	1	2	3	4
Very thin	Thin	Moderately thick	Thick	Full

Fig. 4-134 **Merz Aesthetics Scales (Lip Fullness).**
Copyright© (2009) Merz Pharmaceuticals
Narins, et al. Validated assessment scales for the lower face. Dermatol Surg. 2012; 38 (2 Spec No.): 332-42.

2 Anatomy

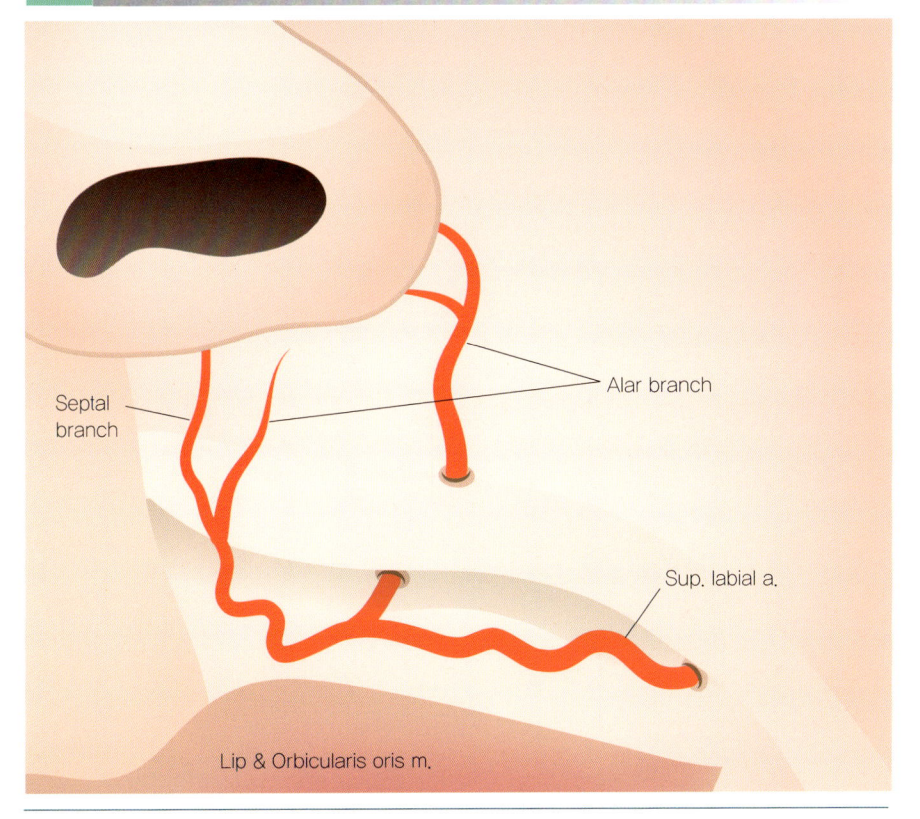

Fig. 4-135 Lips and the sup. labial artery

3 Choice of Filler

- Fillers with moderate viscoelasticity and mid-size particles.
- If cherry-like lips are preferred, biphasic fillers are recommended.
- If even fullness is desired, both monophasic fillers and biphasic fillers can be used.

4 Demonstration of Technique

- Upper lip: Vermilion border enhancement
- Lower lip: Cherry-like lip (volume enhancement)

Safe Filler Injection Technique Demonstration – using live imaging tools

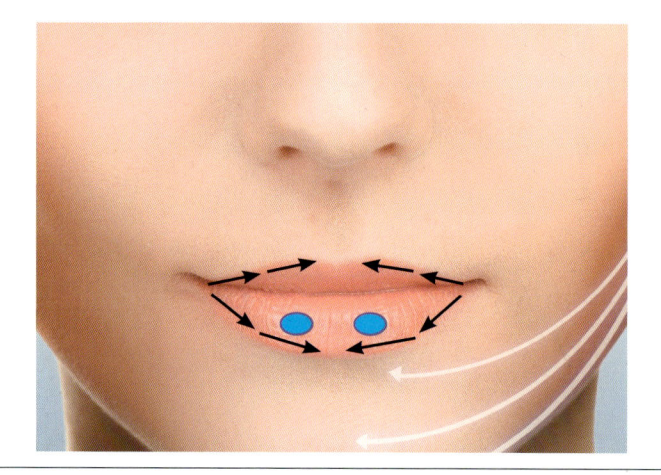

Fig. 4-136   Direction of injection for the lips
Correction of vermilion broder: Using a needle, inject in the direction of the arrows.
Volumizing effect for the lower lip: Bolus injection at one or two points on both sides.

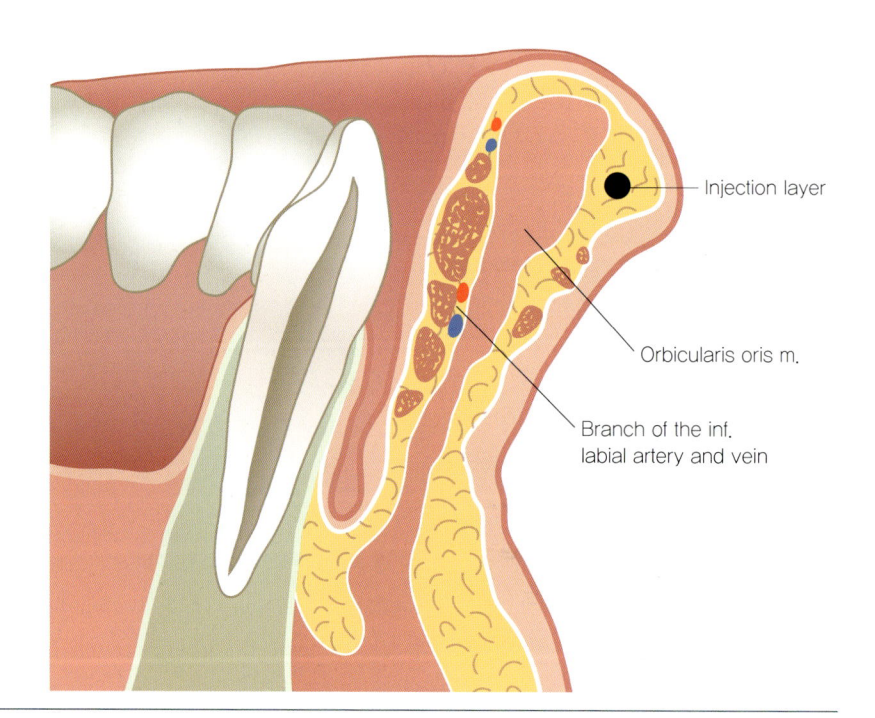

Fig. 4-137   Cross-section of injection

1) Design

- Complex design is unnecessary.
- Prior to the procedure, check the area to be corrected and degree of volume desired with the patient, using a mirror.

2) Anesthesia

- Topical anesthesia.
- Nerve block: For upper lip – infraorbital nerve. For lower lip – mental nerve.

3) Puncture Point

- Needle injection method: Any point on the vermilion border can be an entry point.
- Cannula injection method: Entry point at the oral commissure.

4) Injection Method

- Upper and lower lip lines: Procedure using the retrograde linear thread method.
- Cherry-like lip: Inject bolus.

5) Depth

- Inject above the orbicularis oris muscle.

6) Injection Amount

- Upper lip: 0.2~0.4 cc each side.
- Lower lip: 0.2~0.4 cc each side.

5 Complications

1) Blood Vessel Accident

- Small risk.
- If injection is made too close to the inside of the mucous membrane, there is a risk of reaching the superior and inferior labial artery. Injection must not be placed too close to the mucous membrane layer.

SUMMARY of Lips

A
- Understand the courses of the superior and inferior labial arteries.

B
- The ideal ratio of the thickness of the upper lip to the lower lip is 1:1.5 to 1:1.618 (the golden ratio).
- Make the lower lip fuller and add definition to the ridges of the upper lips.
- Koreans prefer the shape of a cherry for the lower lips (fullness in center of the lower lip, like two beads).

C
- Fillers with moderate viscoelasticity and mid-size particles.
- If cherry-like lips are preferred, biphasic fillers are recommended.
- If even fullness is desired, both monophasic fillers and biphasic fillers can be used.

D
- For augmentation of the lips, enter from the front or perpendicularly and inject after locating the needle tip at the middle depth of the lips.
- To improve the vermilion border, enter the needle in parallel with the lip line and inject while withdrawing.

X
- Other than injections into a very superficial layer or inner layer of the mucous membrane, complications are rare in this area.

Reference

1. Mendelson B, Wong CH. Anatomy of the aging face. Plastic surgery. 3rd ed. Philadelphia: Elsevier Saunders; 2013. p. 78-92.

2. Lee JG et al. Frontal branch of the superficial temporal artery: anatomical study and clinical implications regarding injectable treatments. Surg Radiol Anat. 2015;37(1):61-8.

3. Senem Erdogmus, Figen Govsa. Anatomy of the Supraorbital Region and the Evaluation of it for the Reconstruction of Facial Defects. J Craniofac Surg. 2007;18(1):104-12.

4. Jeffrey E. Janis et al. Anatomy of the Supratrochlear Nerve: Implications for the Surgical Treatment of Migraine Headaches. Plast Reconstr Surg. 2013;131(4):743-50.

5. Hyung-Jin Lee et al. Description of a Novel Anatomic Venous Structure in the Nasoglabellar Area. J Craniofac Surg. 2014;25:633-5.

6. Tomoyuki Yano et al. Usability of the Middle Temporal Vein as a Recipient Vessel for Free Tissue Transfer in Skull-Base Reconstruction. Ann Plast Surg. 2012;68(3):286-9.

7. Xuan Jiang et al. Middle Temporal Vein: A Fatal Hazard in Injection Cosmetic Surgery for Temple Augmentation. JAMA Facial Plast Surg. 2014;16(3):227-9.

8. Jung WS et al. Clinical implications of the middle temporal vein with regard to temporal fossa augmentation. Dermatol Surg. 2014;40(6):618-23.

9. Hun-Mu Yang, Wonsug Jung et al. Anatomical study of medial zygomaticotemporal vein and its clinical implication regarding the injectable treatments. Surg Radiol Anat. 2015;37(2):175-80.

10. Robert M et al. Surgical Anatomy of the Nose. Clin Plast Surg. 2010;37(2):191-211.

11. Hong-San Kim et al. An anatomical study of the risorius in Asians and its insertion at the modiolus. Surg Radiol Anat. 2015;37(2):147-51.

12. Ashkan Ghavami et al. The Orbicularis Retaining Ligament of the Medial Orbit: Closing the Circle. Plast Reconstr Surg. 2008;121(3):994-1001.

13. Philippe Garcia et al. Anatomy and volumizing injections. E2e Medical Publishing.

Safe Filler Injection Technique Demonstration
– using live imaging tools

Part 5

Filler Complications

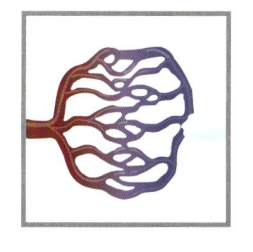

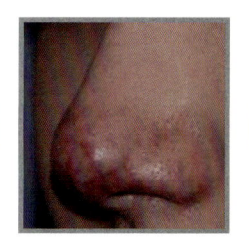

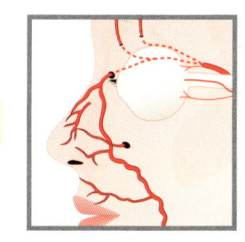

Safe Filler Injection Technique Demonstration
- using live imaging tools

Part 5 Filler Complications

1. Filler Complications and Interventions

1. Bruising and Hematoma
2. Erythema
3. Edema
4. Neovascularization
5. PIH
6. Nodule
7. Infection
8. Skin Necrosis (Blood Vessel Complications)

2. Mechanism and Treatment of Skin Necrosis

1. Predisposing Factors of Skin Necrosis
2. Factors Affecting the Extent of Skin Necrosis
3. Symptoms of Skin Necrosis
4. Treatment of Skin Necrosis
5. Notes for Preventing Necrosis during Procedures
6. Tips for Early Discovery and Treatment of Necrosis
7. Factors Affecting the Prognosis of Skin Necrosis

3. Other Blood Vessel Complications

1. Blindness and Cerebral Infarct
2. Pulmonary Embolism

Part 5

Filler Complications

1. Filler Complications and Interventions

●●● With the increasing popularity of filler procedures and changes in trends, the incidence of adverse events has also increased and the types of filler complications being reported are becoming more diverse. In the past, procedures were performed by unlicensed practitioners. The collagen fillers were associated with a high incidence of granuloma formation. Thereafter, as filler procedures became more popular and accessible, cases of skin necrosis began to be reported. Within the past three, four years filler and autologous fat transfer accidents resulting in blindness and cerebral infarction have been reported. Recently, there have been reports of pulmonary embolism and it is expected that the incidence of such complications will increase.

Other than the severe complications mentioned above, there have been cases of minor adverse events such as bruising, redness, edema, soft tissue infection, pigmentation, over-correction, nodules, etc., all of which can be easily treated in outpatient care.

Table 5-1 Filler complications	
Early onset (within a few days)	Late onset (within a period of a few days to a few weeks)
Bruising	Nodule
Edema	Biofilm
Pain	Migration
Itching	PIH
Infection	Chronic infection
Nodule/Lump	Granuloma
Vascular compromise • Skin necrosis • Blindness • Pulmonary embolism • Cerebral infarction	

Adverse events from fillers can be classified according to the degree of severity or the time of occurrence (early onset vs. late onset). The most important principle in the treatment of filler complications is early detection and early treatment. Therefore it is necessary to have a thorough understanding of the differences between the complications, the onset, and the respective treatments.

1 Bruising and Hematoma

Bruising and hematoma are the most commonly seen filler complications. Regardless of filler type, bruising can occur. If an injection is made into the supraperiosteal layer, the risk of bruising decreases, but when procedures are carried out in the subcutaneous or subdermal layer, there is a higher risk of bruising. Inducing vasoconstriction with cold compress pre- and post- treatment may reduce the risk of bruising. Applying a vitamin K cream to the bruised area helps. If the patient is on medication or supplements that increase the risk of bleeding, he/she may be advised to stop taking it for a maximum of one week before and after the procedure.

1) Factors associated with Bruising and Hematoma

- Needle gauge
- Depth of injection plane
- Patient-specific factors (age, medication, liver disease)
- Medication (aspirin, warfarin, clopidogrel, NSAID, vitamin E, fish oil, etc.)

2) Method of Reducing Bruising and Hematoma during Procedure

- Apply ice pack before and after the procedure.
- Mix epinephrine with lidocaine when performing nerve blocks.
- Inject slowly.
- Perform gently.
- Use a cannula rather than a needle.
- While proceeding with the cannula to procure space, there are cases when the skin bulges. If the skin bulges even though no filler has been administered, vessel injury can be suspected. Immediately withdraw the cannula and apply pressure. Apply pressure for at least five minutes. Even if the bulging has subsided, it is advisable to postpone the procedure.

2 Erythema

After the filler procedure, the appearance of minor redness in the treated area is normal. However, if the redness persists for several days after the procedure, the other conditions must be considered.

1) Factors associated with Erythema

- Pre-existing rosacea
- Depth of injection plane
- Patient-specific factors (age, medication, liver disease)
- Medication (aspirin, warfarin, clopidogrel, NSAID, vitamin E, fish oil)
- Poor product quality
- Hypersensitivity to the filler material

2) Treatment for Erythema

- Must check the presence of inflammation
- In case of erythema only
  - moderate potency topical steroid (long term use is contraindicated as this cause telangiectasia)
  - laser (dye laser, KTP laser)

3 Edema

Immediately after the filler procedure, temporary swelling is normal, and normally subsides within one to two weeks. In such cases, the method of minimizing swelling is the same as the method for minimizing bruising.

Some fillers have a strong tendency to absorb water, causing unexpected swelling. Accordingly, it is advisable to inform the patient about swelling prior to the procedure.

1) Water Retention of Filler

- Depending on the properties of the filler, the filler body can retain up to 300% its volume in water.

2) Delayed Hypersensitivity Reaction (Nonantibody-Mediated)

- Can occur as early as one day after procedure, or as late as many weeks after
- Erythema, edema, itching sense
- Generally does not respond to antihistamines

Treatment methods

- Oral steroids
- In the case of HA fillers, degrade with hyaluronidase. Repeat until it is resorbed. There is no research that clearly indicates the safe daily maximum dose of hyaluronidase. In an area where a nodule can be felt, inject reconstituted triamcinolone. After injecting hyaluronidase into the injected region, massage rigorously. The symptoms will disappear only after the filler has completely resorbed.
- Remove filler

4 Neovascularization

In some cases capillary vessels may form, days or weeks after filler injection. The risk is higher with injections into the subdermis of the superficial subcutaneous layer versus a deeper layer. This forms as a result of tissue trauma due to bolus injection or excessive molding.

Even without intervention, the neovascularization disappears naturally after a few months to one year. However, if laser treatment is required, blood vessel laser can be performed.

5 PIH

Postinflammatory hyperpigmentation can occur in the injected area. Patients with Fitzpatrick Skin Types IV- VI have highest risk for PIH.

Treatment
- Skin lightening ointment (hydroquinone), Q-switched ND: Yag 1,064 nm laser treatment.

Prevention
- Reduce the number of skin punctures made during the procedure.
- Use the smallest gauge needle or cannula possible.

6 Nodule

1) Non-Inflammatory Nodules

Especially in patients with thin skin, visible or palpable nodule/s may form. In contrast to an inflammatory nodule, there is almost no change in size or color in non-inflammatory nodules.

Cause

- Uneven injection
- Injection of an excessive amount
- Injection that is too superficial
- Insufficient massaging

Treatment

- In the case of HA filler, inject hyaluronidase.
- In the case of non-HA filler, nodule may flatten if pressure is applied early enough. (However, this depends on the properties of the filler.)
- If the filler cannot be removed with hyaluronidase, disrupt nodule with lidocaine or saline injection followed by vigorous massage.
- If there is no improvement despite forementioned interventions, low dose intralesional steroids (diluted triamcinolone) can be attempted (be cautious of skin atopy).

2) Granuloma

- Granuloma may be a complication associated with filler quality.
- If the granuloma forms immediately after the procedure or within a few days, this may be an issue related to the filler quality. In such a case, it is possible to recognize whether the filler is of high or low quality.
- If the granuloma forms after a number of years, it is difficult to determine if this adverse event is related to filler quality.
- In the past, a few semi-permanent and permanent fillers caused serious problems number of years after the procedure. Filler must be selected cautiously, and only products that have demonstrated a high safety profile must be used.
- If there is a long latency period between time of filler administration and granuloma formation, it can be concluded that filler quality may not be the issue and the filler in question may be used.
- Granuloma is a longstanding inflammatory nodule. It is a chronic inflammatory state and means the filler body is enclosed in a capsule made up of mainly macrophages and giant cells.
- It can appear after latent period which can be several months after injection. Its mechanism of formation has not been accurately determined.

Contributing Factors
- Properties of the filler. (All filler substances can potentially cause granuloma, but they are rare with HA fillers and CaHA fillers.)
- Injection of excessive amounts.
- Intramuscular injection.
- Infection or wound in treated area.
- Repetitive injections.
- High impurity levels.
- Particle size.
- Particle surface charge.

Treatment
- The granuloma that forms with hyaluronic acid fillers are usually cystic granulomas. First line treatment is removal of filler substance by aspiration.
- Hyaluronidase.
- Intralesional steroids (triamcinolone).
- Surgical excision (Performed only if aspiration fails).
- Antibiotics medication.

7 Infection

1) Bacterial Infection

Infection can be suspected with edema, localized heat, and a change in color in the treated area that occurs within two to three days post procedure. Infection rarely appears within one day of the procedure.

Prevention
- Sterilize the injection site with effective topical disinfectant (before and after procedure).
- Strict wearing of gloves during procedures.
- Wipe excess filler substance on needle or cannula tip with sterile gauze.

Differential Diagnosis
- Hypersensitivity reaction (accompanied by pruritus without fever)

Treatment
- Oral antibiotics
- Area should not be massaged as massaging may spread infection to surrounding tissue.
- In case of abscess: incision, drainage, and culture

2) Herpes Infection
- There is possibility of reactivation of herpes virus infections around the perioral area. (If similar symptoms occur in areas other than the area where herpes usually occurs, necrosis may be suspected.)

Prophylaxis
- Valacyclovir (500 mg bid, for three days)

Treatment
- Valacyclovir (2,000 mg bid, one day)

8 Skin Necrosis (Blood Vessel Complications)

Skin necrosis occurs when there is a compromised circulation and shortage of oxygen supply. After filler procedures, skin necrosis occurs from time to time, and its mechanisms can be classified as follows.

1) Intravascular Emboli

Skin necrosis occurs with inadvertent intravascular filler injection. When the filler embolus completely occludes a vessel, it cuts off blood circulation and oxygen supply to the tissue. In the case of a terminal artery, the symptom occurs immediately after the procedure and irreversible injury can occur. Even if the artery in question anastomoses with the surrounding arteries, there may still be an insufficient supply of blood, which results in the formation of a lesion that becomes progressively larger. If filler is injected into a vein, pulmonary embolism can occur through venous drainage.

2) Extravascular Compression

In the event that the injected filler body compresses nearby arteries, skin necrosis can occur via a slow process of ischemia. If the filler lump presses against a vein, venous congestion occurs and arterial pressure decreases. Accordingly, there is a decreased oxygen supply to the tissue and necrosis progresses slowly. In this case, the symptoms are minor.

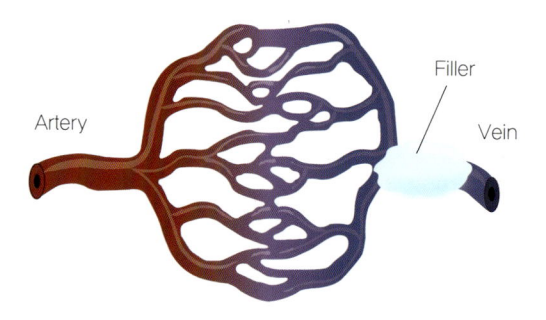

Fig. 5-1 Extravascular compression mechanism

Table 5-2 Complication by Type of Vascular Obstruction

	Intravascular emboli	Extravascular compression
Artery	Skin necrosis Blindness Cerebral infarct	Skin necrosis
Vein	Pulmonary embolism	Skin necrosis

3) Types of Intravascular Complications and the Regions Affected

Skin necrosis, blindness, and embolism, which are vascular complications, can occur anywhere on the face. Cases of skin necrosis were reported before fillers became as popular as they are now, because filler procedures were performed mainly on the nose and the nasolabial folds at that time. The most frequently reported condition recently is skin necrosis and occurs most frequently in the nose and nasolabial fold area. There has been increased reports of blindness in the last three to four years, caused most frequently by injections into the forehead and glabellar region. Blindness is caused by the inadvertent injection into the supratrochlear artery, supraorbital artery, or dorsal nasal artery, which all anastomose with the central retinal artery (see Blindness, 3-1, Part 5).

Pulmonary embolism is rarely reported. It has occurred during treatments on the temples. This is the region where the sentinel vein and the middle temporal vein, the biggest veins of the face, are located.

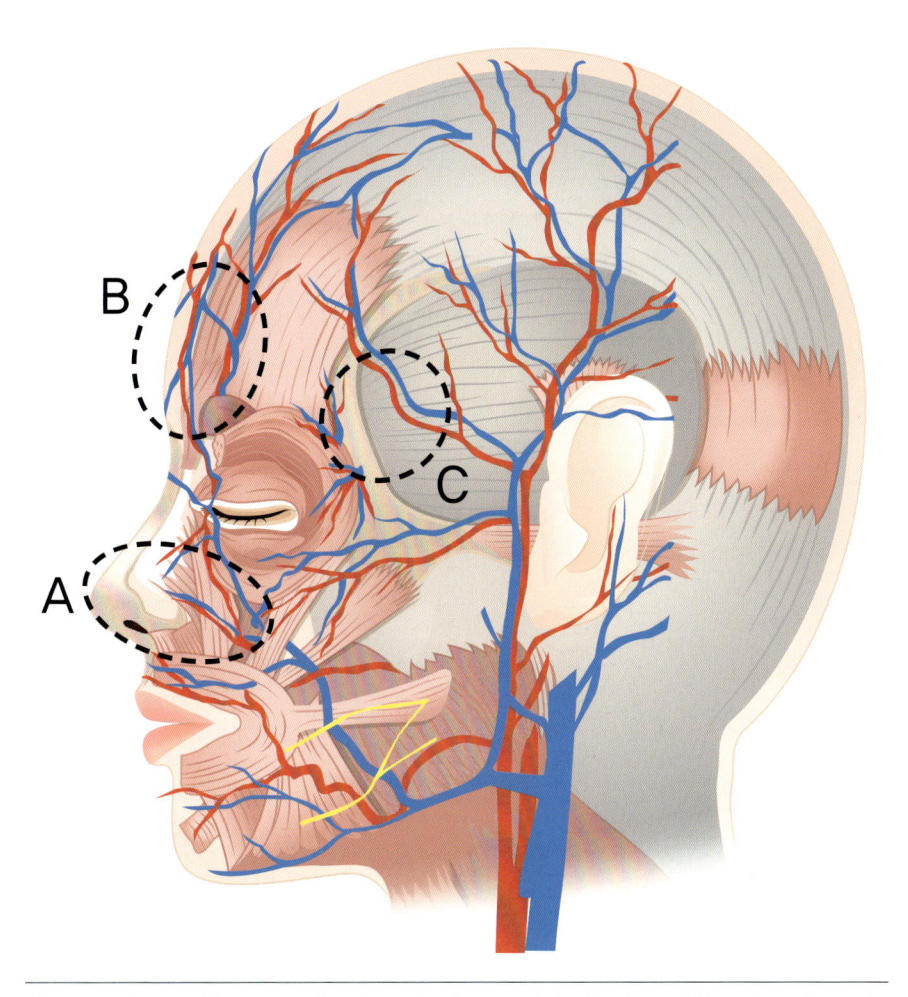

Fig. 5-2 Types of Intravascular Complications and the Regions Affected. A: Necrosis. **B:** Blindness. **C:** Pulmonary embolism.

2. Mechanism and Treatment of Skin Necrosis

1 Predisposing Factors of Skin Necrosis

- **Skin thickness**

    As thick skin has a higher risk of compressing blood vessels than thin skin, areas with thick skin are associated with a higher risk of skin necrosis.

- **Injection technique**

    Injection amount: If an excessive amount of filler is injected in one place, the chance of compressing blood vessels is higher.

- **Entry point/injection plane**

    If an entry point is made in a region where the vessel is located superficially, there is higher risk of puncturing and injecting filler into the vessel.

- **Ejection force**

    When injection is made incorrectly into a blood vessel and injection pressure is higher than the arterial pressure, the filler can move in a retrograde manner into the terminal branches of the internal carotid artery.

- **History of filler/fat injection**

    In cases where patient has a history of autologous fat transfer or filler injections, scar tissue reduces the mobility of the blood vessels. As a result, there is an increased risk of extravascular compression and blood vessel puncture. Care must be taken.

1) Needle vs Cannula

Many people think that for filler procedures, use of a needle results in more blood vessel complications than use of a cannula. Based on a research paper reporting vascular complications, the incidence rate of complications that arose in procedures using needles did not exceed that of procedures using cannulas. On the contrary, there are more complications that resulted with the use of cannula.

Theoretically speaking, it is true that a sharp needle has a higher possibility of damaging a blood vessel. In reality however, as physicians using a cannula think it relatively safer, they tend proceed more aggressively, and it is considered that this is associated with the higher incidence of vascular complications with cannula use.

2) HA Filler vs Non-HA Filler

Opinions vary on whether the filler type affects severity and prognosis of complications. Filler emboli, regardless of filler type, are difficult to remove. The most important step in the treatment of skin necrosis is early detection and early treatment. HA fillers have an advantage in that they can be hydrolyzed with hyaluronidase. But hyaluronidase must be accompanied by other treatment measures depending on the filler complication. Regardless of filler type, early detection can reduce the severity and improve outcomes.

2 Factors Affecting the Extent of Skin Necrosis

- Degree of blockage of blood vessels
  - Intravascular emboli vs. extravascular compression
  - Partial obstruction vs. complete obstruction
- Thickness of blood vessels
- Whether there is collateral circulation
- Current smoker

3 Symptoms of Skin Necrosis

Symptoms of necrosis vary significantly. As treatment differs greatly depending on the stage, proper treatment is possible only after accurate assessment. Symptoms for different stages are as follows.

1) Impending Necrosis

- Stage before scab forms on the skin.
- Progresses slowly as part of blood vessels are compressed (Symptoms occur approximately two to three days after the procedure.)

- Skin: Purple in color with reticular pattern.
- Symptom: Pain, accompanied by minor edema.

2) Dry Necrosis

- A crust forms, accompanied by a obvious infection and wound healing process.
- Severe state of ischemia and more susceptible to bacterial infection; breakdown of skin barrier.
- Skin: Vesicle, pustule, crust, eschar.
- Symptoms: Severe pain and edema.

3) Scar Formation

- Skin defect.
- In moderate to severe cases, scar tissue forms.

> **Differentiating with Connective Tissue Infection**
> - Bacterial infection: Skin color turns red in gradation pattern, skin is warmer than skin affected with necrosis
> - Viral infection: Vesicle and crust are similar to necrosis

Table 5-3 Symptoms and treatments depending on the timing of necrosis

Impending Necrosis – Hypovascularized state	Dry Necrosis – Infection – Wound healing state	Scar Formation – Skin defect
Reticular pattern Purple color Pain, swelling	Vesicle Eschar	Redness Depressed scar

• Decompression
  – Hyaluronidase
  – Puncture & Drainage (if possible)
  – Warm massage
• Revascularization
  – PGE1 IV
  – NTG patch
  – Hyperbaric O_2
  – Aspirin
	• Infection control
	  – PO antibiotics
	  – Remove vesicle
	• Dressing
	  – Antibiotics gauze
	• Growth factor
	  – EGF (PDRN)/PRP/stem cell
		• Scar Treatment
		• Skin graft

4 Treatment of Skin Necrosis

1) Decompression

Symptoms of skin necrosis do not appear immediately after the procedure. Patients usually return to the practice two to three days after the procedure. With the ischemia due to vascular obstruction by filler lumps or edema there is no oxygen being supplied to the tissues. Decompression, the initial treatment, focuses on removing the cause of the occlusion. Without addressing the cause, focusing on other methods of treatment can be said to be meaningless. If, symptoms of necrosis occur right after HA administration, hyaluronidase is injected with subsequent massage of the area. In case of non-HA fillers, incision and removal of filler material must be performed immediately.

(1) Puncture & Drainage

If an injection is made not into a deep plane but into a superficial to medium plane, the most certain decompression method is puncture and drainage of filler material.

(2) Warm Massage

Massaging helps decompression by pressing and spreading the filler lumps that are pressing on the blood vessels (Apply for 5~10 minutes every 1~2 hours). Applying a massage cloth with warm water and saline solution over affected area induces vasodilation. In the case of CaHA filler, which does not react to hyaluronidase, inject lidocaine or saline and massage to disrupt the filler material. However as vigorous massage can cause injury to the already vulnerable vasculature, it should be performed gently. After the impending necrosis stage, in case of severe skin infection or eschar, massaging is contraindicated.

(3) Hyaluronidase

Decompression can be achieved by breaking down the HA with hyaluronidase. Based on our experiment on hyaluronidase, not only the concentration but also the volume of hyaluronidase solution are important. If an excessive volume is injected, the pressure around the lesion can increase temporarily before the HA material gets a chance to dissolve. Accordingly, a moderate amount must be used and consider more injection of hyaluronidase as to the pressure and state of the ischemic lesions. If necessary, it can be repeated the next day. Also, it must be carried out together with massage. As hyaluronidase is a high-particle substance it must be spread by massaging to flatten the surface in order for it to exert its effect properly. An experiment demonstrated that hyaluronidase diffuses through the walls of the blood vessels. Therefore, in the event of a suspected vessel occlusion, injection of hyaluronidase around the entry site can be considered.

(4) Oral Steroid

- This can be used to reduce edema around the lesion.
- Prednisone 10~20 mg per day for 2~3 days.

2) Revascularization

Revascularization is a treatment to help blood circulation. If it is carried out after decompression is performed as an initial treatment, it makes treatment more effective.

(1) PGE1 IV Vasodilator

IV vasodilators that promote blood vessel expansion are commonly used for treatment of pressure ulcers and necrotic tissue. It can also be used to treat tissue necrosis from fillers. It is to be mixed with 500 cc N/S. because rapid infusion of vasodilators may cause headaches, it is to be injected slowly over approximately a two-hour period. It is administered for 3~5 days until there is visible clinical improvement.

(2) NTG Patch

This is applied as a cream in other countries, but in Korea, the NTG patch is commercialized. It is used to treat patients with coronary artery disease but can be used for off label indications. The patch is applied on the lesion. The patch is applied for 3~5 days and because NTG tolerance can developed, it should be worn for only 12 hours at a time and removed. In cases of impending necrosis, namely, when there is a skin color change, this can be used. It should not be used when there is eschar or pustules. In such a case, an IV vasodilator is to be used instead. Patients may report burning sensation in the area treated but as this is not a side effect it does not need to be treated. (Angiderm® Patch, diluted 0.2 mg/hr nitroglycerine, Samgyang Bio Pharm).

(3) Aspirin

Aspirin lowers blood viscosity and helps blood circulation in the narrowed blood vessels. (Aspirin 1T (100 mg) daily, for three to five days.)

(4) Hyperbaric Oxygen Therapy

With embolism or ischemia due to external pressure, the affected tissue becomes prone to infection. At this time, if hyperbaric oxygen is supplied, the sterilizing action of the white blood cells is activated and the supply of fibroblast and collagen necessary for generation of new blood vessels increases. However, such treatment is being recommended as a supplementary measure for treating infection of tissue necrosis. In case of necrosis after filler injections, as a first line treatment, decompression and infection control must be performed. As a supplementary treatment, hyperbaric oxygen therapy can be considered. In most cases, the equipment for hyperbaric oxygen is not available. The oxygen inhaler used during surgery can be used in place of hyperbaric oxygen equipment.

3) Infection Control & Dressing

If a vesicle or pustule appears after the skin color change, it is good to remove this using sterile technique. It is recommended to dress the area using antibiotic gauze at least once a day and preferably as often as possible. If it is not serious, oral antibiotics can be used for treatment.

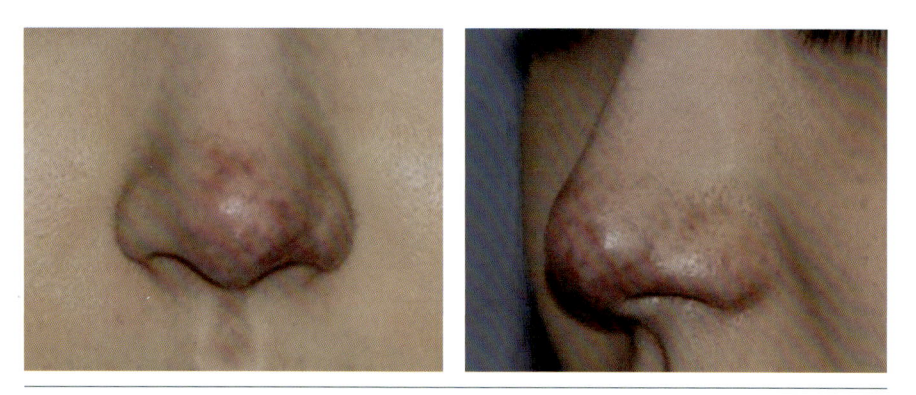

Safe Filler Injection Technique Demonstration – using live imaging tools

Fig. 5-3   Nasal tip skin necrosis

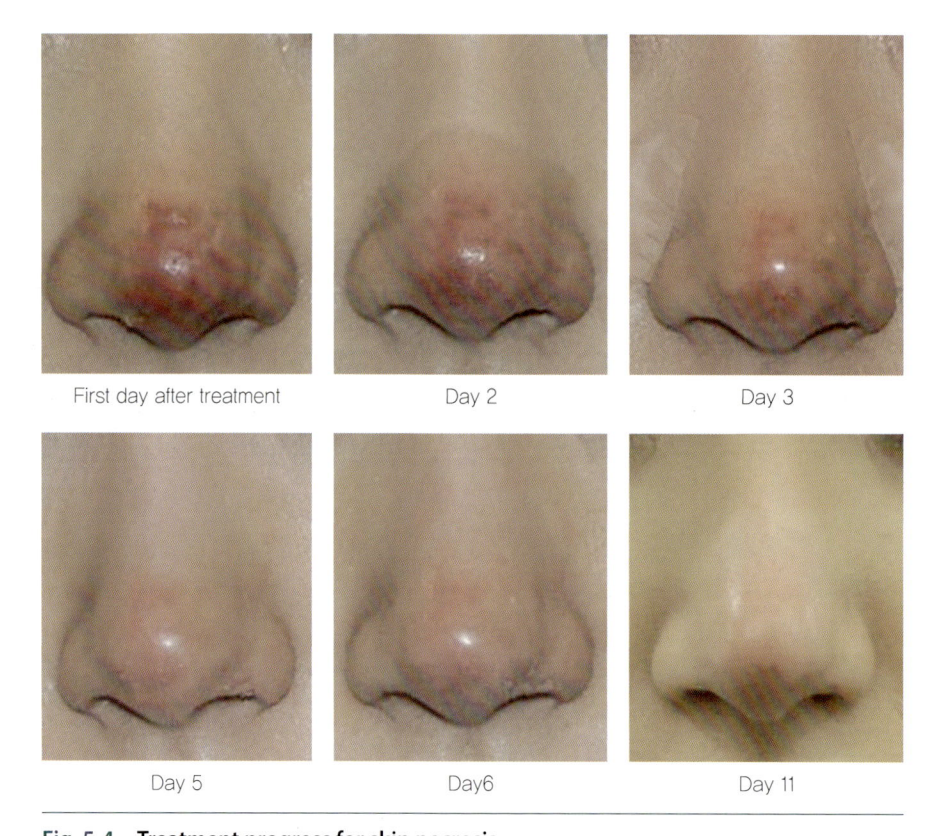

First day after treatment   Day 2   Day 3

Day 5   Day6   Day 11

Fig. 5-4   Treatment progress for skin necrosis

4) Growth factors

As the wound healing progresses, synergistic treatment effects can be obtained by topically applying or injecting growth factor solution in the necrotic lesion. Prior to decompression, if an excessive amount is injected into the lesion, edema can worsen due to the increase in pressure from the substance itself and damage from the needle. This must only be performed after decompression has been achieved. In case of a serious infection, it can be injected in the marginal areas of the lesion only. If the infection is not serious, it can be injected in both the central and marginal areas of the lesion (EFG, PDRN, stem cell).

5) Scar Treatment

If the treatment for impending necrosis is implemented appropriately, recovery without eschar or scar formation is possible. However, in a case of serious infection, or an infection not treated early, a scar may form. Treatment of indented scar is very challenging to doctors . The depression that forms after eschar falls off indicates that the wound healing is still in progress so treatments such as growth factors that promote collagen regeneration should be implemented. In the past, scar treatment was initiated once the scar had settled which was 1~2 months after the occurrence of skin necrosis. Treatment as recommended for general scars such as fractional laser was performed over a long period of time. Recently, a view has grown that it is to better to start active scar treatment as soon as the eschar falls off. In serious cases, a skin transplant may be necessary.

5 Notes for Preventing Necrosis during Procedures

- Retrograde technique
- Vasoconstriction pretreatment (epinephrine + lidocaine)
- Regurgitation (needle, cannula)
- Caliber of needle/cannula
  The smaller the gauge of the needle and higher the viscosity of the filler, ejection pressure increases. High ejection pressure increases the risk of filler reaching one of the branches of the internal carotid artery via retrograde flow.

Safe Filler Injection Technique Demonstration – using live imaging tools

- Understanding of facial anatomy
  Entry point/injection plane
  Caution required in case of thick skin
  Caution required in case of subcutaneous placement (injection into the layer right above periosteum is relatively safe).
- Inject a moderate amount. Consider edema that may arise from the filler.
- Gentle technique
  - Low pressure, slow injection

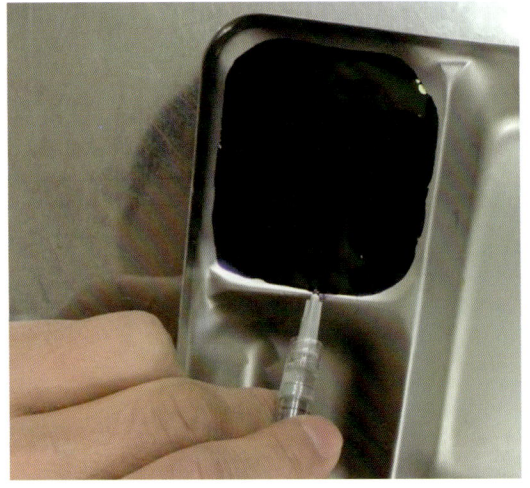

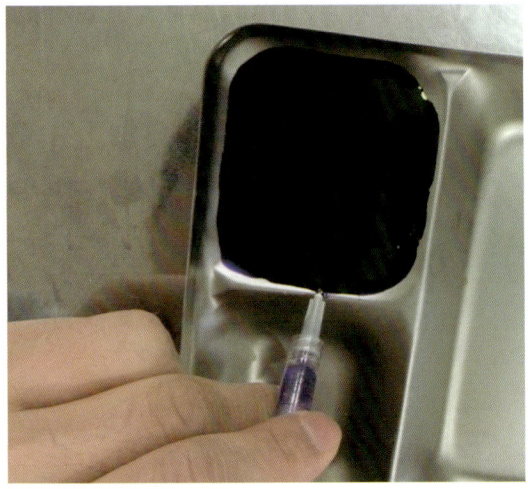

A. No pressure

B. Negative pressure

Fig. 5-5 Regurgitation test (1). Apply negative pressure by pulling on the plunger of the syringe containing the filler. GV solution flows right into the syringe.

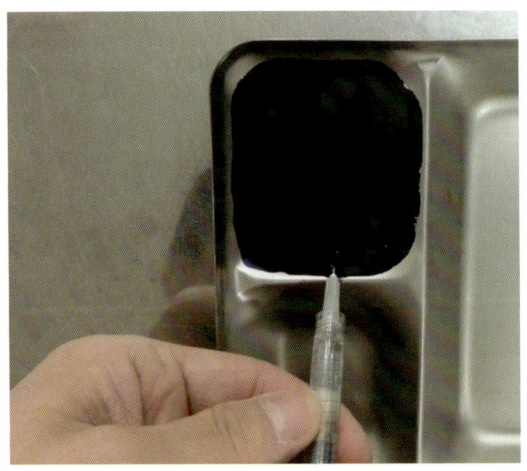

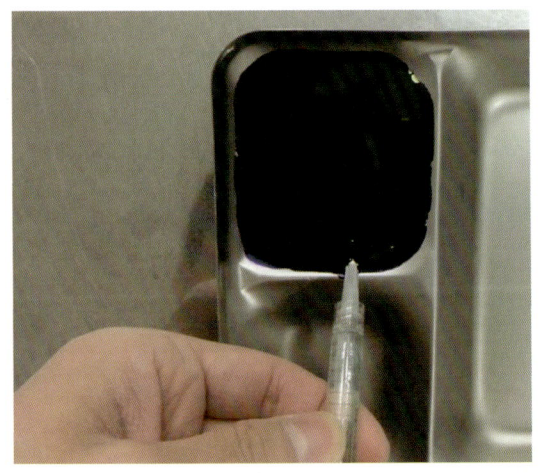

A. No pressure

B. Negative pressure

Fig. 5-6 Regurgitation test (2). With a different type of filler, applied negative pressure did not result in regurgitation of the GV solution. Depending on the viscosity of a filler and gauge of the needle/cannula, despite the applied negative pressure regurgitation may not occur. Even if a needle is inside a vessel, no blood may be regurgitated. This type of test must be performed with fillers and the injection tools used in the clinical practice before administration.

6 Tips for Early Discovery and Treatment of Necrosis

- Follow up call one day after the filler procedure (routine)
- In case of suspected event, repeat follow up call
- If patient reports symptoms, decide if patient needs to come in for check-up after examining photographs (especially if symptoms of necrosis occur after two to three days)
- Prepare emergency kit (NTG patch, PGE1 IV, Hyaluronidase, Dressing)
- Emergency call for advice

7 Factors Affecting the Prognosis of Skin Necrosis

- Vascular obstruction: Partial vs. complete
- Decompression and revascularization time
- Infection control
- The most important factors in treating necrosis are early detection and immediate treatment. Symptoms of necrosis may be misdiagnosed as infection but the distinction must be made carefully.

3. Other Blood Vessel Complications

1 Blindness and Cerebral Infarct

Blindness that occurs as a complication after filler procedures is disastrous. This is a consequence of retinal artery occlusion. In the ophthalmic artery, there are various branches. When filler material is accidentally injected into a vessel and flows in a retrograde manner and occludes one of these branches, blindness results.

- Retrograde flow from the supratrochlear/supraorbital artery
    - → Ophthalmic artery (originates from the internal carotid artery)
    - → Occlusion of retinal artery (blockade of blood circulation to the retina)

Another blood vessel that must be examined is the angular artery which is connected to the dorsal nasal artery. (Refer to External and Internal Carotid Artery, 1-5 Part 3) Blindness occurs when filler is injected at a pressure that exceeds the pressure of the normal arterial flow and results in filler flowing in the opposite direction to the natural blood flow.

Right after the procedure, partial or complete visual loss occurs. If such symptoms appear, a request must be immediately made to the ophthalmology clinic, but recovery of sight has been very difficult despite active treatment. In cases of complete visual loss, recovery is not normally seen. In serious cases, complete bilateral blindness occurs or is accompanied with cerebral infarction.

Prevention

Fillers should be placed at the supraperiosteum level (above the periosteum) where there are no blood vessels (See External and Internal Carotid Artery, 1-5 Part 3). When you want volumization of face.

- Use of a cannula does not guarantee safety. According to literature, a significant number of blindness occurred after fat implants using cannula, and also in which 2 mm cannulas were used.
- Use of HA fillers does not guarantee safety and there is no foolproof treatment method. Vision loss has been reported with various other filler materials such as corticosteroids, paraffin, silicone oil, and bovine collagen.

High risk areas

The glabella and forehead regions are affected more than other areas.

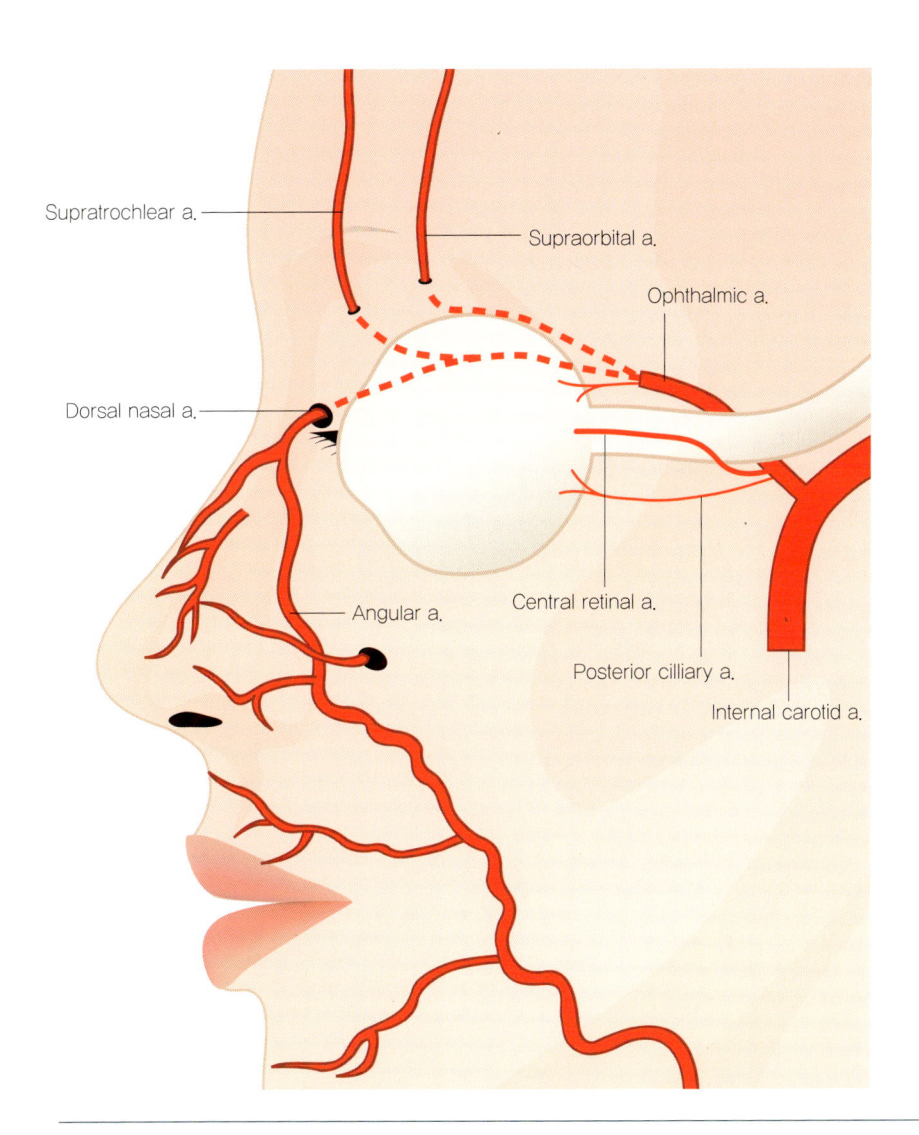

Fig. 5-7   Blindness mechanism after intravascular injection

2 Pulmonary Embolism

So far, blindness and cerebral infarction have been emphasized as severe complications associated with fillers. These events occur when filler substance or autologous fat is injected into the artery. A serious complication that can arise from venous injection is pulmonary embolism. Recently, cases of pulmonary embolism from filler administration have been reported, one of which resulted in death. This patient had received autologous fat in the temporal area.

The temporal area has many layers of fascia, superficial and deep temporal arteries and veins, and the big veins including the sentinel vein and the middle temporal vein. (Refer to Anatomy of the Temples, 3-2 Part 4.)

The sentinel vein and middle temporal vein have thicknesses of approximately 2 mm and 5 mm respectively. When autologous fat or filler material are injected into them, the material moves from the ext. jugular vein to the heart and finally to the pulmonary artery resulting in pulmonary embolism.

Prevention method
- Study the depth and courses of the sentinel vein and middle temporal vein in the temple areas.
- Be careful about the entry point, injection direction, and injection layer (Refer to Injection into the Temples, 3-4 Part 4).
  - Sentinel vein: Move in the layer above the TPF and penetrate through the TPF and DPF.
  - Middle temporal vein: Exists in the layer between the superficial layer and deep layer of the DTF.

Reference

1. David Funt, Tatjana Pavicic. Dermal fillers in aesthetics: an overview of adverse events and treatment approaches. Clin Cosmet Investig Dermatol. 2013;6:295-316.

2. Claudio DeLorenzi. Complications of Injectable Fillers, Part 1. Aesthet Surg J. 2013;33(4):561-75.

3. Claudio DeLorenzi. Complications of Injectable Fillers, Part 2: Vascular Complications. Aesthet Surg J. 2014;34(4):584-600.

4. Massimo Signorini et al. Global Aesthetics Consensus: Avoidance and Management of Complications from Hyaluronic Acid Fillers—Evidence- and Opinion-Based Review and Consensus Recommendations. Plast Reconstr Surg. 2016;137(6):961e-71e.

5. Kyu Hyung Park et Al. Iatrogenic Occlusion of the Ophthalmic Artery After Cosmetic Facial Filler Injections-A National Survey by the Korean Retina Society. JAMA Ophthalmol. 2014;132(6):714-23.

6. Jean D. A. Carruthers et al. Blindness Caused by Cosmetic Filler Injection: A Review of Cause and Therapy. Plast Reconstr Surg. 2014;134(6):1197-201.

7. Katie Beleznay et al. Avoiding and Treating Blindness From Fillers: A Review of the World Literature. Dermatol Surg. 2015;41(10):1097-117.

8. Jong Geol Jang et al. A Case of Nonthrombotic Pulmonary Embolism after Facial Injection of Hyaluronic Acid in an Illegal Cosmetic Procedure. Tuberc Respir Dis (Seoul). 2014;77(2):90-3.

2nd Edition

Safe Filler Injection Technique Demonstration
- using live imaging tools

Copyright © 2017 by Daehan Medical Book Publishing, Inc.

All rights reserved. No part of this book may be reproduced or transmitted in any form or by any means, electronic mechanical, including photocopying, recording, or any information storage and retrieval system, without permission in writing from the publisher.

Permissions may be sought from Daehan's Rights Department:
1209, 288, Digital-ro, Guro-gu, Seoul, Republic of Korea
Tel : (822) 921-0653
Fax : (822) 925-5769
medbook1@medbook.co.kr
www.medbook.co.kr

Printed in Republic of Korea.
ISBN : 979-11-5590-066-6 93510